Essentials of Health Care Marketing

Eric N. Berkowitz, PhD

Chairman
Department of Marketing
The School of Management
University of Massachusetts
Amherst, Massachusetts

JONES AND BARTLETT PUBLISHERS

Sudbury, Massachusetts

BOSTON   TORONTO   LONDON   SINGAPORE

World Headquarters
Jones and Bartlett Publishers
40 Tall Pine Drive
Sudbury, MA 01776
978-443-5000
info@jbpub.com
www.jbpub.com

Jones and Bartlett Publishers
Canada
2406 Nikanna Road
Mississauga, ON L5C 2W6
CANADA

Jones and Bartlett Publishers
International
Barb House, Barb Mews
London W6 7PA
UK

Copyright © 2004 by Jones and Bartlett Publishers, Inc.
Originally published by Aspen Publishers, © 1996.

Library of Congress Cataloging-in-Publication Data
Berkowitz, Eric N.
Essentials of health care marketing / Eric N. Berkowitz
p. cm.
Includes bibliographical references and index.
ISBN 0-7637-3268-0
        1. Medical care–Marketing. I. Title.
RA410.56.B46   1996
362.1'068'8–dc20
95-40372
CIP

Production Credits
Publisher: Michael Brown
Associate Editor: Chambers Moore
Production Manager: Amy Rose
Associate Production Editor: Renée Sekerak
Production Assistant: Jenny L. McIsaac
Associate Marketing Manager: Joy Stark-Vancs
Manufacturing Buyer: Amy Bacus
Printing and Binding: RR Donnelley Harrisonburg
Cover Printing: RR Donnelley Harrisonburg

Printed in the United States of America
07 06 05 04 03   10 9 8 7 6 5 4 3 2 1

To

Sandra, Annie, Julie,
and my parents

TABLE OF CONTENTS

PREFACE

Over the past 20 years, health care marketing has become an accepted function in the management of health care organizations. During this same time, health care itself has gone through a dramatic change in reimbursement, competition, and structure. In 1976, when marketing began to be used in health care as a new tool, the major purpose of health care providers, organizations, and suppliers was to provide the necessary services to deliver care. More volume was viewed as better for the provider and for the organization, since providers and hospitals were reimbursed based on the volume of the service provided. The longer the hospital stay, the more money the hospital would receive from the insurance company or the federal government. So, too, for the physician—the more services provided in terms of diagnostic tests or invasive surgical procedures, the more money the physician would receive. In this setting, the goal of marketing was to generate demand for services. As a result of this goal, the focus of marketing centered primarily on promotional tools to build awareness of preference for the services of a particular provider. For suppliers of health care products, the focus of their efforts was to sell as much product as possible to their customers, the providers. In this setting, the industry structure was rather simple. Most providers operated within their local community, and strategies were developed within this rather narrowly defined geographic location.

As this book goes to press, the reimbursement, competition, and structure of health care is undergoing a massive change. Today's health care environment is governed by the concept of efficient deliverance of care. Providers and suppliers must develop strategies within the concept of managing the patient's care in a cost-effective manner. In this world, necessary services are delivered, but no longer without regard to the cost of such services. Now, hospitals often contract with health insurance plans to provide service for a prepaid amount of money and it is the hospital's responsibility to deliver that quality service in an efficient manner. Physicians, too, now operate in this environment. Most doctors today find an increasing proportion of their business accounted for by a managed care arrangement in which they are given an amount of money to take care of the health care needs of an individual. In this setting, having more volume through longer hospital stays or more diagnostic tests might lead to expending the financial resources allocated before any profit is made. For health care suppliers that, in the past, found selling more to the customer was acceptable, today's customer—the hospital, doctor, or health plan—is asking for ways to use products efficiently. And, suppliers are being paid in a way in which they must share the risk of these product purchases. The less that is used, the more financial reward the supplier will receive. More volume is now an undesirable outcome.

In health care today, the competition and industry structure is also undergoing a massive change. While 20 years ago the competitor was viewed as the other hospital in town, or the other physician who specialized in the same procedure, today's competitor can be a large national organization headquartered in another state with vast economic resources at its disposal. The health care industry of the 1990s is characterized by massive consolidation among hospitals, physician groups, insurance entities, and suppliers. While the health care environment once was viewed as a marketplace of relatively equal-sized, small, local competitors, today's marketplace is dominated by large, national entities that have vast economic resources with which to fight competitors.

In this changing health care world, marketing is increasingly important. Moving from the early days of promotion to generate demand, marketing in health care today is far more similar to what is involved in traditional consumer and industrial industries like food products, automobiles, or aviation equipment. Knowledge of the customer—whether an individual or another company—is the key to developing effective marketing strategies. Understanding product strategies along with the concerns of pricing and distribution are now relevant in a marketplace where organizations have realigned to capture a large number of patients into a health plan that covers all of their medical needs. Promotion, which was the primary focus of marketing in the past, is still of importance, but has grown increasingly complex. Now, a full range of promotional tools are necessary to competitively market a product or service.

In this book, the essential aspects of marketing are discussed. The purpose of this book is to provide a thorough understanding of the principles and concepts of marketing as they apply to health care organizations. Because readers of this book will be in markets composed of varying degrees of managed care, this book will discuss applications from both a traditional fee-for-service approach and a managed care framework. This book examines the essential elements of marketing in the hope that readers will recognize the application of marketing tools and strategies in today's dynamic health care environment.

ACKNOWLEDGMENTS

As any author of a textbook knows, often one name is listed on the cover yet the development and actual outcome of the project are the result of the valuable input of many individuals. Over the past 20 years in which I have been interested in health care marketing, several individuals and organizations have contributed to my understanding and education in this field. At the risk of leaving some people unmentioned, I express particular appreciation to William Flexner, now president of Options Technologies, Inc., of Mendota Heights, Minnesota. Bill and I first collaborated while Assistant Professors at the University of Minnesota. At that time, Bill was a research professor in the Center for Health Services Research at the University of Minnesota where he had a particular interest in applying marketing to health care and I was an assistant professor in the School of Management. Together, Bill and I published some of the first articles on health care marketing. At this time, I acknowledge my appreciation for the early role Bill played in introducing me to an exciting industry.

Secondly, I express my great appreciation to the American College of Physician Executives and its Executive Vice President, Roger Schenke. The American College of Physician Executives is the largest and fastest growing organization of physicians in management. Since 1978, I have had the opportunity to be a regular faculty presenter in the College's education programs. And, in 1985, I was made an honorary member of the College. As a faculty member, I realize that I have learned far more from my association with this organization than any knowledge I will ever be able to transmit to its membership.

Additionally, I recognize the Alliance for Health Care Strategy and Marketing and its President, Carla Windhorst. This organization is the largest association of individuals engaged in health care marketing. My association with the people within this organization continues to show me the value and contribution that marketing has made, both within health care and to the customers of the health care industry.

In developing and preparing this book, several other individuals have been of great help. First, I acknowledge Elizabeth Kempisty, my administrative assistant and the person who truly runs the marketing department that I have chaired for 11 years. For many months she has endured my frustrations about textbook writing and watches with good humor as I enter another project. Several people at Aspen have been helpful throughout this project: Sandy Cannon, Amy Martin, Neal Pomea, Ruth Bloom, and Jack Bruggeman. Each has listened to the concerns and thoughts of another author, for what I am sure is the one-hundredth time, with great consideration. And, while there may be errors within this text for which I take full responsibility, final polishing of this manuscript could not have been accomplished without the consistent focus and dedication of The Fresh Eye, Cathy Frye. As project manager, Cathy worked diligently in prodding me to improve every aspect of this book.

Finally, I express my appreciation to my family, who most often had to endure directly the pressures that I felt in bringing this project to completion. While my daughters have little desire to enter marketing, it is for them that I undertook this project. My best friend and partner of more than 20 years, my wife, fortunately again has tolerated my anxieties as another text is completed.

INTRODUCTION

This book is divided into three main parts. Part I, "The Marketing Process," looks first at what marketing is, the nature of marketing strategy, and the environment in which marketing operates. Chapter 1 provides a perspective on the meaning of marketing and the market planning process. Additionally, this chapter outlines how marketing health care is changing in light of the restructuring that is occurring in this industry. Chapter 2 provides an overview of marketing strategy and an understanding of the strategic options available to a health care organization. Chapter 3 focuses on the environment in which health care strategy is formulated and the implications of the environment on marketing decisions.

Part II of this book is "Understanding the Consumer." At the core of marketing is the focus on the consumer. In today's health care world that consumer might be an individual patient, or another organization such as a company buying health care for its employees, or an insurance company deciding with whom they should contract for health care. Chapter 4 provides an overview of the consumer decision-making process as it pertains to both consumers and organizations. In order to assess the consumer, marketing research is an important tool. Chapter 5 describes the market research process and the alternative methodologies used within marketing research. Finally, it is important to recognize that not all consumers or organizations make decisions in the same way. Marketing strategies must often be tailored to groups of consumers or particular types of companies. This refinement of marketing strategy often occurs as a result of market segmentation, which is the focus of Chapter 6.

The last section of this book, Part III, is "The Marketing Mix." The Four Ps of product, price, place, and promotion form the basis around which all organizations develop their marketing plans and strategies. Chapter 7 reviews concepts and marketing strategies involved in the product or service being delivered. Chapter 8 discusses pricing objectives and strategies and how decisions on prices change in a world in which prices are set by contract negotiation. Chapter 9 presents the place concept of marketing, which is often referred to as distribution.

In today's health care marketplace, there are middlemen who can control the access of hospitals or physicians to a patient. Understanding the strategies of distribution assumes greater importance today. Chapters 10, 11, and 12 involve the promotional element of marketing. Understanding the communication process and the range of promotional elements are the focus of Chapter 10. Chapter 11 discusses the advertising component of marketing, while personal sales is presented in Chapter 12. Chapter 13, the final chapter, provides an overview of monitoring and controlling marketing activities. Measuring the outcome of marketing decisions is necessary in order to continue to refine effective marketing strategies.

Chapter Organization

Readers of this book will find that six sections appear in each chapter. These are: Learning Objectives, Conclusions, Key Terms, Chapter Summary, Chapter Problems, and Notes. Whenever a Key Term appears, it is presented in bold print for easy identification in the text. All Key Terms appear with their definitions in the Glossary. At the end of the book, an Index is provided for the reader's convenience.

Part I
The Marketing Process

THE MEANING OF MARKETING

LEARNING OBJECTIVES

After reading this chapter you should be able to:

- Define marketing and differentiate between a marketing-driven and non-marketing-driven process

- Distinguish among marketing mix elements

- Delineate between health care needs and wants

- Understand the dimensions of the environment that have an impact on marketing strategy

- Appreciate the ongoing restructuring of the health care industry

Primary care satellites, integrated delivery systems, managed care plans, and physician-hospital organizations (PHOs) are but a few of the elements that dominate the structure of the health care industry today, as the government, employers, consumers, providers, and health care suppliers deal with a new health care market. This marketplace is typified by massive restructuring in the way health care organizations operate, health care is purchased, and care is delivered. Competing in this new environment will require an effective marketing strategy to deal with these forces of change. This book will focus on the essentials for effective marketing and their implementation in this new health care marketplace. This discussion begins with an examination of what marketing is and how it has evolved within health care since first being discussed as a relevant management function in 1976.

MARKETING

For anyone involved in health care during the past ten years, the term *marketing* generates little emotional reaction. Yet, health care marketing—a commonplace concept today—was considered novel and controversial when first introduced to the industry two decades ago. In 1975, Evanston Hospital, in Evanston, Illinois, was one of the first hospitals to establish a formal marketing staff position. Now, more than 20 years later, marketing has diffused throughout health care into hospitals, group practices, rehabilitation facilities, and other health care organizations. In this book, fundamental marketing concepts and marketing strategies are discussed. Although health care is undergoing significant structural change, the basic elements of marketing will be at the core of any organization's successful position in the marketplace.

The Meaning of Marketing

There are several views and definitions of marketing. The most widely accepted definition is that of the American Marketing Association, which is the professional organization for marketing practitioners and educators, defines **marketing** as "the process of planning and executing the conception, pricing, promotion, and distribution of ideas, goods, and services to create exchanges that satisfy individual and organizational objectives."[1]

Central to this definition of marketing is the focus on the consumer, whether that be an individual patient, physician, or organization such as a company contracting for industrial medicine. This definition also contains the key ingredients of marketing that lead to consumer satisfaction. Increasingly in health care, customer satisfaction is the key issue.

The Joint Commission on Accreditation of Healthcare Organizations, the industry's major accrediting agency for operating standards of health care facilities, required—in its 1994 accreditation manual—that hospitals improve on nine measures of performance, one of which is patient satisfaction. This focus on patient satisfaction for hospital accreditation is an overt recognition of the need for health care facilities to be marketing oriented, and, thus, customer responsive.

Prerequisites for Marketing

This book's definition of marketing includes several prerequisite conditions that must exist before marketing occurs. First, there must be two or more parties with unsatisfied needs. One party might be the consumer looking to fulfill certain needs; the second, a company seeking to exchange a service or product for economic gain. A second prerequisite for marketing is the desire or ability of another party to meet those needs. Third, parties must have something to exchange. For example, a physician has the clinical skills that will meet an individual patient's need to have a torn meniscus repaired. A consumer must have the health insurance or financial resources to exchange for the receipt of these medical services. Finally, there must be a means to communicate. In order to facilitate an exchange between two parties, each party must learn of the other's existence. It is this last aspect of health care that has formally evolved in recent years.

Until 1975, advertising and promotion really did not exist within health care. Communication to facilitate exchange occurred by word of mouth. One would consult with a physician, and that individual in turn recommended the physician to other consumers who would then seek out that particular doctor. Prior to 1975, the American Medical Association had within its codes of ethics a prohibition against advertising. That very year, the U.S. Supreme Court ruled that professional associations were subject to federal antitrust laws. The American Medical Association revised its code of ethics to be less stringent regarding advertising. Further legal actions between the Federal Trade Commission (FTC) and the American Medical Association had, by 1982, removed even those restrictions. The FTC believed the restriction on advertising deprived consumers of the free flow of information regarding health care alternatives and services. The FTC and the federal courts recognized the value of communications to consumers. Communication is a prerequisite for marketing. It is only in the last two decades that more formal means of communication have evolved within health care and that marketing strategies have become more visible.

Who Does Marketing?

Traditionally, only for-profit commercial businesses in consumer or industrial settings conducted marketing. In this text, they will be referred to as traditional businesses. Yet, the application of marketing broadened in the late 1960s.

In 1969, two marketing academics—Philip Kotler and Sidney Levey—at Northwestern University in Illinois, published an article about broadening the concept of marketing. Their writing was the first attempt to recognize that for-profit and nonprofit businesses engaged in marketing activities. They recognized that marketing activities occurred in both service and product businesses. At the core of these organizations' activities was the notion of "exchange."[2]

Viewing the concept of exchange as the core of marketing allowed people to consider other areas where marketing might also be useful. Fine arts centers and museums, hospitals, and school districts began to see the relevance of marketing strategies and tactics to their settings. A consumer exchanges time and money for the pleasure of seeing a display of fine art. A patient pays for medical services provided by a free-standing diagnostic clinic, while a school district provides education in exchange for public support through tax levies.

The scope and nature of who markets has broadened considerably. Marketing is conducted by individuals and organizations. Marketing is relevant to for-profit and nonprofit entities. Throughout this book, examples of marketing programs at businesses such as General Motors or Johnson & Johnson will be discussed, along with the marketing programs of health care providers such as the Geisinger Health System in Danville, Pennsylvania or the Mayo Clinic in Rochester, Minnesota. While there are distinct aspects within any industry that require the modification of marketing principles to fit particular needs, the core of marketing and the marketing mix is relevant for almost every organization.

THE ELEMENTS OF SUCCESSFUL MARKETING

Marketing Research

Within the definition of marketing is the discussion of a process of planning and executing to meet consumer needs. Marketing requires an understanding of consumer wants and needs. This understanding is derived through an assessment of these needs. Within this book, Chapter 5 focuses on marketing research. **Marketing research** is a process in which there is a systematic gathering of data from customers to identify their needs.

The Four Ps

The heart of marketing strategy is the development of a response to the marketplace. As noted in the definition, marking is the "execution of the conception, pricing, promotion, and distribution of the goods, ideas, and services." To respond to customers, an organization must develop a product, determine the price customers are willing to pay, identify what place is most convenient for customers to purchase the product or access the service, and finally, promote the product to customers to let them know it is available.

Product, price, place, and promotion are referred to as the **four Ps** of marketing strategy.[3] It is these four controllable variables that a firm uses to define its marketing strategy. The mix of these four controllable variables that a business uses to pursue a desired level of sales is referred to as the **marketing mix**. The definitions of the four major elements of marketing as discussed below provide the focus of this book.

Product

Product represents goods, services, or ideas offered by a firm. In this text, the term "product" also will be used interchangeably with health care services and ideas. In health care, the nature of the product has changed dramatically. Twenty years ago, one could define the product simply as a medical procedure or as an orthotic device to correct a physical disability. In today's climate, the discussion of the health care product includes not only these traditional products, but also products and services such as prepaid health insurance plans offered by health maintenance organizations (HMOs), or a group purchasing contract such as that offered by the Premier Health Alliance of Westchester, Illinois, a nationwide association of hospitals.

Price

Price focuses on what customers are willing to pay for a service. What price represents is addressed in the definition of marketing in terms of exchanges. A company provides a service and customers exchange dollars for receipt of a service that satisfies their needs. An employee paying an annual premium to an HMO or an insurance company reimbursing a physician's fee are both exchanges involving some determined price.

As will be discussed in Chapter 8, the issue of pricing for health care services has become a major concern of marketing strategy as the health care environment changes. Several factors are contributing to the greater role that the pricing variable is playing in developing marketing strategy. On one level, more employers are requiring employees to pay a greater percentage of their health care insurance premiums. Many insurance companies also now require consumers to make a co-payment for medical services, whereas in the past, insurance companies paid the full medical bill. As mentioned earlier, companies that historically have paid the full premium for health care costs have become concerned about the price of medical services. These employers are now looking for ways to become more efficient buyers of their health care coverage. Finally, within the health care system itself, new structural organizations such as HMOs have begun to contract with providers and hospitals for services. These organizations are seeking discounts from providers in return for their subscribers' business. These same managed care organizations must determine how to price their prepaid health care plans to attract companies to offer them to their employees, and to stay competitive with other health care plans in the marketplace. For marketers, the issue of price is understanding what level of dollars a customer is willing to exchange for the receipt of some want-satisfying services or products. In the current health care climate, determining the value of these services—represented by the price—is the major challenge facing health care organizations.

Place

Place represents the manner in which goods or services are distributed by a firm for use by consumers. Place might include decisions regarding the location or the hours a medical service can be accessed. Chapter 9 reviews the marketing considerations for place that have assumed greater importance in today's managed care environment.

Increasingly, as more health care organizations establish managed care plans to enroll consumers in an insurance option that provides for all their health care needs, the place variable assumes a more critical role. Companies offering prepaid health care plans must consider location and primary care access for potential enrollees. While 40, 20, or even 10 years ago, a physician would establish an office in a location convenient for the doctor, today the consumer dictates this variable element of the marketing mix.

Promotion

The final P represents promotion. For many people this has historically meant advertising, and advertising has meant marketing. Yet, as can be seen in the definition, promotion is just one part of marketing; promotion alone is not marketing. **Promotion** represents any way of informing the marketplace that the organization has developed a response to meet its needs, and that the exchange should be consummated. Promotion itself involves a range of tactics involving publicity, advertising, and personal selling, which are described in Chapters 10, 11, and 12, respectively.

As discussed earlier, formal communication in the form of advertising was not allowed as recently as 1975. Yet while the past 20 years has seen a change in terms of the amount of advertising, other promotional tactics such as personal selling have become more relevant to compete effectively in today's marketplace. Health insurance companies and HMOs all employ sales forces. A national health care organization, Continental Medical Systems of Harrisburg, Pennsylvania, has a sales force to generate referrals to its specialized rehabilitation hospitals located around the country. Even local acute-care hospitals now often have physician referral staff who call on physicians to ensure that their needs are being met at the facility where they admit patients.

THE DILEMMA OF NEEDS AND WANTS

One of health care marketing's major concerns pertains to the issues of needs and wants. Health care professionals often speak of the fact that what consumers want may not be what they need. Clinical and professional responsibility demands treatment of the need. A **need** has been defined as a "condition in which there is a deficiency of something, or one requiring relief."[4] A **want** is defined as the "wish or desire for something."[5] A consumer *needs* to have medication for hypertension. A person may *want* medication to suppress the appetite and thus lose weight. To which need or want should the health care marketer respond?

Underlying any response in health care must be whatever constitutes providing quality care for the patient. Meeting medical needs must be the primary purpose of the system. Yet wants should not be ignored. For the health care professional, consider the just-cited dilemma of a pill for weight reduction. Should the system respond to this want? A marketer's response would most likely be yes, but the response must be medically appropriate. In fact, the marketer would try to understand more closely what it is the consumer wants (or is buying). In this instance, it is less likely to be a pill and more probably a more attractive appearance through weight reduction. The request for medication might be met more appropriately with creation of an eating disorders program or a wellness center that helps establish an exercise and fitness regimen. The ultimate want that the customer has can be satisfied, but the methodology must observe appropriate practice standards.

Identifying the Customer

In health care, this need/want dilemma often masks the major question, "Who is the customer?" Consider recent trends in the field of obstetrics. For many years, the consumer—the expectant mother—wanted to have her significant other with her in the delivery room. The medical community responded by claiming that this want was inappropriate. It would compromise good standards of care. In fact, the issue had less to do with standards of care and more with standards of convenience for the provider. Now, in most delivery rooms in the United States, a woman in labor will be accompanied by her significant other, a nurse midwife, and possibly, the obstetrician.

The medical community argued that the need to restrict access to the labor suite was for "good standards in obstetrical care." In reality, medicine lost sight of who the customer was and how her needs and wants could be met. In the delivery process, the physician may be viewed as part of the production line, not as the customer. Medical needs are not compromised in modern labor rooms, but customer needs are being more closely addressed.

While the composition of people present in the labor and delivery room has been resolved, a new conflict between needs and wants has arisen within obstetrics again as organizations try to control costs. Many managed care plans have moved to a 24-hour discharge practice for mothers who have an uncomplicated delivery. Plans like Maryland's Blue Cross & Blue Shield follow up with a home visit by a nurse the next day. The health insurers want more cost-effective deliveries. Yet the American College of Obstetricians and Gynecologists (ACOG) does not believe this policy meets the needs of the patients and the newborn babies. In May 1995, the ACOG called for a moratorium on such discharge practices until further study. The college recommends stays of 48 hours for routine deliveries and 96 hours for Caesarian sections. Here, the wants of one group and the needs of another are in conflict and still to be resolved.[6]

In our current health care marketplace, most health care organizations have multiple markets or customers to whom they must be attentive. Figure 1–1 shows an array (but probably not all-encompassing) of potential markets for a health care organization. An organization offering a mental health or substance abuse program for adolescents might have to accommodate the needs of judges, probation officers, or social workers. Schools might be the market for a sports medicine program. Long-term care facilities might be the market for a geriatric assessment program. Also included are the more traditional markets represented by physicians, nurses, patients, referral physicians, employee assistance personnel at

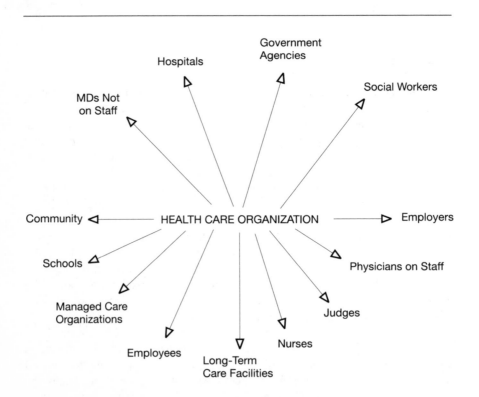

Figure 1–1 Multiple Health Care Organization Markets

companies, managed care plans, and regulators. One increasingly important market includes employers. For many years, this segment was considered of secondary importance, since companies paid the full insurance premiums for their labor force. Now, however, companies are controlling rising health care costs (a factor discussed further in Chapter 3) by dealing directly with providers to meet their employees' health care needs.

As the topic of markets is discussed in this book, it is important to be aware that health care organizations have multiple markets—the importance of each one is a function of the program or issue being addressed.

THE EVOLUTION OF MARKETING

In both traditional businesses and in health care the marketing concept has taken several decades to evolve. In health care this evolution has occurred in a relatively short time period. As previously noted, the first hospital to hire a person with a marketing title was Evanston Hospital in Illinois in 1975. In traditional product businesses, the evolution of the marketing concept took longer.

Production Era

To understand how marketing has evolved, let's consider its development in a corporation such as Pillsbury Company of Minneapolis–St. Paul, long known as a manufacturer of flour, baking goods, and other food products. Let's also trace this same evolution in the typical hospital.

Pillsbury located itself in the Minneapolis–St. Paul, Minnesota, market in the 1800s. The location, along the Mississippi River, offered the company a source of water power. (In that era, the Mississippi River had waterfalls that far north.) This location was also close to the raw materials needed for the production of Pillsbury's product. Robert Keith, a former Pillsbury president, described the company at this stage of its development. "We are professional flour millers. Blessed with a supply of the finest North American wheat, plenty of water power, and excellent milling machinery, we produce flour of the highest quality. Our basic function is to mill high-quality flour, and of course we must hire salesmen to sell it, just as we hire accountants to keep the books."[7]

At this stage of the company's evolution, the primary focus of the business was producing a high-quality product—flour. The sales and even the consumption or purchase of the product were incidental to the firm's focus—it was assumed that people would buy Pillsbury flour because it was high quality.

Many hospitals were and are at this stage in their own evolution. One might rewrite Keith's statements for a production-oriented hospital to say, "Our basic function is to provide high-quality medicine. Accompanied by the highest forms of technology, we have physicians, nurses, and allied health personnel to provide this service. And, we have administrators to keep the books." For a production-oriented hospital or health care organization, the focus is on providing high-quality medicine. As can be seen in Table 1–1, the health care organization's focus is on delivering clinical quality.

Sales Era

For many traditional businesses such as Pillsbury, the production orientation worked well until the early 1900s. By 1920, the automobile became part of our way of life and changed the world for consumers and companies. The federal government began to finance the construction of a roadway system in the United States. Consumers became more mobile in the everyday life of work, shopping, and recreation. For companies, the strategic change was in the hiring of traveling salespeople. Competition heightened as competing sales forces fought for customers who formerly were the domain of manufacturers in their particular region. Robert Keith so characterized Pillsbury's business focus at this stage: "We are a flour-milling company, manufacturing a number of products for the consumer market. We must have a first-rate sales organization which can dispose of all the products we make at a favorable price."[8]

For hospitals, the sales era occurred in the mid-1970s with the change in reimbursement. Under cost-based reimbursement, competition with other hospitals was not a major concern. Hospitals had patients, lengths of stay were not an issue, and occupancy rates were high. Hospitals treated patients and passed along the actual cost, along with an appropriate profit margin, for reimbursement by the third-party payers. The focus for a hospital administrator in the sales stage was twofold. The first and top priority was to get as many patients as possible. Traditionally, this goal was accomplished by attracting as many physicians as possible to admit patients to the hospital. Since this era preceded the days of utilization reviews, hospitals had no concerns about attracting efficient physicians

Table 1–1 The Evolution of Marketing

Business Orientation	Pillsbury	Hospital
Production	Product quality focus	Clinical quality focus
Sales	Generating volume	Filling beds
Marketing	Satisfying needs and wants	Identifying health care needs and meeting them

who could care for patients in some limited time period. The hospital wanted to ensure that as many patients as possible wanted to be admitted into the facility who were so directed by their doctors.

Changing Mr. Keith's statement, one might characterize the focus of a sales-oriented hospital as: "We are a high-quality hospital providing numerous medical services to the market. We must attract physicians in the community to want to admit to our facility. And, we must encourage patients to want to come here." This stage of marketing evolution focused on sales. Hospitals tried to entice doctors to admit to a particular facility. Hospitals built medical office buildings attached to their facilities offering doctors the convenience of admitting patients at the hospital contiguous to their offices. Hospitals developed physician relations programs to bond with the providers. They sponsored seminars for physicians, or provided valet parking and attractive doctors' lounges. All these were attempts to build the census, fill the beds.

At this time, hospitals also recognized that the patient might play a role in the hospital selection decision.[9] A second, concurrent strategy of selling to the public also occurred. In the mid-1970s, many hospitals adopted mass advertising strategies to promote their programs, including the use of billboard displays and television and radio commercials touting a particular service. The advertising goal was to encourage patients to use the hospital facilities when the doctor presented a choice, or to self-refer if necessary. In health care, this was the evolution to sales.

Marketing Era

The evolution to marketing occurred after World War II. In the late 1940s, many companies found that their level of technological sophistication had increased dramatically as a result of their wartime efforts. Moreover, consumers were returning from the war and establishing households, escalating the demand for products and services. For many companies the major question became one of deciding which products or services to offer. Pillsbury's perspective changed to: "We are in the business of satisfying the wants and needs of consumers." With this focus, it is the customer who drives the production process and directs the organization's efforts.

So, too, in health care, a similar perspective can and is being achieved. Health care providers can offer any number of services by reallocating their financial resources. The underlying question, however, becomes, which service to offer? This is where a marketing-oriented perspective is valuable. In health care, the focus of a marketing-oriented institution can be viewed as "We address the health care needs of the marketplace." Such a marketing-oriented focus might lead to a product or service line that includes home health care, geriatric medicine, after-hours care, or wellness centers. The trend toward integrated delivery systems (a concept discussed in greater detail later in this text) is a response to a marketplace that does not want to deal with a fractionated health care system of providers, free-standing medical centers, a hospital, and an insurance firm. The integrated system formation can deliver a seamless health care product to the buyer that involves not only delivering the clinical care, but also accepting the risk for the cost of that care through a managed care product. It is a focus that begins with the consumer; the organization responds to this demand.

THE MARKETING CULTURE

Some organizations achieve a final level of evolution, where marketing becomes part of the corporate culture, diffused throughout all levels of the organization. The focus of marketing no longer lies solely under the responsibility of the marketing department. Rather, in the health care setting, marketing is performed by the clinical nurse administrator for the neurology program. The admitting desk clerks and the house maintenance staff understand and appreciate the need to maintain a customer orientation.

The evolution to this stage may be seen in organizations that have adopted a patient-focused system. Sentara, an integrated delivery system in Hampton, Virginia, and Lakeland Regional Medical Center, a large tertiary hospital in Lakeland, Florida, are two such institutions. These organizations have made the customer the central focus of all their activities. Admitting is accomplished on the floor where the patient is assigned a bed, employees cross-train for skills that allow them to be the most patient-responsive possible without compromising the quality of care delivered. Whenever possible, certain diagnostic equipment is brought to the patient rather than having the patient move through the hospital. It is the primary responsibility of each employee to respond to customer needs first. The development of patient-focused care in such organizations is the transference of a marketing culture throughout the organization. Rather than having the patient (customer) go to the provider (such as when the patient moves through the delivery system for treatment or clinical testing), the provider goes to the patient whenever possible to administer the necessary clinical interventions.

For organizations at this stage, the concept of a marketing orientation has taken hold. A **marketing orientation** has five distinct elements: *you need to be:*
to be a market culture you need to be:

1. Customer orientation: having a sufficient understanding of the target buyers to be able to create superior value for them continuously
2. Competitor orientation: recognizing competitors' (and potential competitors') strengths, weaknesses, and strategies

3. Interfunctional coordination: coordinating and deploying company resources in a manner that focuses on creating value for the customer
4. Long-term focus: adopting a perspective that includes a continuous search for ways to add value by making appropriate business investments
5. Profitability: earning revenues sufficient to cover long-term expenses and satisfy key constituencies.[10]

THE NON-MARKETING-DRIVEN PLANNING PROCESS

While the patient-focused health care approach represents the diffusion of a marketing orientation throughout a health care institution, such an approach has not always been the perspective taken by health care providers. Most health care organizations have been characterized by a non-market-driven culture and planning process. In no place is the difference between being marketing-oriented and non-marketing-oriented more apparent than when a health care organization goes about its long-range planning process.

To understand the difference between a marketing-driven and non-marketing-driven process, it is important to recognize the implications of the difference between the two concepts on long-range planning.[11]

Figure 1–2 shows the sequence involved when a non-marketing-driven organization conducts long-range planning. In most health care organizations, long-

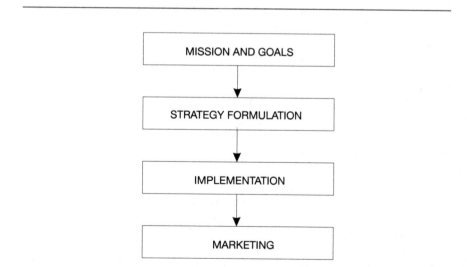

Figure 1–2 Non-Marketing-Based Planning Sequence

range planning is assigned to a committee comprising administrators, key members of the hospital's board of directors, and a few influential physicians. Typically, the first step involves a review of the organization's mission and goals. A hospital might reaffirm its mission "to provide high-quality health care regardless of race, creed, religion, and [in small print] ability to pay."

The second step of the planning process—strategy formulation—is often difficult and time-consuming. At this point, members of the long-range planning committee debate what objectives should be included in the hospital's five-year plan. Now, the real implications of the non-marketing-driven approach become evident. Often, a senior physician stands up at the strategy formulation stage and makes a speech such as the following. "I've been at this hospital since the day I entered the medical profession. This hospital is my life and I never even admitted a patient to another facility. Of course, I'm also being recognized as an expert in the future of medicine. I've been invited to conferences to speak on the future of medicine and I've just published an article in the *New England Journal of Medicine*. As I think about what services we need to provide in the new ambulatory care wing of the hospital, it's clear to me that we need a sports medicine program." Usually, the physician making this recommendation appears to be a self-serving orthopedic surgeon.

At this stage in the planning process, several committee members become dismayed. Some think the hospital should, instead, offer an expanded geriatric medicine program; other committee members want to get into rehabilitative medicine. Yet this physician is very influential and has lined up committee votes in favor of a sports medicine program before the committee met. The vote is taken and the final tally is seven to five in favor of a sports medicine program, which becomes part of the strategic plan.

The next stage of the long-range planning process—implementation—is more difficult. The hospital realizes it has no staff members trained in sports medicine. The hospital hires a physician recruiting firm to find a new medical director for sports medicine. The position is filled and it is at this stage of the process where conflict often occurs within the organization. Many committee members opposed opening a sports medicine program, yet now, the new director and new program require resources. Other services within the hospital find their budgets for the coming fiscal year are reduced in order to reallocate dollars to sports medicine. Other program directors are upset because they lose space in the new ambulatory care wing due to the needs of the sports medicine service. The new sports medicine director has an aggressive agenda. She has hired her staff, purchased the necessary equipment, and is setting up shop.

A state of anxiety soon takes hold of the hospital's administrators. As the date moves closer to the grand opening of the sports medicine program, they ask, "Who is really going to use the service?" Recognizing the need for patient volume, they attempt to market the program. But what happens is not marketing but sales.

The hospital administrator typically places a frantic call to the public relations director requesting an open house for the new sports medicine program. Advertisements are placed in the local community paper. Invitations to tour the facility are distributed to influential people. The goal is to attract visitors to the new program. On the day of the open house, attendance is disappointing. Four months later the finance committee convenes to review the performance of the sports medicine program. It is a failure. Why?

The first response is to blame public relations; the PR director didn't promote the service well. This may be a possible explanation. A second hypothesis suggests the failure is the fault of the new sports medicine director, whose interpersonal style is discouraging other physicians from referring patients to the program. Yet, there may be a third, more viable explanation—the sports medicine program wasn't needed. The program differed little from the competition's offering, hence, patients had no reason to switch facilities.

This scenario is a common result of a non-marketing-driven planning process. The problem with a non-marketing-driven process is that it requires a group of people (or one powerfully persuasive committee member) to have insight into what kinds of health care service the marketplace wants, how it wants that service configured, and what it is willing to pay for it. This approach to delivering a service or health care product to the market is an internal-to-external development process. The product is sold first. The challenge then is to find enough buyers willing to use the service or product at a level sufficient to make a profit. This approach is risky at best in that it relies on the market forecasting ability of a few people within the organization.

It is this limitation of the internal-to-external perspective of the non-marketing-driven approach, as well as overcoming the political power of a few people within the organization, that are addressed by taking a marketing-driven approach to planning.

A MARKETING-DRIVEN PLANNING SEQUENCE

A marketing-driven planning sequence is dramatically different from a non-marketing-driven process, as illustrated in Figure 1–3. The first step is the same; every organization has the right to determine its mission and goals. Yet the marketing-driven approach is substantially different at step two. It is at this stage of needs assessment where market research, as will be discussed in Chapter 5, begins to make its contribution. The hospital conducts a survey to determine which services are most needed. Should sports medicine, geriatric medicine, or women's health services be offered in the new ambulatory care wing of the hospital?

When determining the most needed service, it is essential to examine the competition. If there are existing competing services in the market, the necessary

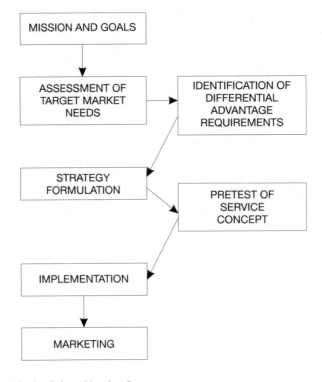

Figure 1–3 Marketing-Driven Planning Sequence

differential advantage for these new offerings must be identified. While the sources of a differential advantage are discussed later in this chapter, a **differential advantage** is the incremental benefits of a product relative to competing products that are important to the buyer and perceived by the buyer. In our example, the hospital's survey reveals that 20 percent of the market wants sports medicine, 25 percent would like to see a new geriatric program, and 50 percent wants women's health. Further research shows that the major differential advantages that would lead women to use this service over their existing providers are convenient location and hours.

With the market research completed, the strategy is clear. A conveniently located, accessible women's health program is written into the hospital's long-range plan. Prior to full-scale implementation, however, market research is employed again in the form of a pretest. Pretesting involves returning to the market with a product sample to ensure that the specifications meet customer expectations. In a service business such as health care, the pretesting stage is particularly difficult. Unlike many product businesses that can manufacture a prototype without incurring major fixed costs, a new health program might require a redesign of physical space, the hiring of trained personnel, and acquisition of new technologies. Pretesting must still be done, however, without the addition of all these costs.

To pretest a service in health care effectively, the personnel involved with the program and with customer relations must develop a detailed concept description of the service. They then assemble a sample of potential female patients similar to those in the target market and walk them through a concept test of the service. Consumers can be questioned about hours, service location, and appointment procedure. Reactions to the concept generate appropriate modifications. Full-scale implementation then begins. At this point, the hospital needs to market—not sell—the program. Market research has determined the product, the price customers are willing to pay, and how the service should be distributed (i.e., locations, hours). All that remains for the hospital is to inform the target market about the availability of the desired new service through the appropriate promotions.

Is a Marketing Planning Approach Needed?

A comparison of Figures 1–2 and 1–3 shows that using market research can lead to a dramatically different result in long-range planning. Yet, is a marketing-driven planning process needed in health care? Twenty or 30 years ago, a non-marketing-driven process was sufficient. Competition wasn't a prime factor. In most communities, including major metropolitan areas, demand exceeded supply. A hospital would offer a new service and the major issue was how to meet demand for it. Twenty or 30 years ago most health care organizations were in a reasonably strong financial position due to cost-based reimbursement and unrestricted lengths of stay. Efficiency and financial prudence were nonissues.

The present competitive health care environment has prompted many organizations to adopt a marketing-driven planning approach. Health care providers find themselves facing significant competition. In many instances, and for many subspecialties, the problem is one of supply exceeding demand. The challenge is to encourage demand for your service at the expense of your competitors. Organizations must find a differential advantage to encourage buyers to use their services. Health care organizations today must be fiscally astute. Few have the excess financial resources to afford the mistake of offering a service that is not needed in the marketplace. A marketing-driven planning process is one tool to help minimize such mistakes.

We have described a non-marketing-driven approach to planning as an internal-to-external methodology.[12] That is, members inside the organization try to foretell or dictate what the market wants and how the service should best be configured to meet those wants. In comparison, a marketing-driven approach follows an external-to-internal methodology. First, there is an assessment of what the market wants, then the organization's response. Health care providers must realize that a marketing-driven planning process does not guarantee success; but it does, however, minimize the probability of failure.

THE STRATEGIC MARKETING PROCESS

The marketing-driven planning model just discussed is devised within the context of a more macro setting. Figure 1–4 shows the setting in which marketing occurs. An organization must develop a marketing strategy that is sensitive to three factors: (1) important stakeholders, (2) environmental factors, and (3) society at large.

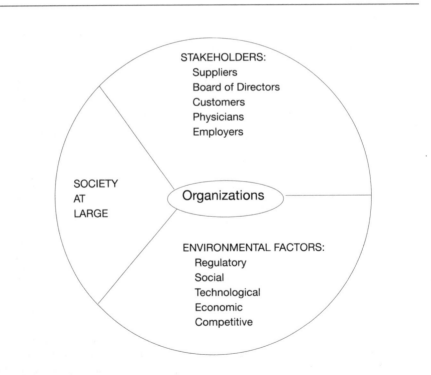

Figure 1–4 Environment and Marketing Strategy

Stakeholders

Stakeholders represent any group with which the company has, or wants to develop, a relationship. As seen in Figure 1–4, the stakeholders can represent customers. For health care organizations, these customers might be patients, physicians who refer to the organization, social workers for an adolescent chemical dependency program, payers, managed care providers with whom contracts are developed, or companies that contract for an industrial medicine program.

Many organizations such as hospitals or proprietary chains also have boards of directors that serve an oversight function. Organizations develop their marketing strategy in light of the direction and values provided and communicated by this constituency. A third major stakeholder group includes suppliers. In health care, suppliers can represent companies that provide laboratory testing or maintenance services, or they again can represent physicians. For many hospitals, physicians are customers. In a group practice setting, physicians represent the shareholders or owners. In other organizations, physicians, by providing coverage of the emergency room, might actually be suppliers.

Uncontrollable Environment

Any marketing strategy is developed within the context of a broader environmental perspective. The **environment** pertains to regulatory, social, technological, economic, and competitive factors to which the organization must be sensitive when developing a strategy. These elements, which are discussed in greater detail in Chapter 3 (and briefly described below), are uncontrollable, but impact marketing strategy. For example, a company cannot change the uncontrollable trend that society is aging. Yet a company can develop a strategy to respond to marketplace needs resulting from this trend. Between 1990 and 1993, the number of adult day-care centers nationwide increased almost 50 percent to 3,000 such facilities. Forecasts predict that 10,000 such centers will be needed by the year 2000 in response to an aging marketplace.[13] Building planned retirement communities or developing long-term care facilities are just two strategies for dealing with this trend.

Regulatory Factors

Regulatory factors include legal issues and requirements. In many health care communities, programs cannot be instituted without prior government approval. Some strategies, such as paying physicians for referrals, are illegal.

Social Forces

Social forces include demographic and cultural trends to which organizations must be sensitive. An aging population, a changing work ethic, and a culturally diverse marketplace are some of the issues to consider when developing marketing plans.

Technological Factors

Technological factors affect few industries more dramatically then they do health care. It is these technological forces that can change the viability of any service. Until the 1950s, the treatment of polio victims constituted a major revenue stream for many hospital facilities. As we know, this disease was all but eliminated by the technological achievement of the Salk vaccine in the 1950s.

Economic Factors

Economic factors include changes in income distribution or fiscal conditions such as borrowing rates that can determine any company's investment plans. As will be discussed in Chapter 3, the rising cost of health care has led one major customer group—corporations—to work more aggressively with their health care providers in seeking solutions to rising costs.

Competitive Forces

Competitive forces are the final uncontrollable element in any marketing plan. Strategies and programs must be developed in light of this constraint and should reflect the considerations that exist in the marketplace.

Society

Ultimately, all marketing programs and strategies are developed within the context of a broader societal perspective, a context that requires an ethically responsible decision-making process. For example, many companies have become more keenly aware of and responsible for the impact of their products and programs on the environment. The broader societal market represents all the individuals, groups, businesses, and other entities that affect, are related to, or derive benefit from the health care organization, as seen in Exhibit 1–1.

TARGET MARKET

At the core of the marketing program is the **target market**, the group of customers whom the organization wishes to attract. In the development of a

Exhibit 1–1 Organizations in the Health Care Environment

Organizations That Plan for and/or Regulate (Primary and Secondary Providers)	Organizations That Provide Health Services (Primary Providers)	Organizations That Provide Resources (Secondary Providers)	Organizations That Represent Primary and Secondary Providers	Individuals and Patients (Consumers)

• Federal Regulating Agencies
  – Health Systems Agencies (HSAs)
  – Department of Health and Human Services (DHHS)
  – Health Care Financing Agency (HCFA)
• State Regulating Agencies
  – Public Health Departments
  – State Planning Agency (CON)
• Voluntary Regulating Groups
• Joint Commission On Accreditation of Healthcare Organizations
• Other Accrediting Agencies
	• Hospitals
	  – Voluntary (Barnes Hospital)
	  – Governmental (VA Hospitals)
	  – Investor Owned (Humana, AMI, NME)
	• State Public Health Departments
	• Long-Term Care Facilities
	  – Skilled Nursing Facilities (Beverly Enterprises)
	  – Intermediate Care Facilities
	• HMOs and IPAs (Care America)
	• Ambulatory Care Facilities (National Rehab Services)
	• Hospices (Hospice Care, Inc.)
	• Physicians' Offices
	• Home Health Care Institutions (VNA, Upjohn Healthcare Services)
		• Educational Institutions
		  – Medical Schools (Johns Hopkins)
		  – Nursing Schools
		  – Health Administration Programs
		• Organizations That Pay for Care
		  – Third-Party Payers
		  – Government (Medicare)
		  – Insurance Companies (Blue Cross)
		  – Social Organizations (Shriners)
		• Pharmaceutical and Medical Supply
		  – Drug Distributors (McKesson)
		  – Drug & Research (Merck, Eli Lilly)
		  – Medical Products (Johnson & Johnson, Bausch & Lomb)
			• American Medical Association (AMA)
			• American Hospital Association (AHA)
			• State Medical Associations
			• Individual Professional Associations
				• Independent Physicians
				• Nurses
				• Allied Health Professionals
				• Technicians
				• Patients

Source: Reprinted from Ginter, P.M., Duncan, W.J., Richardson, W.D., and Swayne, L.E., Analyzing the Health Care Environment: You Can't Hit What You Can't See, *Health Care Management Review*, Vol. 16, No. 4, p. 44, Aspen Publishers, Inc., © 1991.

marketing strategy, the target market is within an organization's control as a function of the effectiveness of the marketing mix developed by the health care providers.

The notion of controlling the target market, however, is an idea that is often lost on health care providers. Whom a health system attracts to its facilities and whom it targets may be two different populations. Too often in the past, health care organizations have defined their market by simply identifying who walked into their facility or used the emergency room. Health care organizations developed profiles of their patients and developed strategies based on the users. Yet the central issue to marketing strategy is to decide whom you want to attract and then determine what this group's needs are. The organization that defines a target market, such as "all consumers with incomes above $75,000 who have private insurance and live in a particular area," can then focus its market research on identification of an appropriate strategy to meet the needs of the targeted group. Sharp Health Care of California has decided that one of its target markets will include Mexican patients. Sharp Health Care, a large health care system that includes various health care subsidiaries and five hospitals in San Diego, California, opened a hospital under the Sharp name in Mazatlan, Mexico in December 1994. Sharp also hopes to capture referrals from this target market by an affiliation agreement with Hospital Notre Dame in Tiajuana, Mexico. To support this effort, Sharp will provide continuing medical education programs for that hospital's medical staff.[14] Determining the target market resulted in several strategies to attract this consumer population.

ORGANIZING FOR MARKETING

Establishing the marketing function within an organization can be accomplished in one of several ways. The two most common organizational structures for marketing are by product and by market.

Product-Oriented Organization

The product management structure has been increasingly common in health care settings, structured as shown in Figure 1–5. In this setting, the responsibility, authority, and accountability rests with the product line manager. Nursing, pharmacy, laboratory, and other departments coordinate their services across, and in support of, the product lines. In the true **product-oriented organization**, each distinct product or related set of products has its own marketing organization.

The product manager is responsible for developing and overseeing the marketing strategy for the product or **strategic business units**, which are businesses operated as separate profit centers within a large organization. In a product management structure, individual managers commonly share staff resources, such as marketing research, as well as operational personnel, such as the sales force. The product manager approach is of value when a product has such unique requirements that it demands the commitment of a separate individual.

Product line management has two major advantages for health care organizations. First, having someone responsible for all aspects of a product line helps to refine the service area and to meet needs more easily. This structure

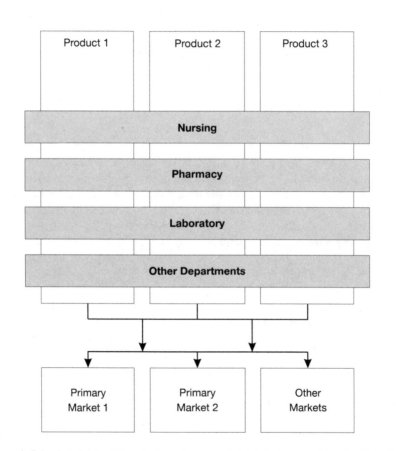

Figure 1–5 Product-Oriented Organization. *Source:* Reprinted from Zelman, W.N. and Parham, D.L., Strategic, Operational, and Marketing Concerns of Product-Line Management in Health Care, *Health Care Management Review,* Vol. 15, No. 1, p. 32, Aspen Publishers, Inc., © 1990.

helps combine services and benefits for customers. Second, packaging related services into product lines helps contribute to continuous, rather than sporadic, planning.[15]

A disadvantage with the product management structure in traditional businesses has been the fact that the product manager has no direct control over many operational details—the product manager must negotiate for sales force time or marketing research resources. This same limitation holds in health care. While the product manager has the focus to develop program plans, there is no direct operational control over how the service is delivered within the facility. Often, in many health care organizations, the product manager acts as the salesperson for the program. For health care organizations, there is another consideration that may limit the value of a product organization. If the same customer is targeted for more than one product line, it could lead to significant marketing inefficiencies or customer resistance. For example, a referral physician may be unwilling to see four different product line representatives from one tertiary medical center.

Market-Oriented Organization

The second most common marketing structure is a **market-oriented organization** in which each distinct major market has its own marketing organization, as seen in Figure 1–6. A health care organization might design a marketing organization around its major customer groups (referral physicians, corporations, managed care buyers, and other referral sources) as shown in this figure.

The value of this approach is its focus on customers who have different buying structures and purchasing requirements. For any health care organization, supporting marketing activities can be serviced by the manager of each major market group. The underlying rationale for this approach is that each major customer group has distinct needs.

For decades, IBM Corporation was organized around product lines. In 1994, the corporation concluded that customers demanded solutions to problems, not products. This forced the company to restructure around major markets and industries. In this way, IBM can develop expertise in financial services, telecommunications, or manufacturing and meet the information needs of these respective industries. Whether the solution is provided by a local area network system, a mainframe computer, or a series of independent desktop computers is irrelevant to the customer. This same analogy applies to the health care setting. Corporate expectations and demands differ from the requirements and concerns of a second major market of referral physicians. In each instance, solutions to problems are sought rather than the purchase of a specific clinical program.

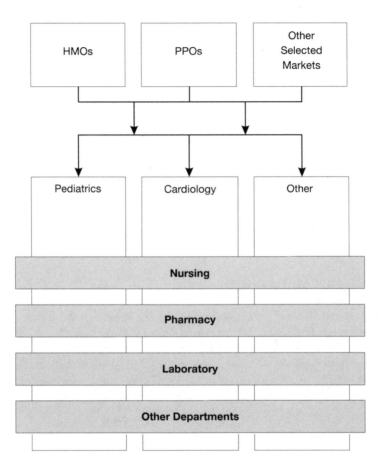

Figure 1–6 Market-Oriented Organization. *Source:* Reprinted from Zelman, W.N. and Parham, D.L., Strategic, Operational, and Marketing Concerns of Product-Line Management in Health Care, *Health Care Management Review,* Vol. 15, No. 1, pp. 29–35, Aspen Publishers, Inc., © 1990.

REQUIREMENTS FOR ORGANIZATIONAL MARKETING SUCCESS

Many hospitals and medical groups have problems making the transition to becoming a market-oriented organization. Often, marketing has not met the expectations of filling hospital beds or generating substantial numbers of new subscribers into the HMO. The disappointment in marketing is due to a lack of appreciation of what it means to be marketing driven, and of what marketing alone can accomplish. There are four prerequisites for successful marketing, as shown in Figure 1–7.[16]

Pressure To Be Market-Oriented

First, there must be pressure to be market-oriented. There must be a shared view that is accepted throughout the organization concerning the need for an improved marketing program. To some extent, this represents the fourth stage in the evolution of marketing that is appearing in organizations previously mentioned, such as Sentara. Not only must senior management want to become more market-oriented, but peer pressure to understand and to respond to customer needs must be strong throughout the organization. Information and reward systems must recognize the value of a customer orientation, and department program objectives and measurement systems must be tied to progress on this goal.

Capacity To Be Market-Oriented

A second criterion for organizational marketing success is the capacity to be market-oriented. The health care organization must have enough staff members who are not only experienced and adequately trained, but also devoted to improving the organization's marketing effort. Management, staff, and clinical personnel must be receptive to ideas on how to become more market-oriented and have a marketing budget to support their efforts. Although Figure 1–8 shows a

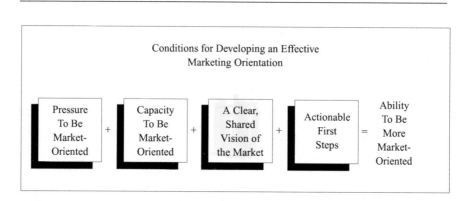

Conditions for Developing an Effective
Marketing Orientation

| Pressure To Be Market-Oriented | + | Capacity To Be Market-Oriented | + | A Clear, Shared Vision of the Market | + | Actionable First Steps | = | Ability To Be More Market-Oriented |

Figure 1–7 Prerequisites to Marketing Success.   *Source:* Reprinted from Diamond, S.L. and Berkowitz, E.N., Effective Marketing for Health Care Providers, *Journal of Medical Practice Management,* Vol. 5, No. 3, p. 198, with permission of Williams & Wilkins, © 1990.

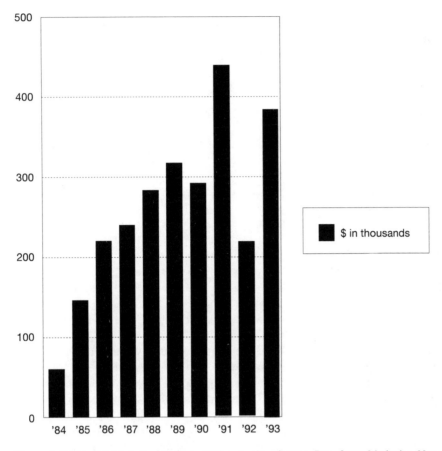

Figure 1–8 Hospital Marketing Budgets: Rising Again. *Source:* Data from *Marketing News,* Vol. 28, No. 1, p. 1, American Marketing Association, 1994.

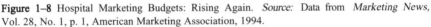

recent drop in hospital spending for marketing, overall, hospital marketing budgets have nearly quadrupled since 1984.

Besides financial support, significant time must be devoted to improving marketing efforts and to developing an understanding of how these efforts integrate with other organizational priorities.

Shared Vision of Market

A clear, shared vision of the market is a third prerequisite to success. Many questions must be answered when developing an understanding of the marketplace: Who are the key customers and stakeholders? What are their needs? What change must the organization make in terms of its marketing mix to meet the needs of these core constituencies? How will this organization differentiate itself from other providers?

Action Plan To Respond to Market

Last, the organization must develop a clear set of actionable steps to respond to market needs. It will need a detailed marketing plan that includes the necessary strategies and tactics along each of the four Ps. This also requires well-defined mechanisms to track the progress of and address minor difficulties in implementation before they become major customer problems.

Missing any one of these elements can lead to marketing ineffectiveness. Figure 1–9 reveals the results of these prerequisite gaps. Without the pressure to be market-oriented, there is a "bottom of the In box" feeling toward marketing. The words are mouthed but there is no pressure to change. Lacking the capacity to be marketing-oriented leads to frustration and anxiety. Attempting to be efficient, many health care providers have pared resources. Yet, marketing personnel and programs must be viewed as an investment to generate additional revenue, not solely as an expense item.

Many health care organizations' marketing efforts have suffered from a fast start that quickly fizzled because of the absence of a clear, shared vision of the market. Well-designed, effective marketing programs require an in-depth understanding of the marketplace. Many hospitals, in the 1980s, began to advertise programs before they even knew what they were advertising.[17] This same problem seems to be reoccurring now as many health organizations rush to promote their integrated delivery systems with little understanding of system definition or market requirements.

False starts, another pitfall for marketing, occur when there are no actionable, first steps in place. Effective marketing requires detailed plans that specify the tactics to be implemented within each of the four Ps. Allocated responsibilities, benchmarks for measuring performance, and timetables are specified at the planning process. With all four components in place, the contributions of the marketing function and resultant strategy to any health care organization's success increase dramatically.

THE CHANGING HEALTH CARE MARKETPLACE

No discussion of marketing in health care can begin without an overview of the dramatic restructuring occurring in the industry today. As this chapter began, it mentioned terms that any reader of health care literature or practitioner in the field

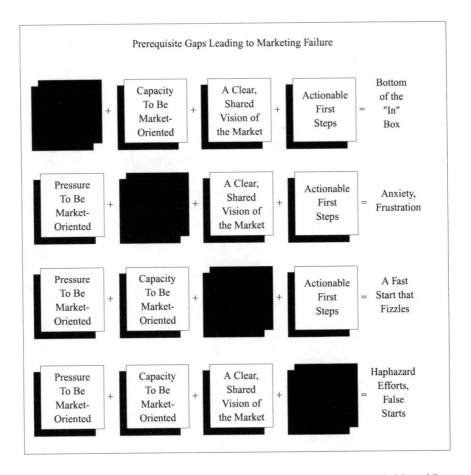

Prerequisite Gaps Leading to Marketing Failure

Figure 1–9 Prerequisites to Marketing Success. *Source:* Reprinted from Diamond, S.L. and Berkowitz, E.N., Effective Marketing for Health Care Providers, *Journal of Medical Practice Management,* Vol. 5, No. 3, p. 203, with permission of Williams & Wilkins, © 1990.

faces daily—integration, satellites, managed care. What are the implications of these changes for marketing? To appreciate the impact on marketing of the restructuring occurring within health care today, it is instructive to reexamine the traditional industry structure from which we are rapidly moving away.[18]

The Traditional Industry Structure

In communities that have not truly experienced the formation of an integrated delivery system, the health care marketplace can be considered fractionated, in that each entity operates independently. Figure 1–10 shows the major components of this traditional health care structure. At the top of the figure is the hospital, then physicians, followed by the community-at-large.

The focus of the hospital's marketing efforts are twofold, represented by the solid arrows. The focus primarily has been on physicians. The key to maintaining a census within the facility is by encouraging doctors to admit to one's own particular facility as opposed to a competitor's. Consider, then, what has been the typical marketing efforts by hospitals in this regard.

Most hospitals today have a physician relations staff who call on physicians to ensure they are satisfied with the facility and to determine whether the hospital can provide any additional services to meet their needs. Other hospitals have built connecting medical office buildings and rented space at attractive rates for doctors' offices, on the premise that physicians will admit to the hospital most convenient to their offices. In any case, physicians are a major focus of marketing efforts.

A second market for the hospital in the traditional industry structure is the community-at-large. Since 1975, hospitals have targeted their advertising efforts at building name recognition within the community for the facility and its programs. The rationale for this strategy is that patients may ask their doctors to refer them to a specific hospital, or they may self-select the facility when they need medical treatment.

The second level of this chart involves physicians and their marketing focus, represented by the dotted lines. Here, too, there have been two markets—other

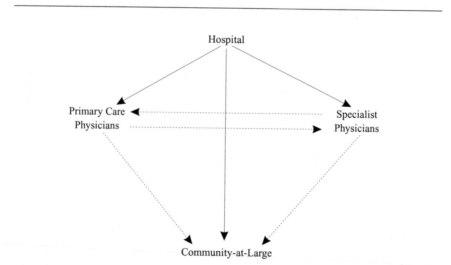

Figure 1–10 The Traditional Industry Structure

doctors and the community-at-large. Specialists focus their efforts on generating referrals from primary care doctors, although in some specialties, such as plastic surgery and dermatology, it's common to see direct appeals to the community-at-large through advertisements. Primary care physicians have historically attracted new patients in the community either through word-of-mouth, or through more formal communication strategies including advertisements or detailed telephone directory listings. This type of market structure is very similar to that faced by consumer product companies. That is, the decision to buy the service is typically made by one individual or a small group of individuals. A doctor decides to admit to a particular hospital, or a family decides to become regular patients at a particular medical clinic. In this type of consumer market, mass communication is vital since there are so many people within the community who could, at any point of time, avail themselves of the medical provider's service. Similarly for the specialist, there is always a large number of primary care doctors who could refer patients to them. The comfort of this world is knowing that individual buyers only represent their own volume of business.

This is a somewhat simplified but macro view of the traditional health care market structure that has existed for many years, and still does in communities with little managed care or little pressure from employers to control health care costs. This world, however, is rapidly disappearing. The health care marketplace of the next decade will be defined as more of an industrial marketplace.

The Evolving Industry Structure

In communities such as Minneapolis–St. Paul, San Francisco, and Phoenix, the health care marketplace is undergoing a massive restructuring. Hospitals and physicians are banding together in new structures in which they will operate as a single entity in the management of health care delivery. These entities are either contracting with HMOs or offering their own prepaid health care plans to provide medical care to the community. In this new health care environment, the structure of the industry has changed and is more typical of that shown in Figure 1–11.

These changes carry tremendous marketing implications. The hospital is still at the top of the figure, but is now joined by physicians. They are one organizational entity that can bring to bear all the necessary resources to meet the health care needs of the community. In a sense, this box can be viewed as the integrated delivery system, representing the hard assets (inpatient beds, surgery centers, laboratory, rehabilitation facility, and long-term care beds), and the personnel (skilled clinicians) that can deliver the expertise, the appropriate technologies, and the setting for needed care.

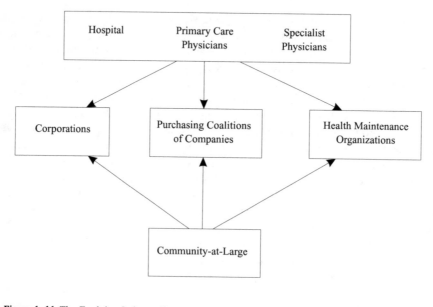

Figure 1–11 The Evolving Industry Structure

At the bottom of the chart is still the community-at-large. These people represent the individuals who will need the services of the integrated delivery system. Yet, access to this care is now affected by a new intermediary shown in the middle of the figure. The community-at-large now goes through the new intermediaries to gain access to a particular health care provider.

The doctors who used to be the market have been replaced by corporations or HMOs. These entities decide which facilities can be used by their employees or by their subscribers. Employers are contracting directly with some providers for particular aspects of care. Many HMOs contract with a particular health care facility, which means that health plan subscribers can only use the contracted provider.

From a marketing perspective, the implications of this restructuring are dramatic. While the traditional health care structure was a consumer market with a large number of potential buyers (doctors who could use the facility or patients who could access the hospital), this new structure is more typical of an industrial marketing setting in which there are a restricted set of buyers for a company's products. Pratt & Whitney in Hartford, Connecticut, for example, is a manufacturer of engines for jet aircraft. There are a limited number of buyers for jet engines. So, too, a hospital in any community may find there are only a handful of HMO plans with which it can obtain a contract, or one or two corporate purchasing coalitions that will contract directly for the care of the employees they represent. In this world, effective marketing becomes essential because each buyer now represents a significant amount of business and potential revenue.

CONCLUSIONS

As the health care industry restructures, so too must the perspective regarding marketing's challenges. Historically, the customer has been either the individual doctor who was free to choose where to admit a patient and send a referral, or the individual patient free to choose where to go for treatment. In the evolving health care marketplace, the customer will be an organization responsible for buying or contracting for the health care coverage of a large group of people. In the traditional marketplace, health care was purchased on an episodic basis. When an individual was sick and received medical treatment, payment for that treatment came from the government or from an insurance company. In the evolving marketplace, health care will be delivered for a contractual amount agreed upon between buyer and provider. It will then be the provider's responsibility to deliver the medically necessary care at that predetermined price for a particular length of time. Buyers are increasingly concerned about the value they receive for their health care dollar.

The restructuring of health care only serves to underscore the importance of marketing. In the traditional industry setting, if one doctor is unhappy and no longer admits to a particular hospital, the hospital suffers from the loss of only one doctor. In this traditional environment, if one patient is unhappy with service received at the medical clinic or in the emergency room and decides never to return to that facility, the loss to the organization is the future revenue from one patient.

The new environment of health care, however, requires that marketing be at the core of the organization's strategy. With only a few major buyers in a marketplace that will be contracting for service, the challenge is clear. A health care provider or supplier cannot afford to lose a customer. That customer—be it the corporation, HMO, or group purchasing alliance—represents significant revenue through its contract agreement. It is important also to recognize that the buyer represents users who must also be satisfied. Dissatisfaction among users can lead the buyers to change providers or suppliers rather than face continual dissatisfaction from their employees or subscribers. As the health care industry restructures, marketing is moving into an age where it will be a functional area of major importance for an organization's survival. Knowing the needs and wants of a smaller core of buyers who hold greater economic influence will be the primary requirement to obtaining new business.

KEY TERMS	
Marketing	Want
Marketing Research	Market Orientation
Four Ps	Differential Advantage
Marketing Mix	Stakeholders
Product	Environment
Price	Target Market
Place	Product-Oriented Organization
Promotion	Strategic Business Units
Need	Market-Oriented Organization

CHAPTER SUMMARY

1. *Marketing is a process that involves planning and execution of the four marketing mix variables: product, price, place, and promotion.*

2. *Effective marketing for health care organizations involves the recognition of multiple customers or markets who often have a diverse array of needs and wants.*

3. *A non-market-based approach to planning is one in which the conception of the service begins internally within the organization. Marketing-based planning is an external-to-internal process.*

4. *The strategic marketing process must consider the broad macro environment consisting of stakeholders, environmental factors, and society at large.*

5. *Health care marketing planning requires identification of the target market, which may differ from the organization's present customer base.*

6. *In a product-oriented organization, services are managed as separate profit centers, or strategic business units.*

7. *In a market-oriented organizational structure, major markets or customer groups are the focus.*

8. *Marketing success has four prerequisites: pressure, capacity, vision, and actionable steps.*

9. *The structure of the health care industry is evolving from a consumer market to an industrial market.*

10. *In the evolving health care industry, the focus of marketing efforts will also change. In the consumer market, marketing efforts were directed at physicians and consumers. In the new marketplace, intermediaries like HMOs, employers, and*

buying coalitions that will control access to patients will be the important target for marketing activities.

CHAPTER PROBLEMS

p 4

1. Several prerequisites are necessary for marketing to occur. Identify each prerequisite in the following examples: (a) a politician running for political office, (b) a consumer seeking physical therapy, (c) a company choosing health coverage for its employees.

2. At a recent hospital planning meeting, the marketing director reports on consumer interest in a women's health center. Hearing strong interest, the planning committee endorses the concept. A group of clinicians is charged with developing the program. Upon introduction, market response does not meet expectations. A senior physician was heard to complain, "What went wrong? We did the survey." Explain the possible reasons for this program's failure.

3. An orthopedic group practice has decided to develop a pediatric sports medicine program. Identify potential target markets for this new service.

4. In developing the new pediatric sports medicine program (described above in question 3), what are some of the uncontrollable environmental factors to consider?

5. A major concern for many health care professionals is the belief that marketing "creates" needs. Explain the complexity of this issue.

6. After reviewing the volume of subscribers to the health maintenance plan, the executive director is dismayed. Projected enrollment is far below the forecasted level for the targeted time period. A decision is made to hire additional salespeople to market the plan more aggressively. Explain the inconsistencies between this decision and an evolutionary marketing perspective.

7. Explain the difference between existing customers, target markets, and stakeholders for an acute-care community hospital.

NOTES

1. AMA Board Approves New Definition, *American Medical News* 15, no. 5 (March 1, 1985): 1.

2. P. Kotler and S.J. Levy, Broadening the Concept of Marketing, *Journal of Marketing* 33, no. 1 (1969): 10–15.

3. This conceptualization of the four Ps was first proposed by J. McCarthy, *Basic Marketing: A Managerial Approach* (Homewood, Ill.: Richard D. Irwin, Inc., 1960).

4. *Webster's New World Dictionary* (New York, N.Y.: Simon and Schuster, Inc., 3rd College Edition, 1994), 906.

5. Ibid., 1504.

6. K. Pallarito, State Legislatures Enter Debate on Mom, Newborn Hospital Stays, *Modern Healthcare* 25, no. 24 (1995): 22.

7. R.F. Keith, The Marketing Revolution, *Journal of Marketing* 24, no. 3 (January 1960): 36.

8. Ibid.

9. E.N. Berkowitz and W. Flexner, The Market for Health Services: Is There a Non-Traditional Consumer?, *Journal of Health Care Marketing* 1, no. 1 (Winter 1980–81): 25–34.

10. J. Narver and S. Slater, The Effect of a Market Orientation on Business Profitability, *Journal of Marketing* 53, no. 4 (October 1990): 20–22.

11. This discussion is based on E.N. Berkowitz, Marketing as a Necessary Function in Health Care Management: A Philosophical Approach, in *The Physician Executive*, ed. W. Curry (Tampa, Fla.: American College of Physician Executives, 1994), 221–228.

12. W.A. Flexner and E.N. Berkowitz, Marketing Research in Health Services Planning, *Public Health Reports* 94, no. 6 (November–December 1979): 503–513.

13. Adult Day Care Is Worth Looking Into, *Briefings on Long Term Care* 2, no. 5 (May 1994): 1–3.

14. L. Kertesz, California-Based Sharp Taps Mexican Market, *Modern Healthcare* 24, no. 35 (1994): 28.

15. E.M. Robertson, Product Line Management Focuses on the Customer, *Health Care Competition Week* 8, no. 23 (1991): 1–2.

16. S.L. Diamond and E.N. Berkowitz, Effective Marketing: A Road Map for Health Care Providers, *The Journal of Medical Practice Management* 5, no. 3 (Winter 1990): 197–204.

17. S. Powills, Hospitals Calling a Marketing Time-Out, *Hospitals* 60, no. 11 (June 5, 1986): 50–55.

18. This discussion is drawn from an unpublished working paper, E.N. Berkowitz and M. Guthrie, The New Health Care Paradigm (November 1994).

2

MARKETING STRATEGY

LEARNING OBJECTIVES

After reading this chapter you should be able to:

- Understand the scope of strategic marketing planning

- Identify broad organizational market strategy alternatives

- Describe the value of alternative portfolio models

- Appreciate the factors that affect the level of competitive intensity within an industry

- Understand the essential components of marketing strategy formulation

STRATEGIC PLANNING PROCESS

In order to respond to the opportunities and challenges of the marketplace, most organizations engage in a process of strategic planning. **Strategic planning** has been defined as a process that describes the direction an organization will pursue within its chosen environment and guides the allocation of resources and efforts.[1] The strategic planning process is shown in Figure 2–1 as containing four steps. It is within the context of this strategic plan that the functional areas of marketing, finance, human resources, and operations develop their own plans, as shown in Figure 2–2.

To develop an effective strategic plan, an organization must first define its mission. Second, it must conduct a situational assessment of the threats and

39

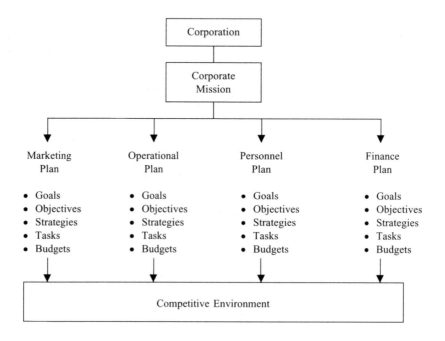

Figure 2–1 The Strategic Planning Process. *Source:* Reprinted from *Health Care Marketing Plans: From Strategy to Action,* 2nd ed., by S.G. Hillestad and E.N. Berkowitz, p. 48, Aspen Publishers, Inc., © 1991.

opportunities to which the organization can respond in light of its mission. At this stage, the organization must also assess its own distinctive competencies. Last, the organization must define its mission and establish a set of priorities based on organizational objectives. Once these steps have been taken, the organization can then determine which strategies to pursue in competing in the broader market.

Defining the Organizational Mission

Organizational mission refers to the organization's fundamental purpose for existing, defining who the organization is, its values, and the customers it wishes to serve. Mission statements are established to set the tone for the organization and provide the management with a purposely broad set of directions for how it should develop further business strategies. Exhibit 2–1 shows two alternative mission statements: one for Cascade Healthcare Alliance in Bellview, Washington; and the other for SwedishAmerican Health System in Rockford, Illinois. These two

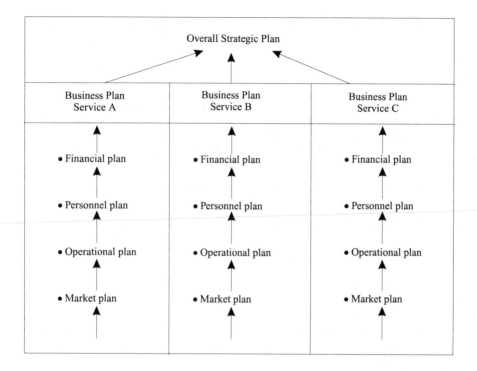

Figure 2–2 Portfolio Model For a Business Plan. *Source:* Reprinted from *Health Care Marketing Plans: From Strategy to Action,* 2nd ed., by S.G. Hillestad and E.N. Berkowitz, p. 48, Aspen Publishers, Inc., © 1991.

mission statements reflect the significant changes that health care providers face today. Cascade Healthcare Alliance is a group of physicians equally comprised of specialists and primary care providers—all of whom are attempting to organize and directly accept risk contracts. SwedishAmerican Health System, which has Swedish Hospital as its major organization, is on the forefront of establishing an integrated health system. SwedishAmerican Health System has a partnership between the physicians on the medical staff and the hospital.

Organizations can establish missions that are either broad or narrow, but it's important to establish a mission with the greatest likelihood of success in a competitive marketplace. Figure 2–3 shows the range of possibilities regarding a health mission statement.

An effective mission statement should clearly articulate most of the following components:

Exhibit 2–1 Alternative Mission Statements

Cascade Healthcare Alliance:

By the year 2000, CHA will evolve into the Eastside multispecialty group practice component of a vertically integrated delivery system aligned with hospitals and physicians and with exclusive contracts for at least 100,000 lives. This practice will be governed by physicians with majority physician ownership, acknowledging the central role of primary care. It will be the benchmark for quality care, with shared accountability for superior outcomes, high patient satisfaction and cost effectiveness through measurable objective standards.

The members of CHA will work cooperatively, have mutual respect, and trust each other and support synergistic process level thinking. CHA adopts a strategy of accepting full risk contracts and providing proper incentives to all. The organization will create, purchase, and network comprehensive services for its members.

CHA accepts the reality of a dynamic, evolving marketplace and will adapt to its customer and member needs.

SwedishAmerican Health System:

The mission of SwedishAmerican Health System is to improve the physical and mental well-being of the individuals we serve. We shall pursue that mission by providing the highest value care to those who are ill and the most effective prevention strategies to those who are well.

We define quality as achieving the best patient care results our resources will allow while minimizing risk and discomfort and maximizing patient satisfaction. We will carry out our mission with compassionate care and respect for the individual as we strive to achieve superior outcomes through continuous quality improvement.

Source: Courtesy of Cascade Healthcare Alliance, Bellview, Washington, and SwedishAmerican Health System, Rockford, Illinois.

---

1. The basic product or service, primary market, and technology to be used in delivering the product or service;
2. Organizational goals, such as growth, profitability, stability, or survival, stated in a strategic sense;
3. Organizational philosophy—the code of behavior that guides the organization's operation;
4. Organizational self-concept—a self-evaluation based on a realistic determination of its strengths and weaknesses; and
5. Public image—how those outside the organization view the particular entity.[2]

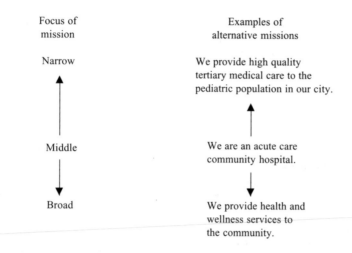

Figure 2–3 Strategic Mission Options. *Source:* Adapted from *Health Care Marketing Plans: From Strategy to Action*, 2nd ed., by S.G. Hillestad and E.N. Berkowitz, p. 21, Aspen Publishers, Inc., © 1991.

Essential to a successful mission statement is the recognition of what the business is and what the customer wants. Levitt described the marketing myopia of some organizations whose definition of their mission failed to recognize the threats and opportunities in the external marketplace. For many years, the railroads described themselves as "railroad companies." In fact, the marketplace was not so interested in railroads as much as it was in transporting goods quickly and saving time. This led other firms such as air transportation companies to supplant the service that could have been provided by a diversified "railroad" company.[3]

The health care industry has suffered a great deal of myopia in the past regarding organizational mission. A modern health care organization today must decide whether providing high-quality medicine or improving societal or community health status should be the organizational goal. If community wellness becomes the mission, this might lead to the recognition of different trends in the environment, and necessitate different responses from the organization. In this greater recognition of health care as opposed to medical care, Riverside Health System in Newport News, Virginia has broadened its focus. Once a four-hospital, nonprofit system, Riverside now also operates five profitable wellness centers. And Springfield Hospital, part of the Crozer-Keystone Health System, of Media, Pennsylvania, is building a 170,000-square-foot athletic club and attached medical office building as another reflection of a broadened mission and a changing health care marketplace. This $40-million project is turning the hospital into a "healthplex" that will offer integrated primary care, rehabilitation services, ambulatory care, diagnostics, outpatient surgery, and a fitness center. The executive director of the hospital believes this new healthplex will provide a lower cost setting in which to do rehabilitation, and by encouraging patients to become healthier, the director believes it will put the hospital in a good position to obtain contracts from managed care organizations.[4]

Situational Assessment

The **situational assessment** is an analysis of the organization's environment and of the organization itself. This process is referred to as the **SWOT analysis** (so named because it examines the Strengths and Weaknesses of the organization, as well as the Opportunities and Threats relevant to the organization's future strategy).

One aspect of this SWOT analysis involves assessing the environment. It is at this stage in the process where the organization must consider the economic, competitive, regulatory, social, and technological changes occurring in the marketplace. Scanning these dimensions of the environment yields insight into the opportunities and threats that exist, to which the organization must respond in its overall strategic plan and in subsequent functional plans.

In reviewing each of these environmental areas, the organization must ask: (1) What are the changes and trends?, (2) How will these changes affect the organization's businesses?, and (3) What opportunities do these changes present? While these changes will be discussed in greater detail in Chapter 3, consider one demographic change—the aging marketplace—and its impact on company strategy.

For many years, the Gerber Products Company of Fremont, Michigan, defined its business as "Babies are our business, our only business." This was a great mission in the early 1950s when the United States was witnessing a rapidly growing birthrate. An aging population, however, as shown in Figure 2–4, might necessitate some revisions to that mission. A review of this environmental position might lead Gerber to make some basic strategic changes.

As the population ages, Gerber must consider this trend, and decide what implications it holds for its business. In what ways must the company respond, and what opportunities does it present? Does an aging population suggest a need for food that is easily digestible, such as baby food? Will an aging population result in a greater number of widows and widowers who will avail themselves of easily prepared food in single-sized servings? What impact will this trend of an aging population have on the future growth of a health care organization whose strength lies in pediatrics?

One other example of demographic change—the competition—highlights its role in corporate marketing strategy. In analyzing business opportunities, a

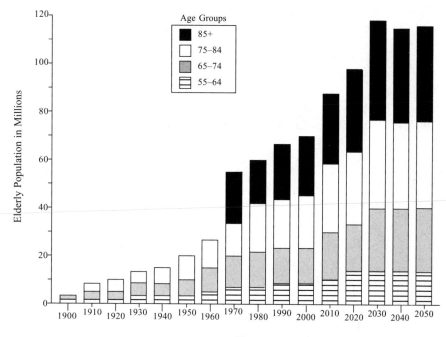

Figure 2–4 Changing Market Demographics: Actual and Projected Growth in the Elderly U.S. Population. *Source:* Taueber, C.M., U.S. Bureau of the Census, America in Transition: An Aging Society, *Current Population Reports* Series P-23, No. 128 (September 1983) (for years 1900–1980); Spencer, G., U.S. Bureau of the Census, Projections of the Population of the United States by Age, Sex, and Race: 1983 to 2080, *Current Population Reports* Series P-25, No. 952 (May 1984) (for years 1990–2050).

Wisconsin health insurance firm found a market that was a direct result of the waiting time for elective surgery in Canada. Wisconsin-based American Medical Services offers a policy that covers the cost of travel for Canadians treated in the United States. The $450 policy pays part of the patient's travel costs, plus food and lodging for a family member. Coverage begins once the policyholder has to wait more than 45 days for the surgery in Canada.[5]

With this situational analysis, it is important for the organization to consider the barriers that exist in the marketplace. In analyzing any business plan, an organization must consider the **barriers to entry**, which are the conditions that a company must overcome in order to pursue a business opportunity. Barriers to entry might be regulatory, technological, financial or strategic. In health care, for example, the regulatory process in many states has provided a strong barrier to entry. To enter certain businesses that require the addition of resources and capital allocations, hospitals must obtain various forms of regulatory approval.

One of the fastest growing segments of the health care industry is subacute care. This level of care is designed for those patients who are sufficiently stabilized to no longer require acute-care services. Subacute care can be provided in a free-standing nursing home or a skilled nursing facility, rather than a hospital. Since these nursing facilities face fewer regulatory hurdles than hospitals do, the barriers to entry are often low. Hence, this new segment of health care is projected to grow from a $1-billion business in 1994 to a $10-billion segment of the industry by the year 2000.[6]

Acquisition of some technology might be a barrier to entry, or the cost of such technological acquisition could represent an effective barrier. Image alone can also be an effective strategic barrier. A competitor may have established a strong reputation and marketplace position regarding a particular service that poses a real challenge—and forms a barrier—for a competing health care organization wanting to enter the market for that service.

In the same regard, the organization must also consider the **barriers to exit**, or the costs of leaving a particular business line. In health care, many services require a large commitment of fixed assets or specialized personnel. This fact alone can make it difficult to move away from a business in spite of the environmental overview provided. This, in fact, might be a weakness highlighted with a SWOT analysis.

For the SWOT to be successful an organization must be able and willing to do the following:

1. Turn the focus of the SWOT analysis away from the organization's products and toward its business processes that meet customer needs.
2. Capitalize on its strengths by delivering better value to customers than the competition.
3. Turn any weakness into a strength by investing strategically in key areas.[7]

These steps serve as a catalyst for corporate strategy, as suggested by Figure 2–5. As seen in this representation, strengths that have no matching opportunities are of little value. A liability exists when a weakness is matched by a competitive threat. Capabilities to capitalize on marketplace potential exists when one can match organizational strengths to market opportunities.

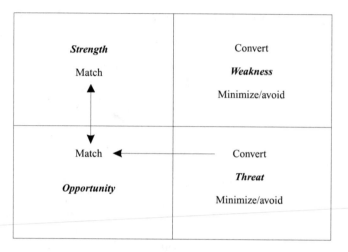

Figure 2–5 Four-Cell SWOT Matrix. *Source:* Reprinted from *Strategic Marketing Management* by O.C. Ferrell, G. Lucas, and D. Luck, p. 46, with permission of South-Western College Publishing, © 1994. All rights reserved.

Differential Advantage

Within this situational analysis, an organization must also consider its own strengths and weaknesses. At this point, an organization should assess what it does that is better than the competition and gives it a differential advantage, which has been defined in Chapter 1 as the incremental benefits of a product relative to competing products that are important to the buyer as perceived by the buyer. This analysis and specification of the differential advantage are based on the core competencies of the firm that are critical to success.[8]

There are three areas in which an organization can seek a differential advantage: (1) product, (2) market, or (3) cost.[9] As shown in Table 2–1, a product-based differential advantage is one in which the company has a unique technological capability or clinical expertise that allows it to establish a competitive position. In health care, the establishment of a product-based differential advantage is difficult. The pace of technological change is such that the advantage goes to competitors who have the resources to acquire a new technology. A distribution network that improves access, however, can be a differential advantage.

A market-based differential advantage is available to those who focus on a particular market segment. For example, in the Cleveland, Ohio metropolitan area, Rainbow Children and Babies Hospital is recognized as a leader in pediatric care.

Table 2–1 Sources of a Differential Advantage

Product-Based	Market-Based	Cost-Based
Technological capability	Targeted segment	Operational efficiency
Clinical expertise	Narrow product line	Expense control
Name/image	Geographic focus	Experience curve
Distribution network		Government subsidy

While other competitors also provide pediatric service, the differential advantage rests with Rainbow Children and Babies and their narrow market focus.

The third area in which to establish a differential advantage is cost. An organization that is highly efficient, either through the use of technology or with tight management control of expenses, can achieve this advantage. Increasingly in health care, as the marketplace focuses on the cost of care, a cost differential advantage is becoming a strong competitive position. The challenge for the organization, however, is that it must strive for large market share in order to receive the margin lost from a cost leadership position. Establishing a differential position in this area is closely tied to the pricing strategies the organization pursues in the market. This issue is discussed in greater detail in Chapter 8.

Each of these respective sources of differential advantage have their own set of inherent weaknesses. In a product-based approach, the challenge is to maintain the product advantage in the face of competitors who take a low-cost position. As low-cost providers enter the market, the consumers must still value the product differential advantage. There is also the risk that the marketplace changes its preferences and no longer values the product's differential advantage. A more realistic possibility is that there is a large number of imitators, which minimizes any perceived differentiation in product.

For a market-based position, competitors might target smaller groups or sub-markets to establish a differential advantage. Or, cost factors could eliminate an advantageous position within the market. In health care, the cost position may be the most difficult to maintain. Technology has a dramatic impact on the cost position of any provider. Exclusive focus on cost can also lead to a failure to recognize market needs or new service opportunities that might present themselves.

Organizational Objectives

The third step in the strategic planning process is the establishment of **organizational objectives**, which are the long-term performance targets the company hopes to achieve. These might include sales, market leadership position, or market share terms. In setting these objectives, it is valuable that, as much as possible, they be stated quantitatively and in realistic terms. General Electric Company, for example, had an organizational objective that related to market share. The company would only operate in business lines in which it could be the number one or number two company in terms of market share. Similarly, a national health maintenance organization might set an organizational objective to only compete in market areas in which it could be the dominant plan in terms of number of subscribers. The organizational objectives set the broad targets for the operating units.

ORGANIZATIONAL STRATEGY

Once it has progressed through the previous planning stages, the organization can then begin to formulate its broad strategies. For any organization, these can include either *growth market strategies* or *consolidation strategies*. With growth market strategies, the organization is attempting to gain more sales from an existing business line or attempting to penetrate new markets. An alternative growth perspective might lead the firm to develop a new product or service that can generate sales from existing customers to new buyers. An organization that implements a consolidation strategy is paring either the services they offer or the markets they serve.

Growth Market Strategies

Exhibit 2–2 shows four broad strategies that can guide an organization's growth; they reflect the internal organization and the external market conditions. Internal capabilities and services are represented by the product dimension. External market factors, a reflection of the situational analysis, are represented by the market dimension. Using this product/market matrix as a guide, there are four broad strategies to consider.[10]

Market Penetration

The **market penetration** strategy involves increasing the sales of present products and services in present markets. This a useful approach when the current market is strong and growing. Fulfillment of this strategy might involve attracting new customers or converting nonusers. For example, a managed care product might attempt to win over subscribers from a competing health plan, or to convert fee-for-service customers to a prepaid plan. A health care organization also might attempt to increase its business from existing customers. A managed care plan, for instance, might try to increase the number of employee subscribers within corporations and other businesses that offer the plan to their employees.

Exhibit 2–2 Product/Market Opportunity Matrix

Product/Market	Present	New
Present	Market Penetration Strategy	Market Development Strategy
New	Product Development Strategy	Diversification Strategy

Source: Adapted from Ansoff, H.I., Strategies for Diversification, *Harvard Business Review*, Vol. 35, September–October 1957, pp. 113–124.

Another way to fulfill a market penetration strategy is through more intensive efforts to distribute the product or service, or through more aggressive promotion. Or, the managed care plan will price itself more competitively to attract more customers.

Market Development

A second growth strategy involves initiating sales of existing products and services in new markets, a **market development** strategy. This strategy is followed when existing markets are stagnant in terms of growth and market share gains would be difficult to achieve because of the existence of strong, dominant competitors. This approach is followed by relocating a service to new locations or regions where it has not previously been offered. There are several variations to this strategy.

A health care organization might enter new geographical markets. For example, a hospital in San Antonio, Texas might establish a clinic in Mexico to attract consumers who might ultimately be referred to the hospital for inpatient tertiary care. M.D. Anderson is a major national cancer center located in Houston, Texas. Recognized as a leader in the treatment of cancer, this organization undertook a market development strategy by offering cancer services in Orlando, Florida.

Alternatively, a health plan can follow a market development strategy of appealing to new market segments that it has been unable to attract before. Many HMOs have established senior programs to enroll more elderly subscribers, such as the Harvard Community Health Plan's First Seniority health care plan in Massachusetts.

Product Development

A third organizational growth strategy is **product development**, which involves providing new products to existing markets. In this situation, a health system has a strong customer base and seeks to retain these customers by offering new services or quality improvements. Organizations pursue this strategy to meet changing customer needs, to take advantage of new technologies, or to meet the needs of some specific segment of the market. This situation is becoming increasingly typical in the health care industry. Many well-known organizations that first entered the marketplace as fee-for-service, multispecialty group practices, such as the Carle Clinic in Champaign-Urbana, Illinois, or the Fallon Clinic in Worcester, Massachusetts, have developed their own managed care products in the form of HMOs. This strategy is a response to changing market conditions and it provides loyal users with another option for receiving care from member physicians. This strategy is ultimately a reaction to a changing competitive marketplace.

In pursuing this strategy, health care organizations will often engage in **vertical integration**, which involves incorporating related services or products that have usually been developed or offered by others to the marketplace. There are two forms of integration strategies. A health care system can use **backward integration**, which entails becoming its own supplier. Increasingly, for example, hospitals have established their own physician-hospital organization (PHO). These entities then offer a managed care product to the market as the PHO accepts risk. Swedish Health System of Rockford, Illinois is actively pursuing risk contracts for their new entity. With **forward integration** a company offers new services or products usually closer to the customer than existing services. Many of these have been previously provided by other intermediaries. PRUCARE of Orlando has its own providers who staff a health maintenance organization at multiple locations in the community. Prudential, which acted solely as an insurance firm, has integrated forward by now providing care directly. Each of these strategies is discussed in greater depth in Chapter 9.

Diversification

The fourth growth strategy, **diversification**, entails developing new products or services for new markets. This strategy is followed when the growth in existing markets is slowing or when environmental changes—be they societal, technological, economic, regulatory, or competitive—make it risky to remain in present markets. Diversification strategies are currently being followed by innumerable health care providers. Hospitals have diversified into long-term care facilities, influenced by several factors such as reimbursement, utilization, and network referrals. Table 2–2 shows several factors influencing diversification and some of their benefits.

Strategic Alliances. For many organizations, it is often difficult—in terms of resources or for strategic reasons—to enter new markets. In such instances, many companies following a diversification strategy have established **strategic alliances** or formal arrangements with other companies to operate in a particular

Table 2-2 Factors Influencing Long-Term Care Diversification

Long-Term Care Option	Market Variables	Risk	Reimbursement Climate	Advantages	Disadvantages
Nursing homes	% of elderly in population, affluence of elderly, competition	High (construction or purchase costs required)	Depends on state	Earlier hospital discharge, referral network, ancillary charges, economies of scale	Reimbursement is often low, requires a great deal of attention
Retirement housing, life care, CRCs	Affluence of elderly	High (need good market survey)	Not applicable	Ties residents to hospital	Very costly to build
Domiciliaries, assisted living, personal care	% of elderly in population, affluence of elderly	High because of construction costs	Not applicable	Referrals, ties residents to hospital, economies of scale	Target market is usually small
Home health care	Degree of market saturation	Medium (low capital intensity)	Good	Flexible staffing, referral network	Potential market saturation
Wellness programs, health promotion	Not applicable except to determine if other hospitals are doing this	Low	Not applicable	Good will, referral network	Poor financial return
Outpatient rehabilitation	% of elderly in population, proximity to industries	Medium (purchase of equipment, employment of staff)	Excellent	Referral network, flexible staffing (if existing therapists can be used)	Potential market saturation

Source: Reprinted from Giardinia, C.W., Fotter, M.D., Shewchuk, R.W., and Hill, D.B., "The Case for Diversification into Long-Term Care, Health Care Management Review, Vol. 15, No. 1, p. 79, Aspen Publishers, Inc., © 1990.

market.[11] Strategic alliances assume many forms. Some strategic alliances involve the establishment of **joint venture businesses**, which are new corporate entities in which both partners hold an equity position. Other strategic alliances can simply be formal agreements that give each partner some access to the distinctive strengths of the other firm. J.C. Penney in Plano, Texas has formed such an alliance with Presbyterian Health Systems. Penney opened a 6,000-square-foot urgent care and occupational medicine facility. The company asked Presbyterian to staff and operate the center with a physician and nurse and to provide medical referrals when necessary.[12]

Hoffman–LaRoche and Millennium Pharmaceutical is a strategic alliance formed in the early 1990s within the pharmaceutical industry. Millennium is a small biotechnology firm that has a differential advantage because of its expertise in genetics research. Hoffman-LaRoche is a large pharmaceutical company that holds a differential advantage in its marketing capabilities and regulatory process knowledge. The two firms have formed a strategic alliance to develop gene-based drugs to treat chronic obesity and adult onset diabetes. In order to enter the Asian market, Sterling Winthrop Inc. of New York, a manufacturer of pharmaceutical preparations, established a strategic alliance with a Chinese partner, Shanghai Melyou Pharmaceutical Company. Marketers at Shanghai Melyou will promote Sterling Winthrop's drugs, but brand managers at Sterling Winthrop will monitor these activities closely to ensure they meet with its worldwide plans.[13]

Consolidation Strategies

Occasionally, when examining marketplace considerations, an organization might establish strategies for **consolidation**, or focusing business on a smaller set of markets, products, or services. There are several ways to accomplish this objective.

Divestment

Selling off a business or product line is called **divestment**. This strategy is often followed when an organization believes there is a weak fit between its major core business and a particular product line. The lack of fit may be due to the management resources required, or the result of a product whose market differs from the core market being pursued by the company. Often, divestment is the result of an unsuccessful diversification growth strategy. In the late 1980s, Hospital Corporation of America (HCA) of Nashville, Tennessee divested itself of its psychiatric hospital business in order to concentrate on the acute-care business.

Pruning

A second consolidation strategy occurs when a firm **prunes** or reduces the number of products or services it offers to the market. The company continues to serve the market, but does so with a reduced set of products. IBM remains in the personal computer business. However, in 1984 it decided not to pursue the low-end user and it dropped its IBM PCjr. model, which was not well accepted. This approach is useful when certain segments of the market are too costly or too small to service.

Retrenchment

In a **retrenchment** strategy a company decides to withdraw from certain markets. This strategy might be considered the opposite of the market development growth strategy. A clinic might decide to close a primary care satellite in a neighboring community. Organizations follow this kind of strategy when certain market areas do not perform well or meet overall corporate objectives.

Harvesting

A fourth consolidation strategy, **harvesting**, involves gradually withdrawing support from a product until there is little or no market demand. In these instances, an organization continues to support a product, but at a decreasing level. A business would follow this strategy as long as the service had some level of profitability, or had a loyal customer base that generated additional revenues through purchases of other services.

DETERMINING ORGANIZATIONAL STRATEGY

Several alternative models have been proposed to help companies develop their organizational strategies. Two well-known approaches are the BCG matrix and the GE matrix. Each of these models has received widespread recognition as useful conceptualizations for formulating organizational strategic direction.

The BCG Matrix

The Boston Consulting Group, a well-known management consulting firm, developed a strategy based on market growth rate and relative market share to focus company strategies in firms with multiple product lines.[14] Figure 2–6 represents the **BCG matrix**. In this model, the underlying assumption is that cash flow and profitability are closely related to sales volume. Products or strategic

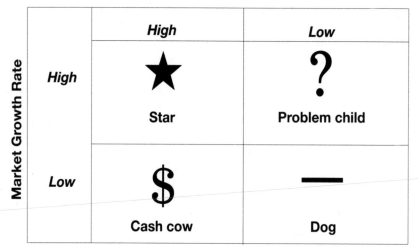

Figure 2–6 The BCG Matrix. *Source:* Reprinted from *Henderson on Corporate Strategy* by Bruce Henderson, with permission of Abt Books, © 1979.

business units are then placed within this matrix according to their position on two dimensions. **Market growth rate** refers to the rate of sales growth in the market, while **relative market share** is the ratio of a product's share of business within the market compared to that of its largest competitor. This second measure is an indicator of market dominance. If the share equals that of the largest competitor the measure would be 1.0. An administrator can then classify the organization's product lines into one of these four quadrants.

In examining the position of businesses in this matrix, it is important to consider the issue of control. A company cannot directly control the market growth rate. This rate is determined by uncontrollable, variable environmental forces. For example, pediatrics may be a declining business, but there is little direct control a provider can have over the overall growth rate of the number of children. A company does have direct control of its relative market share, however, which is a reflection of the success of the organization's strategy, particularly its marketing strategy relative to competitors. A company that places a service in the quadrants representing lower share must reexamine its internal strategy and its implementation.

Products and services are represented in the matrix as one of the following: stars, cash cows, problem children, or dogs. *Stars* are products with high market share and high growth rate. An organization is doing well with these products (represented by their high relative market share) and their future potential is still strong as reflected in the high growth rate. From a cash perspective the revenues generated by these business lines should be reinvested back into services that need additional investment in personnel or facilities in order to capitalize on the market growth rate. Growth strategies are the primary focus of products placed within this quadrant.

Cash cows are products that have a high market share but a low growth rate. These might be seen as mature businesses; but this maturity is not due to any controllable factor. Placing a service in the cash cow position means that, even though the market is maturing, a company has been able to retain a strong share position. These businesses typically generate a substantial amount of cash, in fact, they usually represent the greatest source of cash flow. There is no need to invest in new facilities or other fixed assets. Monies from these product lines should be reinvested or redirected into services whose market position is growing. The major strategy for these products focuses on maintaining share as long as the market exists. When share drops, then consolidation strategies might be considered.

Problem children represent services with low relative market share, but high growth rate. A product could be placed into this quadrant for one of two reasons. First, a product might be classified as a problem child because it is new to the organization, hence its low market share. In that case, a business needs to invest monies generated by cash cows in marketing of the new product. A second, more problematic reason for a product to be labeled a problem child is an organization's inability to establish market dominance in the midst of a growth market situation. This requires a reexamination of the strategy and tactics used to support this service.

Dogs represent those products with low share and low growth. These services typically drain an organization's cash and become targets for consolidation strategy. The simplest recommendation is to drop the product or get out of the market. In health care, however, an organization must often keep one service (such as rehabilitation services) in order to deliver other services (such as orthopedics) to the market. It is important to recognize the dog only because of its resource implications.

The broad nature of the BCG matrix often makes it too limiting for significant strategy formulation. Yet, in health care organizations, it can serve as a valuable conceptual framework to engender strategy discussions. A major source of organizational conflict occurs when everybody views their clinical service in a different market position requiring a different level of resource commitment. The BCG framework is a useful tool for focusing management attention on broad marketplace considerations and for getting participants to discuss the issues of market growth and the requirements for market dominance in a particular clinical setting.

The BCG matrix is also a useful tool for helping a medical organization assess its internal strengths and future direction. Depending on the distribution of services within the matrix, an audit might reveal an organization that needs to redirect resources to generate more new products or services. For example, if a health care organization has a large number of cash cows (60 percent), a reasonable number of stars (25 percent), a few dogs (5 percent), and only 10 percent problem children, it might indicate that the program directors of mature services have succeeded in keeping the cash within their own operations. Little revenue, therefore, has been redirected to generate new opportunities at the low-share, high-growth potential position. Similarly, a business with a large number of problem children relative to the number of cash cows might need to prioritize which problems it will invest in to gain share. To move a service from the problem child to star position often requires redirecting the marketing mix, and infusing financial and management resources in new areas. If too many services are vying for these resources, investment must be prioritized to ensure that at least some services receive the needed support to become successful market competitors.

The GE Matrix

The BCG matrix is limited by the consideration of only two dimensions. Yet, for most products and services, these considerations often require a multidimensional evaluation. Figure 2–7 shows the considerations used in the **GE matrix**, a multidimensional model for focusing corporate strategy in organizations with multiple product lines based on the dimensions of market attractiveness and business strength.

Market attractiveness is an index comprised of nine elements: (1) overall market size, (2) annual market growth rate, (3) historical profit margin, (4) competitive intensity, (5) technological requirements, (6) inflationary vulner-ability, (7) energy requirements, (8) environmental impact, and (9) social/political/legal issues. *Business strength* is an index comprised of 12 elements: (1) market share, (2) share growth, (3) product quality, (4) brand reputation, (5) distribution network, (6) promotional effectiveness, (7) production capacity, (8) production efficiency, (9) unit costs, (10) supply costs, (11) R & D perform-ance, and (12) management talent. Each of these factors within both dimensions are given a weighting of importance. A product is rated on each factor and then multiplied by the weighting. Every product is assigned a value for marketing attractiveness and business strength. Calculation of the value for a product leads to its positioning within the matrix, which includes its relevant strategic direction as well.

The GE matrix has nine cells representing three broad zones of strategic corporate action. The three cells at the lower right represent businesses that are low

Business Strength

		Strong	Average	Weak
Market Attractiveness	*High*	Premium—Invest for Growth: • Provide maximum investment • Diversify worldwide • Consolidate position • Accept moderate near-term profits • Seek to dominate	Selective—Invest for Growth: • Invest heavily in selected segments • Share ceiling • Seek attractive new segments to apply strengths	Protect/Refocus—Selectively Invest for Earnings: • Defend strengths • Refocus to attractive segments • Evaluate industry revitalization • Monitor for harvest or divestment timing • Consider acquisitions
	Medium	Challenge—Invest for Growth: • Build selectively on strengths • Define implications of leadership challenge • Avoid vulnerability—fill weaknesses	Prime—Selectively Invest for Earnings: • Segment market • Make contingency plans for vulnerability	Restructure—Harvest or Divest: • Provide no unessential commitment • Position for divestment *or* • Shift to more attractive segment
	Low	Opportunistic—Selectively Invest for Earnings: • Ride market and maintain overall position • Seek niches, specialization • Seek opportunity to increase strength (for example, through acquisition) • Invest at maintenance levels	Opportunistic—Preserve for Harvest: • Act to preserve or boost cash flow • Seek opportunistic sale *or* • Seek opportunistic rationalization to increase strengths • Prune product lines • Minimize investment	Harvest or Divest: • Exit from market or prune product line • Determine timing so as to maximize present value • Concentrate on competitor's cash generators

Figure 2–7 General Electric Business Screen. *Source:* Reprinted from *Strategic Market Planning* by B.A. Rausch, p. 88, with permission of American Marketing Association, © 1982.

in attractiveness and low in business strength. As suggested within the chart, these represent services for which consolidation strategies must be considered. Services that fall within the cells on the diagonal from lower left to upper right are either weak or average in attractiveness and in business strength. These are businesses where selective growth strategies or some harvesting might be appropriate. Finally, services within the cells in the upper left represent businesses with the most promise. Growth strategies need to be pursued.

The advantage of the GE matrix compared to the BCG model is that it provides consideration of multiple factors. Like the BCG model, however, it ultimately places the services along a two-dimensional framework. Also, many of the elements used within the composition of the matrix values are often considered within the BCG discussion of growth rate. The specification is helpful, yet can often pose a challenge for managers considering both models simultaneously.

ANALYZING THE COMPETITIVE MARKET

Within the context of strategic planning, companies must analyze the competition. Firms must assess not only the existing competition but also potential competition. Porter has developed a widely accepted conceptual model that considers factors affecting the competitive intensity within an industry.[15] As shown in Figure 2–8, competitive intensity is affected by four major forces: (1) the threat of new entrants, (2) bargaining power of suppliers, (3) bargaining power of customers, and (4) the threat of substitute products or services.

Existing Competitors

In analyzing the competitive environment, it is important to first look at the existing competitors. This analysis provides a perspective on the cost of competing and on the bases around which the competition will occur. A major focus of the competitive analysis is also to assess the degree to which competition is cost-based.

Competition is intense among existing competitors when the product is relatively standardized and the competitors are relatively numerous and similar in size. This frequently describes the market for hospitals and medical groups in major metropolitan areas. Competition can also be intense when the cost of switching providers is relatively low. In health care, this is a major factor that managed care companies face. For many employers, the cost of switching health plans is often not a large obstacle. Competition also tends to be intense in industries characterized by overcapacity and among firms still in the market because of a high fixed-asset position. These latter two issues define the competitive setting for inpatient hospital care in the 1990s.

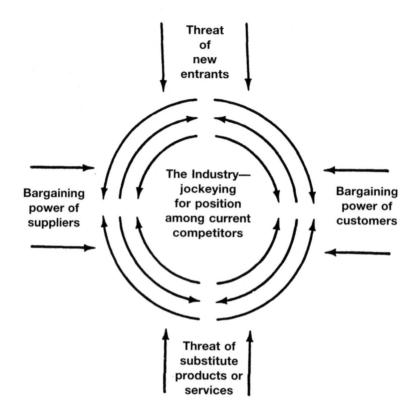

Figure 2–8 Forces Affecting Competitive Intensity. *Source:* Reprinted from *How Competitive Forces Shape Strategy* by M.E. Porter, *Harvard Business Review,* March–April 1979, with permission of the President and Fellows of Harvard College, © 1979. All rights reserved.

New Entrants

While it is essential to consider the existing competition when developing a strategic plan, an organization must be keenly aware of the entry of new players in the marketplace. As the market changes, so does the competition. For example, many medical groups that once competed against other local providers are now finding themselves competing against insurance companies for the provision of care. Large insurance providers, such as Aetna Life & Casualty of Hartford, Connecticut, have recently acquired provider groups in Charlotte, North Carolina; Chicago, Illinois; Atlanta, Georgia; and Dallas, Texas, and are becoming major competitors for the delivery of care in many local markets.

New competitors can come from several sources, such as a segment or market that is underserved. Occasionally, competition comes from either competitors or customers. The academic medical group that used to supply tertiary services to a community hospital might integrate to a lower level of care and establish its own academic group of family practitioners. Many academic medical centers, such as George Washington University in Washington, D.C., actively compete against other providers by offering their own health maintenance plans. Other academic medical centers, such as the one at the University of Minnesota in Minneapolis and University of Michigan in Ann Arbor, have established faculty practice plans as vehicles to attract, process, and organize for patient revenue activities. Similarly, an employer that had purchased outside medical services for its employees might hire its own medical staff and conduct employee health programs in-house.

Threat of Substitution

A second major source of competition is found in the threat of substitution. In traditional businesses, this threat exists when one product class can be substituted for another. For example, plastic can be a major threat to steel as the tensile strength of the product increases.

In health care, the threat of substitution most often occurs due to technological change. Technology can eliminate a particular business line in a short period of time. Figure 2–9 shows how successive new generations of diagnostic imaging technology each affected the usage of preceding technologies in a particular area. The source of suppliers of this technology has also continually changed. Each new technological advance has provided increased performance in terms of scanning and imaging capabilities. The new technology moves the existing product into a mature phase of its life cycle. As can be seen in this figure, there is an ever-decreasing time before new technology with higher performance capabilities appears. Several warning signs have been identified by McKinsey, et al., indicating when a technology may be nearing obsolescence and supplanted by a competing new technology:

1. Greater efforts are needed to produce even small performance improvements.
2. R&D shifts away from product improvement toward process improvement.
3. Sales growth comes from minor product modifications that serve new segments rather than from quality improvements that improve penetration across all segments.
4. There are wide differences in R&D spending among competitors, with minor differences on resultant market shares.

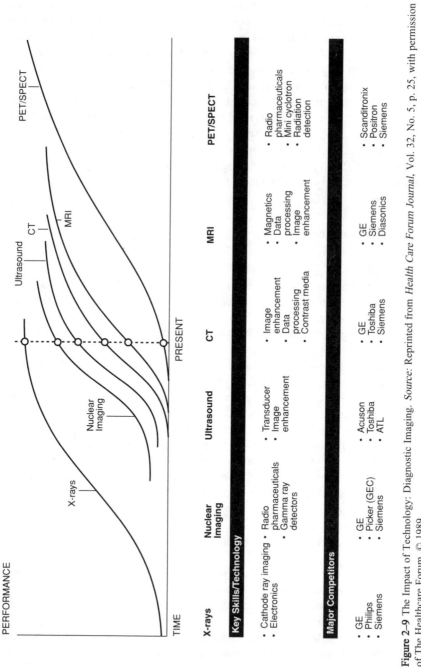

Figure 2–9 The Impact of Technology: Diagnostic Imaging. *Source:* Reprinted from *Health Care Forum Journal*, Vol. 32, No. 5, p. 25, with permission of The Healthcare Forum, © 1989.

5. Some market leaders begin to lose share to small competitors in selected market segments. This shift may indicate that smaller competitors are being more productive with a new emerging technology.[16]

Powerful Customers and Suppliers

Buyers can dramatically affect the competitive intensity in an industry. The more economic power the buyer has, or the greater the source of customer dollars that the buyer represents, or the fewer buyers there are, the more pressure the customer can exert. The Voluntary Hospital Association (VHA), which is comprised of hundreds of hospitals that have joined together to facilitate purchasing and other activities, such as consulting, can wield significant power with health care manufacturers of wound dressings such as Kendall or 3M, since this organization represents all of its member hospitals. Buyers can wield power when the product is relatively standardized, or when they are able to integrate backwards and provide the service for themselves.

Suppliers are also a major threat when they can integrate forward to deliver a service. They also can exert great power when there are few other sources of supply, or when it would be very costly for an organization to shift suppliers.

DEVELOPING THE MARKETING PLAN

After an organization develops a strategic plan, it can then formulate a marketing plan in light of the broad strategies identified by the top corporate management. Similar to the strategic planning process, marketing planning involves the establishment of marketing objectives, formulation of marketing strategies, and development of an action plan.

Establishment of Marketing Objectives

Marketing objectives are quantitative measures of accomplishment by which the success of marketing strategies can be measured. Marketing objectives might include retention, new sales growth, and market leadership in the form of a share gain.

Marketing Strategy Formulation

The next step is the formulation of marketing strategies. This aspect of strategic market planning involves determining the target market, specifying the market strategy, and developing the tactical plans for the four Ps.

Determining the Target Market

As noted in the previous chapter, the basic first step in this process is the identification of the *target market*, specifying whom the organization is trying to attract. Selection of the target market involves assessing the organization's own strengths, the competitive intensity for the target market, the cost of capturing market share, and the potential financial gain in attracting the targeted group.

In selecting the target market, organizations have several options, as presented in Figure 2–10. They can treat the entire market as one homogeneous group of customers, or they can divide the market into segments or subgroups that are homogeneous within a particular dimension. The concept of segmenting a market is described in more detail in Chapter 6.

Treating the entire market as one target market and appealing to the broadest group is referred to as **mass marketing**. Customers are viewed as relatively undifferentiated in what they desire. This strategy tries to satisfy the greatest number of buyers with a single product. Historically, most hospitals in the United States have followed a mass market strategy in their own local areas. The advantage of this approach is that the largest number of people can be targeted. The size of the market alone can increase the likelihood of attracting customers. The

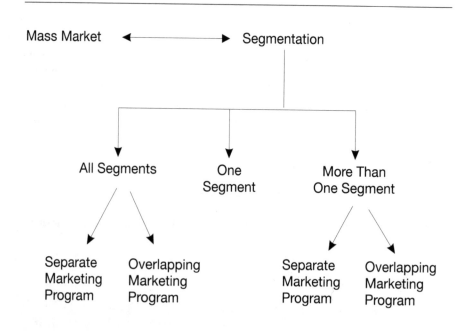

Figure 2–10 Target Market Options

disadvantage of this marketing strategy is that it leaves the organization susceptible to new competitors who might tailor a marketing strategy to particular subgroups that is more closely aligned with the needs of these groups.

Figure 2–10 shows the possibilities of a segmented strategy. An organization might consider targeting all possible segments or a number of different segments. This approach is referred to as **multi-segment marketing**, in which a distinct marketing strategy might be developed for each group. A hospital might target two segments within the female population. One program might address issues and concerns for women of childbearing age, while a second program targets older women, offering education and resources regarding menopause, breast cancer screening, and osteoporosis. Or, a company can recognize differences in market segments yet have an overlapping strategy that uses similar parts of the marketing mix for all groups, but different strategies for particular groups. For example, a medical group practice might have one main office where all services are delivered. Yet, the group has decided to target two different groups: higher income executives and elderly consumers with third-party insurance. While they are offering the same product and services and using the same distribution strategy, they employ different promotional strategies for each group. The group practice might advertise to executives in the metropolitan edition of *The Wall Street Journal*. At the same time, however, the group will send a representative to senior citizens clubs to speak about the health needs and concerns of older consumers.

Another option for some organizations is to pursue only a subset of market segments or just one market segment. Targeting only one segment of the market is referred to as the **market concentration strategy**. In selecting only one segment, an organization must be able to defend its choice in the face of competition. An organization's entire future may be based on its ability to solidify its market share position within this particular group. This strategy does have the advantage of sometimes providing opportunities for efficiencies in production, distribution, or promotion, since a company needs only to tailor its efforts to one segment's requirements.

Specifying Market Strategies

In developing marketing plans, a company must decide which one of several market positions it will take. The options are to be a market leader, market challenger, market follower, or a market niche.[17]

Within a single industry, one organization usually tries to be the **market leader**—the firm that has the largest market share and dominates the competitors in a given market. This leader dictates the pricing strategies of its competitors and is the first to introduce new products. The market leader defends its position against all new entries and will seek to expand the market or expand its current market share. A health care study conducted in 1992 found that hospital return on investment was significantly related to market share. Hospitals that sought and attained large market share had higher profitability than those that did not.[18]

A second market position is that of being the **market challenger**—the firm that attempts to confront the market leader. These companies tend to be smaller than the market leaders, but aggressive in their strategy formulation. They attack the market leader, either through directly vying for the leader's customers, or by trying to attract customers or market segments where the market leader is weak.

A market challenger can follow several approaches that might involve any one or more of the marketing mix elements, such as price cutting, less costly product alternatives, an improved distribution strategy, or a novel promotional approach.

A **market follower** is a business that competes in the marketplace by following the market leader rather than by attacking it directly. These companies try to maintain existing customers and attract new ones. In industries where there is little product differentiation and high price sensitivity, a follower strategy is often useful. By implementing this approach, an organization tries to prevent aggressive price competition. It will gain new customers by offering a quality service at a good value.

A final market position that a firm may try to create is that of a **market niche**, which it achieves by following a strategy of targeting a narrow segment or segments in a large market with specialized products or services. This is a common approach for many small, successful companies. This approach is so common, in fact, that *Forbes* magazine has labelled its listing of the 200 best small companies as its "Niche List."[19] An interesting niche strategy is being developed by Helian Health Group of Monterey, California. This company has set up inns licensed to provide acute care. These small facilities are targeted to handle surgery and recovery for less cost than what is incurred in traditional facilities. California data indicate this recovery center concept can save 28 percent on the cost of recovery from an abdominal hysterectomy and 60 percent on recovery from a cholecystectomy.[20]

Niche strategies are becoming more common in health care, especially among large academic medical centers that historically focused upon the highest level of tertiary care. Yet the movement of technology and the existence of well-trained physicians in a community make that a difficult niche to defend. Consider the situation faced by the University of Minnesota's medical center in Minneapolis. This institution has a history of being the center of significant medical advances. In 1952, it was the site where the first successful open heart surgery was performed, and, in 1977, it pioneered the first full-body CT scanner. While both of these technologies have great market potential, they are available at several facilities in the Minneapolis–St. Paul market. At one time, the University of Minnesota's medical center dominated the transplant surgery niche and was recognized as a world leader in bone marrow transplants. In 1995, five other hospitals in the Twin Cities were performing the identical procedure.[21]

Development of an Action Plan

Once the target market has been selected and the broad strategy determined, an organization can specify the tactical components of the marketing plan. These tactics address each of the marketing mix elements. The tactical plan identifies actions to be taken regarding each aspect of the marketing mix. This plan will address the advertising strategy, pricing strategy, distribution issues, and the nature of the product in terms of quality, range of options, etc.

Evaluating the Plan

The final aspect of the marketing plan involves evaluating its results. The monitoring and evaluation stage is described in greater detail in Chapter 13. Ultimately the success of monitoring depends on the initial quantitative objectives used in the plan's development.

While each health care organization's marketing plan will vary to some degree, an outline of a basic marketing plan is provided in Exhibit 2–3 as a guide.

Exhibit 2–3 Marketing Plan Outline of Fidelity Bank, Philadelphia, Pennsylvania

---

Marketing Plan Outline

For each major bank service:
   I. MANAGEMENT SUMMARY
      What is our marketing plan for this service in brief?
      This is a one-page summary of the basic factors involving the marketing of the service next year along with the results expected from implementing the plan. It is intended as a brief guide for management.
  II. ECONOMIC PROJECTIONS
      What factors in the overall economy will affect the marketing of this service next year, and how?
      This section will comprise a summary of the specific economic factors that will affect the marketing of this service during the coming year. These might include employment, personal income, business expectations, inflationary (or deflationary) pressures, etc.
 III. THE MARKET—qualitative
      Who or what kinds of organizations could conceivably be considered prospects for this service?
      This section will define the qualitative nature of our market. It will include demographic information, industrial profiles, business profiles, etc., for all people or organizations that could be customers for this service.
  IV. THE MARKET—quantitative
      What is the potential market for this service?
      This section will apply specific quantitative measures to this bank service. Here we want to include numbers of potential customers, dollar volume of business, our current

---

continues

Exhibit 2–3 continued

share of the market—any specific measures that will outline our total target for the service and where we stand competitively now.

V. TREND ANALYSIS

Based on the history of this service, where do we appear to be headed?

This section is a review of the past history of this service. Ideally, we should include quarterly figures for the last five years showing dollar volume, accounts opened, accounts closed, share of market, and all other applicable historical data.

VI. COMPETITION

Who are our competitors for this service, and how do we stand competitively?

This section should define our current competition, both bank and nonbank. It should be a thoughtful analysis outlining who our competitors are, how successful they are, why they have (or have not) been successful, and what actions they might be expected to take regarding this service during the coming year.

VII. PROBLEMS AND OPPORTUNITIES

Internally and externally, are there problems inhibiting the marketing of this service, or are there opportunities we have not taken advantage of?

This section will comprise a frank commentary on both inhibiting problems and unrealized opportunities. It should include a discussion of the internal and external problems we can control, for example, by changes in policies or operational procedures. It should also point up areas of opportunity regarding this service that we are not now exploiting.

VIII. OBJECTIVES AND GOALS

Where do we want to go with this service?

This section will outline the immediate short- and long-range objectives for this service. Short-range goals should be specific, and will apply to next year. Long-range goals will necessarily be less specific and should project for the next five years. Objectives should be stated in two forms:

(1) qualitative—reasoning behind the offering of this service and what modifications or other changes do we expect to make.

(2) quantitative—number of accounts, dollar volume, share of market, profit goals.

IX. ACTION PROGRAMS

Given past history, the economy, the market, competition, etc., what must we do to reach the goals we have set for this service?

This section will be a description of the specific actions we plan to take during the coming year to assure reaching the objectives we have set for the service in VIII. These would include advertising and promotion, direct mail, and brochure development. It would also include programs to be designed and implemented by line officers. The discussion should cover what is to be done, schedules for completion, methods of evaluation, and officers in charge of executing the program and measuring results.

Source: Reprinted from *The Marketing Plan, Conference Board Report No. 801,* pp. 63–64, with permission of The Conference Board, © 1981.

CONCLUSIONS

Development of marketing strategy begins with defining an organization's mission. Planning of a firm's final marketing strategy must include an examination of the market environment as well as a SWOT analysis. Understanding the nature of the competition allows a health care organization to develop the appropriate response to face the challenges of a changing health care market.

KEY TERMS

Strategic Planning	Divestment
Organizational Mission	Pruning
Situational Assessment	Retrenchment
SWOT Analysis	Harvesting
Barriers to Entry	BCG Matrix
Barriers to Exit	Market Growth Rate
Organizational Objectives	Relative Market Share
Market Penetration	GE Matrix
Market Development	Marketing Objectives
Product Development	Mass Marketing
Vertical Integration	Multi-Segment Marketing
Backward Integration	Market Concentration Strategy
Forward Integration	Market Leader
Diversification	Market Challenger
Strategic Alliances	Market Follower
Joint Venture Businesses	Market Niche
Consolidation	

CHAPTER SUMMARY

1. Marketing plans, along with finance, production, and human resource plans, form the core elements of an organization's strategic plan.

2. An organization's strategic plan is guided by the mission that defines its purpose for existing. The mission must recognize who the customer is and what the customer wants to buy.

3. In developing strategic plans, a SWOT analysis provides a review of internal and external factors that can affect strategic outcomes.

4. In developing strategic plans, an organization must be able to recognize the barriers to entry and exit for any new service venture.

5. An organization can develop a differential advantage that is either product-based, market-based, or price-based.

6. There are four broad growth strategies that any organization can pursue: (1) market development, (2) market penetration, (3) product development, or (4) diversification.

7. The BCG matrix and GE matrix are conceptualizations that can aid an organization in the review of its service portfolio. Both models encompass market and competitive considerations.

8. In any industry, the level of competitive intensity is affected by the threat of new entrants, the bargaining power of both suppliers and customers, and the threat of substitute products and services.

9. In developing a marketing plan, organizations can pursue a mass marketing or a market concentration strategy.

CHAPTER PROBLEMS

1. At a strategic planning retreat of a six-person general surgery group, the senior partner begins by stating, "Our mission is to perform the highest quality invasive surgery procedures in the community." In what ways might this view of the organization's mission suffer from the myopia that afflicted the railroads in an earlier era?

2. Children's Hospital, in Boston, Massachusetts, has long been considered an outstanding medical center specializing in the diagnosis and treatment of pediatric problems. This facility is linked academically to the Harvard University Medical School. Conduct a brief SWOT analysis for Children's Hospital in light of the present health care environment.

3. Describe the possible barriers to entry and exit for: (1) a physician wanting to establish a solo practice office in internal medicine, (2) a company offering a health club facility in the same building where employees work, and (3) a tertiary hospital developing a coronary bypass program.

4. You have recently been hired as the senior marketing officer for a new health maintenance organization (HMO). Two other HMOs have been operating for more than two years, in the same community. The first HMO is a closed-panel medical group with three satellite offices. The second plan is an independent practice association (IPA) with a panel of 125 physicians equally divided along primary care and specialty lines with 20 different locations. Both plans offer dental

coverage. As the third entrant into the market, where can you turn to establish a differential advantage? Provide some examples.

5. Retin–A is a topical ointment originally developed for the treatment of severe cases of acne and related skin disorders. An observed side benefit resulting from use of this product is its effect on aging of the skin. If the manufacturer of this product decided to pursue the latter market, what type of a growth strategy would it be pursuing?

6. Since 1982, there has been a steady decline in the number of hospital inpatient days. How might an acute-care community hospital implement the consolidation strategies of: (1) divestment, (2) retrenchment, and (3) harvesting?

7. Two large multispecialty medical groups have recently asked you to conduct audits using the BCG matrix. For the first group, your analysis reveals the following distribution of services: Cash cows—65 percent; stars—10 percent; problem children—20 percent; dogs—5 percent. In the second group, the distribution is: Cash cows—20 percent; stars—60 percent; problem children—15 percent; dogs—5 percent. Provide your analysis to each group.

NOTES

1. P.D. Bennett, ed. *Dictionary of Marketing Terms* (Chicago, Ill.: American Marketing Association, 1988), 195.

2. J.A. Pearce, II, The Company Mission as a Strategic Tool, *Sloan Management Review* 23, no. 3 (1982): 15–24.

3. T. Levitt, Marketing Myopia, *Harvard Business Review* 38, no. 4 (1960): 45–56.

4. K. Pallarito, Hospitals Strengthen Networks Through New Fitness Facilities, *Modern Healthcare* 24, no. 50 (1994): 45; and Springfield Hospital Fitness Center "Pumps Up" Ambulatory Care, *Inside Ambulatory Care* 2, no. 3 (1995): 1, 5.

5. J.R. Rose, Competition Has No Borders, *Medical Economics* 70, no. 14 (July 26, 1993): 13.

6. A. Waldman, Subacute Care: Spreading the Word, *Healthcare Management Report* 12, no. 8 (1994): 6–9.

7. G. Stalk, P. Evans, and L.E. Shulman, Competing on Capabilities: The New Rules of Corporate Strategy, *Harvard Business Review* 70, no. 2 (1992): 57–69.

8. M.A. Hitt and R.D. Ireland, Corporate Distinctive Competence, Strategy, and Performance, *Strategic Management Journal* 6, no. 3 (1985): 273–293.

9. M.E. Porter, *Competitive Strategy: Techniques for Analyzing Industries and Competitors* (New York, N.Y.: Free Press, 1980).

10. This framework was originally presented by H.I. Ansoff, *Corporate Strategy* (New York, N.Y.: McGraw-Hill Publishing Co., 1965).

11. For a useful reading on strategic alliances see P. Lorange and J. Roos, *Strategic Alliances: Formulation, Implementation, and Evolution* (Cambridge, Mass.: Blackwell Scientific Publications, Inc., 1992).

12. P.J. Henkel, Delivering Corporate Health Services, *Modern Healthcare* 23, no. 23 (1993): 24–27.

13. Kodak Unit's Entry in China, *The Wall Street Journal*, 3 September 1993: A4.

14. Boston Consulting Group, *Perspectives on Experience* (Boston: 1972). See also B.D. Henderson, The Experience Curve Reviewed: The Growth Share Matrix of the Product Portfolio, in *Perspectives No. 135* (Boston, Mass.: The Boston Consulting Group, 1973).

15. Porter, *Competitive Strategy.*

16. R.N. Foster, *Innovation: The Attacker's Advantage* (New York, N.Y.: Summit Books, 1986), 162.

17. P. Kotler, *Marketing Management: Analysis, Planning, and Control,* 8th ed. (Englewood Cliffs, N.J.: Prentice Hall, 1994), 381–407.

18. W.O. Cleverly and R.K. Harvey, Critical Strategies for Successful Rural Hospitals, *Health-Care Management Review* 17, no. 1 (Winter 1992): 27–33.

19. S. Kirchen and M. Schifrin, Niche List, *Forbes* 138, no. 10 (November 3, 1986): 160–161.

20. R.L. Cohen, Recovery Inns: A Concept Whose Time Has Come, *Healthcare Management Report* 11, no. 5 (1993): 18.

21. L. Page, Playing Catch-Up, *American Medical News* 37, no. 29 (1994): 3, 7.

THE ENVIRONMENT OF
MARKETING STRATEGY

After reading this chapter you should be able to:

- Understand the impact of the five environmental forces on organizational strategy

- Explain how social and economic forces affect marketing strategy

- Describe the impact of technology on health care organizations' survival and competitive environment

- Know the major regulatory requirements that must be followed when formulating health care marketing strategy

Marketing and marketing strategy is formulated in response to consumer needs. As discussed in Chapter 1, consumers can be individuals or organizations. Yet, marketing strategy must be formulated in response to the environmental conditions that affect the market. An effective marketing organization must continually scan the environment to assess and identify trends that its marketing strategy must consider. An organization must focus its environmental scan on five major environmental forces: economic, technological, social, competitive, and regulatory. As shown in Figure 3–1, environmental scanning is conducted to assess the trends in each of these five areas for their potential impact on the organization's target market. In this way, the health care organization can appropriately adjust its marketing mix strategy.

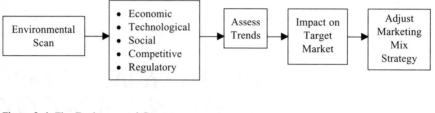

Figure 3–1 The Environmental Scan

This chapter will present a brief overview of each of these environmental factors and their potential implications for health care marketing.

ECONOMIC FACTORS

For any organization, the prevailing major macroeconomic conditions must be a major concern. Whether the marketplace is experiencing inflationary or recessionary conditions affects the willingness and ability of consumers to pay. **Inflation** is the decline in buying power when price levels rise faster than income. The cost of borrowing is also affected during an inflationary period. As the cost of borrowing rises, a health care provider who might find the opportunity to offer new services is constrained by the cost of capital.

Inflation and Health Care

A major factor contributing to President Clinton's 1994 attempt at health care reform, and all related discussions of restructuring health care throughout the United States, has been the rising cost of medical care during the past decade. Figure 3–2 shows two curves representing the rise in all the items that comprise the consumer price index and the corresponding rise in the cost of medical care. The **consumer price index** (CPI) measures monthly and yearly price changes for a broad range of consumer goods and services. The base year of the CPI is 1980, and except for 1990 when the CPI rose more than 5.5 percent, it has risen less than five percent annually since the base reporting year. Examining Figure 3–2, one can see the dramatic rise in the cost of medical care since the early 1980s. The cost of health care has outstripped increases in overall consumer costs in spite of a recent slowdown in yearly increases. The rising cost of health care has forced corporations to explore alternative health care plans to cover their employees. Many alternative systems such as health maintenance organizations and preferred

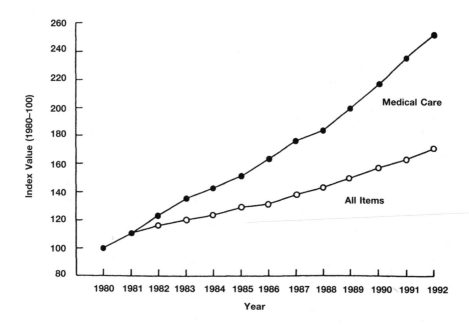

Figure 3–2 The Rising Cost of Medical Care. *Source:* Reprinted from *Journal of Medical Practice Management*, Vol. 8, No. 4, p. 229, with permission of Williams & Wilkins, © 1993.

provider organizations were developed as a mechanism to control cost through more closely managing care.

Consumer Income

There are three dimensions to any consumer's income: (1) gross income, (2) discretionary income, and (3) disposable income. **Gross income** is the total amount of money earned by a person or family in one year. Figure 3–3 shows the change in median consumer income from 1970 to 1992. While the typical family earned $29,760 in 1970, by 1992 that figure had only risen to $30,786. As can be seen in the chart, differences exist between ethnic and racial groups. The gross income of African-Americans and Hispanics has declined since 1990.

Disposable income is the amount of money a consumer has left for food, clothing, and shelter after paying taxes. During the 1990s, many politicians have felt that taxes are rising faster than wages for the middle-income class. The end result has been a decline in disposable income. The last component of income is

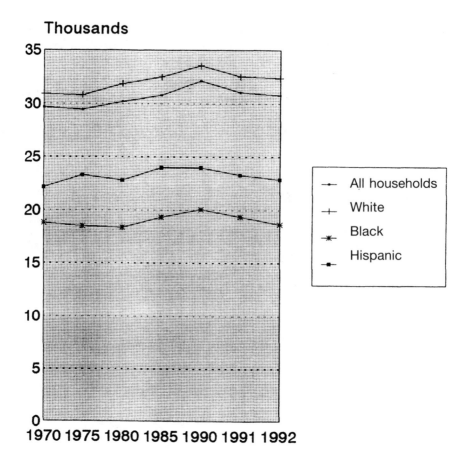

Figure 3–3 Consumer Income: Looking Below the Average. *Source:* Adapted from *Statistical Abstract of the United States,* 114th ed., p. 464, U.S. Bureau of the Census, Department of Commerce, 1994.

discretionary income, which is the income left after paying for taxes and necessities. Discretionary income is what the consumer uses for entertainment, recreation, or luxuries.

TECHNOLOGICAL FACTORS

Few industries are more greatly affected by technology than health care. **Technology** refers to the innovations or inventions from applied science and research. As new technology enters the market, existing products or services are pushed out. Consider the data in Figure 3–4, which show the decline in inpatient days at community hospitals compared to the dramatic corresponding increase in outpatient surgery. This trend was greatly affected by advances in medical technology that increased the ease of performing many medical procedures and reduced patient recovery times.

The impact of technology in health care is threefold. In the short term, new technology results in increasing costs. Each new generation of imaging device has required hospitals to upgrade their equipment. Yet, in the same regard, technology can also contribute to a decrease in cost. Consider the technological changes affecting one of the top 10 surgeries performed in hospitals—hysterectomies. The conventional abdominal hysterectomy involves a three- to four-day hospital stay and costs approximately $7,000, excluding the anesthesiologist's charge. Increasingly, this procedure is being performed as an outpatient vaginal surgery, involving at most one overnight stay. The cost is about $3,000.[1]

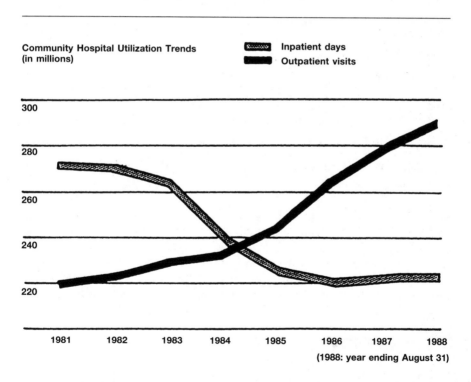

Community Hospital Utilization Trends (in millions)

Inpatient days
Outpatient visits

Figure 3–4 The Changing Demand of Inpatient vs. Outpatient Stays. *Source:* Reprinted from *Vision, Values, Viability: Environmental Assessment 1989–1990*, p. 9 with permission of American Hospital Association, © 1988.

The third competitive consideration for technology is that as each new generation of equipment enters the market, the preceding generation or model becomes cheaper. This factor allows smaller competitors to offer a service by acquiring the slightly older technology or a less expensive version of the new technology. As noted in the previous chapter, academic medical centers such as the one at the University of Minnesota are now facing the competitive realities of the widespread availability of technology. No longer are these facilities the exclusive providers of sophisticated tertiary services.[2] The marginal potential market for the hospital with the new technology depends heavily on how significantly the new generation equipment improves upon the preceding version to capture or shift market share.

Technology may well have a dramatic impact on how care is delivered or managed in the doctor's office. Telemedicine is the source of new advances and directions in the creation of the information super highway. In 1994, the federal government earmarked at least $25 million for investment in telemedicine projects. **Telemedicine** is the delivery of health care through interactive audio, video, or data communications. According to a 1992 study by Arthur D. Little, a consulting firm, advances in telemedicine may help cut the nation's health care bill by $36 billion, with savings achieved across four areas:

1. electronic data management and transport of patient information
2. electronic processing of health care claims
3. electronic inventory management systems
4. teleconferencing for professional training and remote conferencing.[3]

This last benefit of telemedicine is already being realized. The native American reservation in Pine Ridge, South Dakota is linked by satellite to the Mayo Clinic in Rochester, Minnesota. The state of Georgia has financed a telemedicine project linking the Medical College of Georgia hospitals and clinics to 59 health care sites around the state.[4] Similar versions of this program are running in Texas and Iowa.

The true potential and cost-effectiveness of telemedicine has yet to be realized, and is still being debated. There is little doubt, however, that the information super highway advances will affect the future of health care, and greatly affect both the product and distribution components of the health care marketing mix.

SOCIAL FACTORS

The social dimension of the environment includes the demographic characteristics of the population, its culture, and its values. Income, also a factor, was reviewed in a previous section titled Economic Factors.

Demographics

Demographics are statistics that describe members of a population in terms of who they are, where they live, and the types of jobs they have.

The Population

   The population of the United States is changing in two major ways. First, population growth in the country is declining and our population is aging. In 1960, only 9 percent of the population was over age 65, but by 1993 this percentage had increased to 12.5 percent. As Figure 3–5 shows, this more mature market will grow dramatically into the next century.
   Health care organizations are becoming more attentive to this group. Senior care programs, adult day-care centers, Alzheimer clinics, and long-term care facilities are potentially growing business opportunities in light of this aging marketplace. With Alzheimer disease alone, the predicted increase in patients is dramatic. Presently, 3.8 million Americans are diagnosed with this illness. The number is expected to grow to 7 million people by 2030, and slightly over 10 million by 2050.[5] The mature household headed by people over the age of 50 is becoming a

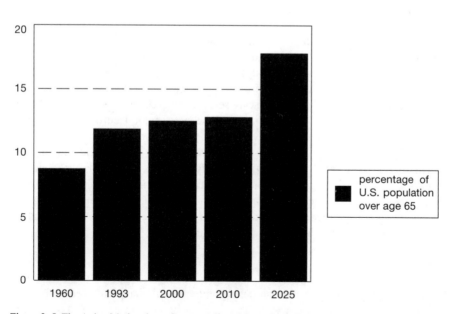

legend: ■ percentage of U.S. population over age 65

Figure 3–5 The Aging Marketplace. *Source:* Adapted from *Statistical Abstract of the United States,* 114th ed., p. 24, U.S. Bureau of the Census, Department of Commerce, 1994.

statistically more significant group. In 1990, these households represented 28 percent of the U.S. population, but will increase to 34 percent by the year 2010, and to 38 percent by the year 2025.[6] In a recent study of 301 hospitals, 62 percent plan to develop clinical quality improvement programs related to care of the elderly, and 35 percent are developing institution-wide strategic planning projects to focus on servicing the elderly American consumer.[7]

The growing senior market is also attracting HMOs. Pacificare Health Systems, Inc. of Cypress, California has 36,000 seniors enrolled in HMOs in California, Washington, Oregon, Oklahoma, and Texas. In 1994, Pacificare also teamed up with Tufts Health Plan, a Massachusetts HMO, to offer a new senior plan called Secure Horizons. This HMO provides all the benefits seniors now receive under Medicare, plus some additional ones.[8]

Baby Boomers

Another potentially explosive market for health care services are those Americans who were born between 1946 and 1964, referred to as the **baby boomers**. This segment of the population is now entering middle age and accounted for 11.3 percent of the population in 1993. These consumers are now increasingly involved in the health care decisions for their aging parents as they play the role of decision maker and, often, caregiver. Companies are beginning to realize the role being assumed by their employees. A 1993 survey of almost 2,000 employees of Transamerica Life Companies of San Francisco found that the firm lost 1,600 workdays, or about $250,000, due to employees taking time off from work to care for elderly relatives. These data, coupled with the fact that the percentage of elderly living with their children declined from 7.5 percent in 1980 to 4.8 percent in 1991, suggest a growing market for elder care services and residential facilities.[9] Within a 10- to 15-year period, this large group will become major users of more intensive health care services themselves.

The baby boomer generation also represents an interesting market segment in terms of its own health care needs. A study conducted in 1991 by David M. Eisenberg, et al., of Harvard University Medical School in Boston found that more than one-third of Americans had turned to alternative medicine therapies. The use of such nonwestern medicinal approaches was most likely among well-educated, white, baby boomers who live in western states.[10]

The Family

Few elements of the American demographic profile have changed more than those representing the family. In the 1950s, 70 percent of U.S. households consisted of a stay-at-home mother, a working father, and one or more children. By 1990, only 20 percent of U.S. households would present this profile.[11]

Increasingly in the United States, marriages are ending in divorce. As a result, we are witnessing the rise of the **blended family**, which is the joining together of two households through remarriage.

Geographic Shifts

Not only is the U.S. population changing in terms of age and family structure, it is also moving. The decade of the 1980s saw a major movement of Americans predominantly to the western states. Major traditional population centers of the northern, eastern, and midwestern United States are experiencing little growth. Figure 3–6 shows this changing population base.

To help analyze geographic markets, the federal government has created a three-tiered description of communities that reflect their population density. Data are gathered and reported according to the following classifications:

1. *Metropolitan Statistical Areas.* These include cities having a population of at least 50,000, or an urbanized area with a total metropolitan population of at least 100,000.
2. *Primary Metropolitan Statistical Area* (PMSA). The second largest category is an area that has a total population of more than one million. It must also include counties that have a total population of at least 100,000, a population

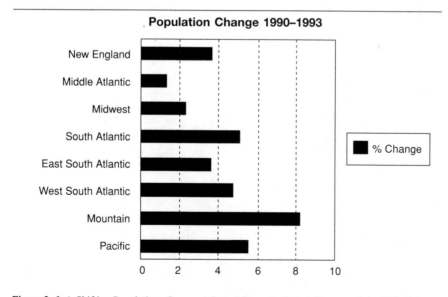

Figure 3–6 A Shifting Population. *Source:* Adapted from *Statistical Abstract of the United States,* 114th ed., p. 29, U.S. Bureau of the Census, Department of Commerce, 1994.

that is at least 60 percent urban, and have fewer than 50 percent of its residents commuting outside the county for employment.

3. *Consolidated Metropolitan Statistical Area.* This is the largest geographical categorization in terms of geographical area and market size. It is comprised of PMSAs that total at least one million people.

Racial and Ethnic Distinctions

The face of the United States is rapidly changing. Increasingly, African-Americans, Hispanics, and Asians are representing a larger percentage of the population. This demographic shift is particularly noticeable in the major metropolitan areas and in some parts of the southwest. In 1992, the U.S. Census Bureau reported that 75 percent of the population was white, 12 percent was African-American, 9 percent was Hispanic, 3 percent was Asian and Pacific Islander, and 1 percent was Native American. The Bureau predicts that by the year 2050, the composition of the population will be 53 percent white, 21 percent Hispanic, 15 percent African-American, 10 percent Asian and Pacific Islander, and 1.2 percent native Americans.[12] Almost one third of all Americans under age 35 are now minorities.[13] In some metropolitan areas there is a heavy concentration of certain ethnic and racial groups. Eighteen percent of all Hispanic Americans live in Los Angeles and 12 percent live in New York City.[14] Health care marketers must recognize and respond to the changing American population. Further discussion about appealing to these market segments is presented in Chapter 6 on market segmentation.

Culture

A second dimension of the social environment is the **culture**, which incorporates the values, customs, and conforming rules passed from one generation to the next. Several cultural changes are occurring in the marketplace, which health care marketers must heed.

The Roles of Women and Men

A significant cultural change that has occurred over the past 20 years is the large number of women who are pursuing higher education and working outside the home. Women are not only working in larger numbers than ever before, they are also heading households in greater numbers. In 1970, slightly more than 20 percent of U.S. households were headed by women, yet that number will grow to 30 percent by the year 2000.[15]

As women work outside the home in greater numbers, organizations must respond to their needs. Pediatric hours may need to be extended to evenings or weekends for appointments. And, as will be discussed in Chapter 4 on buyer behavior, the educated woman who works outside the home plays a different role in terms of household decision making. In these instances, health care organizations are beginning to appreciate the woman's role in the health care decision process.

Changing Providers

The increasing number of women working outside the home has changed the face of medicine, itself. Figure 3–7 shows the increasing percentage of women represented in health care professions. Interestingly, the percentage of women in the traditional profession of nursing is declining, but the percentage of female physicians is increasing. The number of female physicians increased 310 percent between 1970 and 1990. And, in 1992, women represented 42 percent of applicants to U.S. medical schools.[16] Many health care organizations recognize the importance of having clinicians who are sensitive to and representative of the market

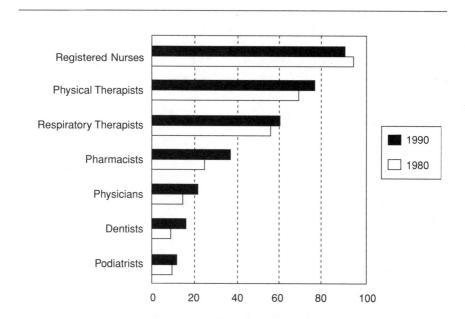

Figure 3–7 Percentage of Women in Health Professions, 1990 vs. 1980. *Source:* Adapted from Braus, P. How Women Will Change Medicine, *American Demographics* magazine, Vol. 16, No. 11, pp. 40–46, with permission of American Demographics, copyright 1994.

they serve. Attracting female practitioners is an important priority for many medical groups in their recruiting efforts.

Changing Attitudes

Attitudinal changes within American society are also significant. Consumers have begun to reconsider the Puritan work ethic of, "I live to work," and are adopting a new perspective that reflects concerns with the quality of one's life. Today's ethic for many could be more appropriately recast as, "I work to live." It is this shift in attitude that might well account for the increasing receptivity of younger physicians to accept salaried positions with a defined number of work hours and a limited number of hours or evenings on call.

A related attitudinal shift affecting health care is the growing health consciousness of American consumers. Fitness, diet, and alternative medicines are all ways for Americans to be more proactive regarding health. Consumers more willingly seek chiropractors, acupuncturists, and even herbalists, as they adopt a more holistic approach to managing their health care status. In 1990, American consumers spent $10.3 million on unconventional medical therapies compared to $12.8 billion spent on hospital care. Grant Hospital in Chicago has developed a "Section of Holistic and Preventive Medicine" that will offer an array of holistic medicine including acupuncture and yoga.[17] Hospitals have also begun to respond with a changing product line. According to the Association of Hospital Health and Fitness, the number of fitness centers affiliated with hospitals and physician groups has doubled since 1991 to a total of 221 such facilities in 1994.[18]

COMPETITIVE FACTORS

A fourth major component of the environment pertains to the competition, the alternative providers of the health care service. There are four basic structural forms of competition that can be arrayed on a continuum as shown in Table 3–1: pure competition, monopolistic competition, oligopoly, and monopoly.

At one end of the spectrum lies **pure competition**, a situation in which every company has the same product. This might be the case of a number of solo-practice, primary care internists who all work in a small community that has no managed care plans. The competitive advantage is difficult to establish, but it is often based on distribution. Whose office is more conveniently located, or who offers extended hours needed by the patient might be the difference in attracting more patients. Other aspects of marketing are of little relevance in this competitive setting.

The second point on the continuum is **monopolistic competition** in which many sellers compete and have substitutable products. Such a situation might exist

Table 3–1 The Continuum of Competition

Pure Competition	Monopolistic Competition	Oligopoly	Monopoly
Many sellers	Many sellers	Few, large sellers	One seller
Substitutable product	Substitutable product	Similar product	Unique product
Little differentiation	Price a key	Little price cutting	Regulatory oversight

in a community where two alternative managed care plans are available. Many of the community's physicians participate on the panels of both competing plans. In this case, small price changes might lead to a consumer shift from one plan to the other.

A third competitive market structure is **oligopoly**, where a few companies control a majority of the industry sales. This is the structure that has dominated the airline industry over the past two decades. Increasingly, this structure is becoming representative of some local and regional health care markets. Columbia/HCA Healthcare Corp., the world's largest hospital chain, based in Louisville, Kentucky, now controls one of every four hospital beds in the state of Florida.[19] If, in fact, the other Florida hospitals are aligned in one or two other systems—Sun Health or the Voluntary Hospitals of America—it might decrease the price competition. With a few large firms dominating the market a price-cutting environment would lead to quick retaliation by one of the other competitors. These strategies would lead to reduced profits for all the competitors. This behavior— one firm engaging in an aggressive promotion tactic—is often seen in the airline industry. The other companies quickly retaliate and the market and fare offerings soon return to a regular basis.

Some oligopolistic markets are considered differentiated, in which buyers perceive a difference among the few competitors. The automobile industry can be viewed as a differentiated oligopoly. The few major manufacturers try to protect their differentiation by focusing on the product component of the marketing mix.

The final position on the continuum is **monopoly**, in which there is only one firm that sells a product. This is quite common for certain natural resources such as water and energy. Usually, government agencies have been established to offer the service or to review the rates and service levels. In health care, monopolies have often been created through a patent, which gives the manufacturer exclusive right to the manufacturing and selling of a product. Because of the high cost of research and development in the pharmaceutical industry, patent protection is a valuable reward, and an incentive to help recoup costs. At the same time, as is true with many monopolies, it often has led to the appearance, or actuality, of abuse. Critics have charged that pharmaceutical companies price their patented drugs too high.

Health Care Competition

The nature of competition within health care is a function of who is defining the competitive set. So, it is useful to consider some of the global environmental trends among the major providers of service within the industry. In recent years, the nature of the health care marketplace has changed within each region of the country as a function of the restructuring among the competitors. Exhibit 3–1 describes the continuum of change and the factors that characterize each stage of evolution as the health care environment moves from a traditional fee-for-service market to a managed care world.

The stage-one market has been termed "unstructured." As can be seen, HMO penetration is rather low—at less than 10 percent—and the marketplace can be described as fragmented with solo practices still viable. Consumers are provided with choice as employers purchase traditional indemnity plans for coverage.

The second stage, termed "loose framework," is characterized by an overcapacity of hospital beds and some physician consolidation with the formation of IPAs. The HMO penetration rate extends to 30 percent of the market. At this stage, companies become more aggressive in seeking cost-control solutions.

Consolidation occurs in the third stage. HMO penetration climbs upwards of 50 percent as the price of care is defined by the marketplace. There are strong incentives to manage care, as alliances form between providers and payers.

The last stage of market evolution is that of managed competition. The incentives are clearly built around accountable quality, and competition exists among only a few large regional networks. This condition now characterizes the market place of Minneapolis–St. Paul—a few large networks dominate and physicians are aligned with only one of the provider systems. At this point, HMO penetration is greater than 50 percent of the market. Table 3–2 shows how states are characterized according to HMO penetration in terms of this topology. Within each state, there often are metropolitan areas further advanced in terms of marketplace evolution.

Hospitals

The environment of the traditional acute-care hospital has changed dramatically in the past 10 to 15 years. Since 1980, an average of 47 hospitals a year have closed, the majority being facilities with less than 100 beds.[20] Several factors account for these closings: changes in reimbursement, an increase in managed care, and the changing location for care delivery.

Exhibit 3–1 The Changing Health Care Market

Market Evolution Indicators

	Unstructured (Stage I)	Loose Framework (Stage II)	Consolidation (Stage III)	Managed Competition (Stage IV)
Employers	• Purchase from indemnity plans • No purchase power	• Form coalition to evaluate providers • Limited power	• Strong managed care incentives • Real managed care demands	• Direct contracting • Some limits on provider intervention • Employers form conditions to purchase
Physicians	• Independent solo, small group practice • Fee-for-service	• Large network formation • Managed care small % of income	• Restricted networks • Significant % of income from managed care • Specialist revenue declines • Group formation	• Integrated system formation • Managed care bulk of income
Hospitals	• Inpatient focused • Financially sound • Independent	• Overcapacity • Price pressure • System formulation	• Moves to outpatient • Hospitals close	• Integrated system formation • PHO structure • Acceptance/share risk
HMO	• 0% to 10% penetration	• 11% to 30% penetration • Market leaders emerge	• 31% to 50% penetration • Marginal HMOs close	• More than 50% penetration • Few HMOs in each regional market

Source: Information from Voluntary Hospitals of America and University Hospital Consortium.

Table 3–2 HMO Penetration Rate by State

Under 5%	5%-15%	16%-25%	25%-35%	Over 35%
Alaska	Maine	New Hampshire	Rhode Island	Massachusetts
West Virginia	New Jersey	Connecticut	New York	California
Wyoming	Virginia	Pennsylvania	Delaware	
Vermont	North Carolina	Florida	Maryland	
Montana	Georgia	Ohio	Arizona	
Idaho	Tennessee	Michigan	Colorado	
North Dakota	Kentucky	Wisconsin	Oregon	
South Dakota	Alabama	Illinois	Minnesota	
Arkansas	Oklahoma	Hawaii	Washington,	
South Carolina	Texas	New Mexico	D.C.	
Mississippi	Kansas	Utah		
Iowa	Nebraska	Washington		
	Nevada	Missouri		
	Indiana			

Source: Information from *Business & Health*, Vol.13, No.1, p.18, Medical Economics Publishing Co., Inc., January 1995.

Regarding the last issue, consider just the shift to outpatient surgery alone. It is estimated that within three years nearly 70 percent of all surgeries will be performed on an outpatient basis.[21] According to the American College of Surgeons, the number of invasive diagnostic and surgical procedures performed on an outpatient basis is rising dramatically. In 1983, there were 377,266 such outpatient procedures, while, by 1994, the number was expected to grow to 18.9 million.[22] As HMO enrollment growth continues, the number of inpatient bed days declines. As noted earlier in this chapter, enrollment of seniors in managed care plans is growing. The impact on hospitals will be serious, since the over-65-year-old customer spends five times as many days in the hospital than does the under-65-year-old patient. The typical hospital relies on senior citizens for 35 percent to 55 percent of its business. HMOs can dramatically reduce these bed days. The national annual average for hospital days per 1,000 Medicare enrollees is 2,835. Yet the average for that same target population among seniors in HMOs is 1,150, with some HMOs in California reporting annual bed days under 900 for 1,000 Medicare enrollees.[23]

Managed Care Providers

The prepaid segment of health care continues to grow. At the end of 1994, the number of HMO enrollees grew to 50.5 million members, a 10 percent increase from the previous year. This growth is the largest recorded since 1987.[24] The fastest-growing segment of the managed care market is point-of-service (POS) plans. In 1991, POS plans had only about 3 percent of all HMO enrollees. By 1995, 15 percent of all HMO enrollees were in POS-type plans.[25]

The market penetration of HMOs varies greatly by state, as evident in Table 3–2. While HMO enrollments are growing, however, the number of operating HMOs are declining from a high of 707 in 1987 to 540 at the beginning of 1994.

Industry Consolidation

The most obvious environmental trend within health care is the consolidation and the resultant appearance of large-scale competitors in many segments of the industry. Columbia/HCA, EPIC/HealthTrust, and Beverly Enterprises, Inc. are but a few of the large, national health care organizations emerging within the industry.

In the nursing home industry, Beverly Enterprises, Inc. of Fort Smith, Arkansas owns 752 nursing homes and controls 80,000 licensed beds. Hillhaven Corporation of Alameda, California and Manor Healthcare Corporation of Silver Spring, Maryland claim control of 33,529 and 21,822 licensed, long-term care beds, respectively, in several states.[26]

In the hospital industry, restructuring has been equally dramatic. During 1993, two of the largest hospital mergers occurred when the EPIC Healthcare Group joined with HealthTrust, and Columbia merged with HCA. The EPIC/HealthTrust consolidation brought together 125 hospitals across 21 states, representing $3.5 billion in revenue, while the Columbia/HCA arrangement resulted in an organization with 192 hospitals generating $10 billion in annual revenues.[27] In April 1995, Columbia/HCA and HealthTrust merged, creating a company with control of 60,000 beds in 31 states. In Texas and Florida alone, this new entity will control 20 percent to 40 percent of the hospital beds in many major market areas. In Florida alone, Columbia now controls 57 percent of the state's 92 investor-owned hospitals.[28]

Hospital consolidation is also occurring at the regional and state level. In a 1993 survey of 402 hospitals, 35.7 percent of the hospital executives reported that their institution had purchased physician practices, and another 38.9 percent reported that they intended to do so within the next five years.[29] In Tennessee, nine small, nonprofit hospitals are joining together to form a 3,000-bed system to compete against the larger national chains.[30] Similar trends are gripping medical practice groups. Nonprofit UniHealth America of Burbank, California has joined together several practices. UniHealth America owns 10 hospitals and has affiliations with 6 medical groups like the 70-person Harrison Jones Medical Group in Long Beach, California.[31] Nationally, the mean size of group practices has increased by a total of four doctors over the last four-year period.[32]

REGULATORY FACTORS

The final aspect of the environment to consider is the regulatory component. **Regulation** consists of the rules or restrictions placed on companies by federal or state governments. Within health care, there are a wide array of regulations pertaining to the delivery of care. In this section, we will review those aspects of major federal legislation that have an impact on the marketing mix.

Competition

There are several key regulations protecting competition that have been in place more than a century. Initiated in the late 1800s in the face of monopolies, they continue to be applied today with increasing frequency in health care.

Antitrust Legislation

Two major antitrust laws are the Sherman Antitrust Act (1890) and the Clayton Act (1914). The **Sherman Antitrust Act** forbids any contracts, combinations, or conspiracies in the restraint of trade. Actual monopolies or attempts to monopolize any part of trade or commerce is also forbidden. The **Clayton Act** supplemented the Sherman Antitrust Act by forbidding certain actions that were likely to lessen competition, even if no actual damages had occurred. In 1950, the Clayton Act was amended by the **Antimerger Act**, which broadened the power of the federal government under Section 7 of the Clayton Act to prevent intercorporate acquisitions that would substantially reduce competition.

This issue of mergers is increasingly a factor in health care. In 1994, for example, Minneapolis Children's Medical Center announced a merger with Children's Hospital in St. Paul. This merger of the two facilities would result in the hospitals controlling 88 percent of the pediatric inpatient care market in Minneapolis–St. Paul. As a result, the state attorney general filed a suit saying it would violate Section 7 of the Clayton Act. The state agreed to withdraw the suit only after the two institutions agreed to several conditions, such as the provision that they would acquire no other hospital; nor would they manage the inpatient pediatric care of another facility. The newly merged facility also cannot enter into an agreement with a physician that would prevent him or her from also practicing at another hospital.[33]

Similarly, the Federal Trade Commission (FTC) intervened in Punta Gorda, Florida, a town north of Fort Meyers. Columbia/HCA proposed to buy a hospital in that community. The FTC denied the acquisition because it would have given the corporation control of two of the three hospitals in the local market.[34]

With the increasing formulation of networks and mergers throughout health care, the federal government released new guidelines on September 27, 1993 clarifying six antitrust "safety zones":

1. The FTC and the Department of Justice will not challenge any merger between two general acute-care hospitals in which one has averaged fewer than 100 licensed beds, and an average daily census of less than 40 patients for the past three years. An additional requirement is that the hospital must be more than five years old.
2. No joint venture will be challenged regarding an agreement among hospitals to purchase, operate, or market the services of high-tech or other expensive medical equipment, providing the number of hospitals are needed to support the cost of the service. A joint venture will not be challenged that includes additional hospitals if these hospitals could not support the cost of the equipment.
3. The agencies will provide a "rule of reason" in the antitrust review of joint ventures that fall outside the antitrust "safety zones." The concern is whether the joint ventures will reduce competition. Even if the result is such, the examination will consider whether procompetitive efficiencies are produced to outweigh this concern.
4. The agency will not challenge the collective provision of medical data by physicians which may improve the purchasers' resolution of mode, quality, or efficiency of treatment issues.
5. The agencies will not challenge hospital participation in written surveys of price for hospital services, wages, or benefits for personnel. The survey must, however, be administered by a third party and contain data more than three months old. A minimum of five hospitals must report the data. No one hospital's data can represent more than 25 percent of the information.
6. The agencies will not challenge any joint purchase agreement among health care providers as long as two conditions are met: (a) the purchase accounts for less than 35 percent of the total sales of the product purchased in the relevant market, and (b) the cost of the product and service purchased jointly accounts for less than 20 percent of the total revenue from all products and services sold by each joint venture participant.[35]

In recognition of this 20 percent requirement, the FTC and the Department of Justice applied the "rule of reason" and cleared a venture by a group of Denver-area cardiologists whose proposed Rocky Mountain Cardiovascular Affiliates would have represented 22 percent of the cardiologists within the market.[36]

The federal government strove to protect competition further with passage of the **Robinson-Patman Act** (1935). This law makes it illegal to discriminate in prices between different buyers of the same product, where the effect may be to lessen competition and create a monopoly.

Product Legislation

In terms of the marketing mix, several laws have also been passed that affect the product and, in varying instances, protect the company or the market. As mentioned earlier, a major form of federal legislative protection is the granting of a patent.

A second major law protecting companies is the **Lanham Act**, which provides for the registration of a company's trademarks—in other words, its brand name. When this law was initially passed, it provided trademark protection to the first user of the trademark. Then, in 1988, the trademark law was updated with the **Trademark Law Revision Act**, which granted a company trademark protection prior to actual use.

A trademark is a valuable asset for a company (more on the value of brand names is described in Chapter 8), but the trademark law does not give a company ownership of the trademark. A company can lose its trademark if the name becomes so generic that it applies to the entire product class. "Aspirin," for example, used to be a company's trademark, so too was "elevator." Now companies such as Xerox and FedEx, both registered trademarks, work to protect against any trademark infringement, but also to ensure that their names are not used as nouns or verbs—which would classify them as generic terms. When you think you are xeroxing a memo, the Xerox Company will tell you that you are photocopying.

Pricing

In health care there are several regulations related to issues of reimbursement. At the macro level, issues of price fixing and price discounting were addressed by the Sherman Act. Although this law did not specifically outlaw price fixing, the courts have ruled that price fixing is, *per se*, illegal and will restrain trade. In terms of discounting, the law allows for discounts to be offered to buyers, providing cost savings can be demonstrated in dealing with a particular buyer. Promotional allowances can also be granted differentially to buyers, but they must be offered on an equal proportionate basis to each buyer based on volume purchased.

Distribution

In this third aspect of the marketing mix, the government has three major areas of concern. The first pertains to **exclusive dealing**, in which a buyer is required to handle only the products of one manufacturer but not a competitor. This requirement is considered a violation of the Clayton Act.

A second area of concern pertains to **requirement contracts**, in which a buyer is required to purchase all or part of its needs for a product from one seller for a defined period of time. The justice system has examined each instance of a requirement contract separately. A third area involves **tying arrangements**, where the seller of a product requires that the purchaser also buys another item. These arrangements are considered illegal when they result in restraining trade in the tied product.

In health care an increasingly important area of government regulatory investigation pertains to vertical integration. Although not specifically illegal, the courts evaluate issues of vertical integration with regard to the Clayton Act to ensure that the result of this activity neither lessens competition nor creates a monopoly. This issue of vertical integration is becoming more important as hospitals establish integrated delivery systems and acquire primary care practices.

Within health care, there is a separate set of regulations pertaining to the issue of patient referrals. In 1991, the Health Care Financing Administration published regulations for the Ethics in Patient Referrals Act, referred to as "Stark I" (for the congressman who sponsored the legislation). This law prohibited physician referrals to entities in which they held a financial interest. This law was broadened in the Omnibus Reconciliation Act of 1993. The new law, known as **Stark II**, also prohibits physician referrals to entities in which they hold a financial interest, and applies to both Medicare and Medicaid. Effective January 1, 1995, no physician or physician family member who has a financial interest in an entity may refer a patient to that entity for health services. This law not only puts restrictions on the physician but also on the entity to which the patient is referred. That organization cannot present a claim or a bill to any individual or third party for reimbursement. While there are degrees of interpretation and exceptions to this legislation, it greatly determines the strategies used to control the channel of distribution for patient referrals.[37]

Promotion

The last element of the marketing mix—promotion—is also subject to various government regulations. The majority of promotional activities are closely monitored and regulated by the **Federal Trade Commission Act of 1914**. This law, which created the Federal Trade Commission, forbids deceptive or misleading advertising and unfair business practices. The FTC has the power to issue cease and desist orders and it can order any company to conduct **corrective advertising**, a means of communication by which the company must correct misimpressions formed in the marketplace.

In 1975, the issue of advertising for professional services underwent a dramatic turnaround. At this time, the U.S. Supreme Court ruled that professional associations were subject to antitrust laws, which were designed to protect competition. In order to comply with this judicial view the American Medical Association and other professional medical and legal associations loosened their restrictions that prohibited their members from advertising. Later U.S. Supreme Court decisions in 1980 and 1982 ruled that restricting advertising was illegal, and since then, advertising has become very common in both the health and the legal professions.

In 1993, the federal government also put into effect the Medicare and Medicaid antikickback law, which affects certain promotional programs. The government recently investigated programs that give physicians frequent flyer miles each time they complete a questionnaire for new patients prescribed the company's product. According to government requirements, a payment or gift may be considered illegal under the kickback law if: (1) it is made to a person who is in a position to generate business for the paying party, (2) it is related to the volume of business generated, (3) it is of greater than nominal value and exceeds free-market value, or (4) it is unrelated to any service other than the referral of a patient.

Self-Regulation

In response to this more active government role, the medical and health professions are stepping up their self-policing efforts. The American Medical Association has developed a set of guidelines which were adopted by the Pharmaceutical Research and Manufacturers of America (PhRMA), a pharmaceutical manufacturers trade group headquartered in Washington, D.C. The PhRMA's members produce almost 90 percent of all the brand-named drugs in the United States. These guidelines restrict drug company gifts to physicians to those that have only nominal value or those with direct educational or patient benefit. The PhRMA also publishes a 700-page book detailing government and private-sector standards on drug promotion.[38]

CONCLUSIONS

Marketing plans and strategies are developed in the context of, and in response to, the broader macroenvironment. While the environment cannot be controlled, organizations must recognize ongoing trends and factors that will likely affect their market success. Because the environmental factors are dynamic, a health care organization must maintain a continual monitoring process and adjust its marketing plans accordingly.

KEY TERMS

Inflation	Regulation
Consumer Price Index	Sherman Antitrust Act
Gross Income	Clayton Act
Disposable Income	Antimerger Act
Discretionary Income	Robinson-Patman Act
Technology	Lanham Act
Telemedicine	Trademark Law Revision Act
Demographics	Exclusive Dealing
Baby Boomers	Requirement Contracts
Blended Family	Tying Arrangements
Culture	Stark II
Pure Competition	Federal Trade Commission Act of
Monopolistic Competition	1914
Oligopoly	Corrective Advertising
Monopoly	

CHAPTER SUMMARY

1. Marketing strategy must be developed in response to and in concert with the broader macroenvironment. Economic, technological, social, competitive, and regulatory forces can all determine the effectiveness of any organization's marketing program.

2. In recent years, the rise in the cost of medical care has dramatically outstripped the rise in cost of consumer goods. This increase has caused employers and other health care buyers to take more aggressive actions to control their health care expenses.

3. Health care is a technologically driven industry. New technological advances dramatically affect the institutions and providers who deliver health care and determine how that care is delivered.

4. The changing demographics of U.S. population represent significant opportunities for health care providers. Older consumers—a fast-growing segment—are major utilizers of health care services and products. Baby boomers are often attracted to alternative medical approaches.

5. Changing marketplace demographics, related to gender, ethnicity, and race, require health care providers to be more responsive to the needs and

46 to Baby Boomers

concerns of women, Hispanics, and African-Americans. In many metropolitan areas, Hispanics and African-Americans represent a significant proportion of the market.

6. The competitive market can be defined as either a pure competition, a monopolistic competition, an oligopoly, or a monopoly. The differences represent the number of sellers in the marketplace.

7. Health care markets are evolving through four competitive environments. Each stage is characterized by greater consolidation among the providers and the buyers.

8. Prepaid health care is a rapidly growing segment of the health care industry. There is significant consolidation occurring among hospitals, which is bringing large-scale, national hospital chain competitors into many local markets.

9. A wide variety of federal (and state) regulations exist that affect each aspect of the marketing mix. In recent years, major federal regulatory attention in health care has been paid to mergers and acquisitions of hospitals and providers by competitors. The government has provided some guidelines pertaining to health care mergers and acquisitions.

10. The issue of provider referrals has also come under scrutiny of federal regulators. While the laws are not exact, in general, it is illegal for physicians to refer to a facility in which they have a financial interest.

CHAPTER PROBLEMS

1. The major on-line computer services such as America Online Inc., CompuServe, and Prodigy provide health news and medical and health forums where users can access medical libraries, exchange messages, and discuss health problems. CompuServe also provides a service called Physician Data Query, from the National Cancer Institute, which provides information on cancer types and treatments. In what ways might the growing use of these services by consumers affect future strategies for: (a) family practitioners, and (b) HMOs?

2. What environmental factors would you suggest account for: (a) the rapid growth of—NordicTrack—a premium-priced home fitness equipment company that formerly sold only through direct mail and has now opened retail stores in shopping malls, and (b) the success of after-hours clinics and urgent care facilities in many metropolitan areas?

3. Assume you were hired to design an HMO plan targeted to baby boomers in San Antonio, Texas, a city with a large Hispanic population. How would you make

this service offering unique to respond to the major trends discussed within this chapter?

4. In late 1994, the U.S. Justice Department settled a case involving ClassiCare Network, a joint venture of eight Long Island hospitals. The joint venture was to act as the "exclusive bargaining agent" in negotiations with all HMOs regarding hospital discounts. The agreement reached with the hospitals barred this arrangement. On what grounds and rules was the Justice Department action based?

5. In considering the continuum of the health care market evolution as shown in Exhibit 3–1, how would you describe the relative power of the following three major markets in terms of their importance in the health care competitive market: (a) physicians, (b) hospitals, and (c) large employers?

NOTES

1. Hospital Stays for Hysterectomy Are Dwindling, *Health Technology Trends* 5, no. 9 (1993):7.

2. L. Page, Playing Catch-Up, *American Medical News* 37, no. 29 (1994):3,7–8.

3. R. Shoor, Long-Distance Medicine, *Business & Health* 12, no.6 (1994):39–45.

4. L. Scott, Will Health Care Accept the "Virtual" Doctor? *Modern Healthcare* 24, no. 48 (1994): 34–41.

5. New Troopers in the Alzheimer's War: Mice, *U.S. News & World Report* 118, no. 7 (1995):18.

6. J. Waldrop, Secrets of Age Pyramids, *American Demographics* 14, no. 8 (1992):46ff.

7. K.S. Taylor, Ready or Probably Not: The Elderly Are Coming, *Hospitals and Health Networks* 68, no. 24 (1994):54.

8. C. Stein, HMO Battleground: Elderly, *The Boston Globe*, 17 July 1994, 49,51.

9. P. Braus, When Mom Needs Help, *American Demographics* 16, no. 3 (1994):38–46.

10. S. Mitchell, Healing Without Doctors, *American Demographics* 15, no. 7 (1993):46–49; D.M. Eisenberg, et al., Unconventional Medicine in the United States, *The New England Journal of Medicine* 328, no. 4 (1993):246–252.

11. J. Waldrop, A Lesson in Home Economics, *American Demographics* 11, no. 8 (1989):8.

12. J.R. Evans and Barry Berman, *Marketing* (New York, N.Y.: MacMillan & Co., 1994), 228.

13. The Trend You Can't Ignore, *American Demographics* 16, no. 7 (1994):2.

14. M. Winsburg, Specific Hispanics, *American Demographics* 16, no. 2 (1994):44–53.

15. D. Crispell, Workers in 2000, *American Demographics* 14, no. 9 (1992):27–28.

16. P. Braus, How Women Will Change Medicine, *American Demographics* 16, no. 11 (1994): 40–46.

17. Grant Makes Holistic Link, *Modern Healthcare* 24, no. 30 (1994):10.

18. K. Pallarito, Hospitals Strengthen Networks Through New Fitness Facilities, *Modern Healthcare* 24, no. 50 (1994):44–46.

19. R. Tomsho, Giant Hospital Chain Uses Tough Tactics To Push Fast Growth, *The Wall Street Journal*, 12 July 1994, A1,A6.

20. Hospital Closings Down, *Modern Healthcare* 24, no. 13 (1994):3–8.

21. Hospitals Face Strong Competition in Outpatient Market, *SMG Market Letter* 7, no. 6 (1993):1.

22. Outpatient Surgery: Empires Strike Back, *MedPro Month* 4, no. 3 (1994):37,59–60.

23. Stein, HMO Battleground.

24. Upward Trend, *American Medical News* 37, no. 29 (1994):2.

25. HMO Enrollment Rises and Premiums Fall, *Business & Health* 13, no. 1 (1995):12.

26. Nursing Home Bed Growth Strongest in Chains and Hospitals, *SMG Market Letter* 8, no. 10 (1994):1.

27. With EPIC, HealthTrust Faces 2nd Turnaround Challenge, *Modern Healthcare* 24, no. 3 (1994):2–3; S. Lutz, Industry Followers Fear the Leader, *Modern Healthcare* 24, no. 7 (1994):23–30.

28. Hospital Mergers Continue, *Business & Health* 12, no. 11 (1994):16; D. Burda, J. Greene, and S. Lutz, Columbia Merger Has Big Impact in Florida, Texas, *Modern Healthcare*, 25, no. 18 (1995):6.

29. J. Johnsson, Hospitals Binge on Practice Buy-Outs, *American Medical News* 36, no. 34 (1993):1,7.

30. T. Rudd, Nine TN Not-For-Profit Hospitals Prepare for Battle, *Health Care Competition Week* 11, no. 8 (1994):1–3.

31. Merger Frenzy in California Picks Up Pace, *Modern Healthcare* 24, no. 10 (1994):42,46.

32. J. Montague, Precision Maneuvers, *Hospitals and Health Networks* 68, no. 1 (1994):26–33.

33. Minnesota Hospitals Make Antitrust Pact, *Modern Healthcare* 24, no. 32 (1994):34.

34. Tomsho, Giant Hospital Chain.

35. New Guidelines From the FTC and Justice Department, *Hospitals and Health Networks* 67, no. 23 (1993):28.

36. Justice Dept., FTC Offer More Antitrust Guidance, *Modern Healthcare* 24, no. 40 (1994):34.

37. H.J. Swibel and M.J. Zaremski, Surfing Stark II: Prohibition Against Self-Referrals, *Physician Executive* 21, no. 2 (1995):11–15.

38. D.M. Gianelli, Drug Makers Warned: Some Promotions Are Kickbacks, *American Medical News* 37, no. 33 (1994):9.

Part II
Understanding the Consumer

BUYER BEHAVIOR

After reading this chapter you should be able to:

• Understand the process of consumer and industrial decision making

• Recognize the internal and external factors that influence consumer decision making

• Identify alternative strategies to affect consumer decision making

• Appreciate the different nature of organizational buying and its implication for marketing strategy

The basic purpose of marketing is to meet the needs of consumers. Central to effective marketing strategy then, is to understand how consumers make the decision to buy a product, select a doctor, or join a health plan. As this chapter will discuss in detail, a variety of factors affect the consumer's decision-making process.

DECISION-MAKING MODEL

The **consumer decision-making process** can be represented in six stages (as shown in Figure 4–1): (1) problem recognition, (2) internal search, (3) external search, (4) alternative evaluation, (5) purchase, and (6) post-purchase evaluation.[1]

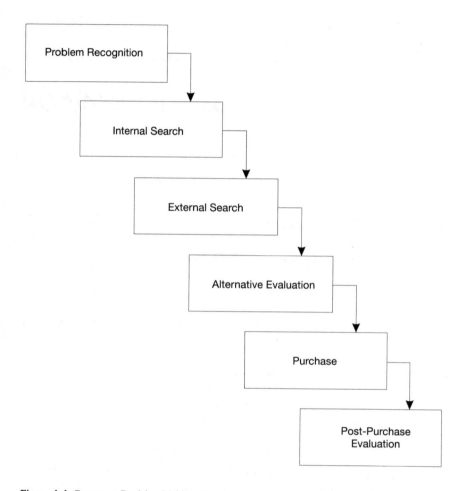

Figure 4–1 Consumer Decision-Making Process

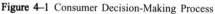

Problem Recognition

The stage of *problem recognition* is where the consumer perceives a difference between the desired and actual state and is motivated to try to close this gap.[2] For example, a consumer begins to notice that he always has difficulty getting an appointment with his primary care physician. This recognition might motivate the individual to explore alternative sources of medical care and seek another physician.

It is critical for an organization to develop marketing strategies to aid the problem recognition stage. For example, an advertisement showing long waiting lines at a competing health plan's office might suggest that consumers need to explore alternatives to using that health plan. Marketing strategy attempts to influence the desired state by trying to alter perceptions of the existing state.

Internal Search

After recognizing the existence of a problem, the consumer often engages in an *internal information search* seeking a solution to the perceived problem. In this example, the individual will try to determine whether he knows of, or remembers, other possible primary care doctors, either those whom he heard about or those he recalls seeing. In traditional industries that manufacture products that are frequently purchased, such as toothpaste or soft drinks, the internal search process is often sufficient for the consumer to make a decision. When internal search does not produce an alternative to solve the recognized problem, the consumer may engage in external search.

External Search

An *external information search* involves seeking information from one or more sources when internal search is insufficient.[3] These sources can be media in the form of advertisements, personal sources such as friends or salespersons, public sources such as government data, or rating organizations such as the Consumers Union, which publishes *Consumer Reports*.[4] Exhibit 4–1 shows a sample of a rating system developed by a coalition of California HMOs and employers. The coalition, called the California Cooperative–HEDIS Reporting Initiative, hired the MedSTAT Group to analyze information from 25,000 medical charts. MedSTAT Group, Inc. of Ann Arbor, Michigan provides consulting expertise in data analysis through prepackaged software and computer-related services. The goal was to provide useful external information to consumers in their decisions regarding which plans to join, by ranking the performance of California HMOs in providing six preventive-care services. This type of information is useful in the external search stage, and it is a valuable testimony for the organization that is favorably rated. A fifth external search alternative is experiential information. A customer derives this information by trying the product in the store, or, in the example of an individual seeking a new doctor, attending an open house conducted by the HMO for potential subscribers.

Exhibit 4–1 External Information on HMOs

Preventive-Care Report Card

California HMOs were rated for their performance in providing six preventive-care services. How the HMOs serving Southern California compare:

○ Above average
◐ Average
● Below average

* Insufficient data submitted by the plan
N/A Not applicable[1]
[1] Health plan was not operational for length of time required for the study.

Health Plan	Childhood Immunization	Cholesterol Screening Ages 40-64	Breast Cancer Screening	Cervical Cancer Screening	Prenatal Care	Diabetes Retinal Exam
Aetna South	◐	◐	◐	◐	◐	◐
Aetna San Diego	○	◐	◐	◐	◐	◐
Blue Shield HMO	◐	N/A	◐	◐	◐	*
CaliforniaCare	◐	◐	◐	○	◐	◐
CareAmerica	◐	◐	●	◐	◐	◐
CIGNA LA IPA	◐	◐	◐	◐	◐	◐
CIGNA LA Staff	◐	◐	◐	○	◐	○
FHP	◐	◐	◐	○	◐	●
Foundation Health Plan	◐	◐	◐	◐	◐	◐
Health Net	◐	◐	◐	○	◐	○
Kaiser Permanente	○	◐	●	◐	◐	○
Maxicare	◐	◐	○	◐	◐	○
MetLife	●	◐	●	◐	●	*
PacifiCare	*	◐	●	◐	◐	*
PruCare	●	N/A	◐	◐	●	◐
TakeCare	○	○	◐	○	◐	○

Data from: California Cooperative-HEDIS Reporting Initiative

Source: Reprinted from Olmos, D.R., ABCs of HMOs: New Study Rates Groups in State, *Los Angeles Times,* February 24, 1995, p. D5, with permission of the Los Angeles Times Syndicate, © 1995.

Table 4–1 shows the external search information sources used by consumers in seeking primary care assistance. Yet, in a 1991 study, women preferred doctors as their primary information source.[5]

Alternative Evaluation

The fourth stage of the consumer decision-making process is *alternative evaluation*, where the consumer compares the various choices that may best meet the individual's need. In this stage, the consumer determines on what criteria the alternative products or services are to be judged. These are termed the **evaluative criteria**. Evaluative criteria can differ in terms of type, number, and importance. Consumers can use tangible and intangible criteria. Tangible criteria might include the cost of joining a particular health maintenance organization. An intangible

Table 4–1 External Search Sources for Primary Care

	Provider Used				
Information Source	Internist (N = 66)	Family Practitioner (N = 174)	OB/GYN (N = 32)	General Practitioner (N = 192)	All Respondents (N = 479)
Friends	19.7	21.4	34.8	26.4	23.4
Family	25.8	27.6	25.0	27.0	26.5
Phone call to provider	16.7	18.4	15.6	9.4	14.1
Observation of office when passing by	3.4	9.8	9.7	3.7	6.4
Another doctor	33.3	17.8	25.0	16.2	19.5
Heard doctor speak (PTA, church, etc.)	7.0	6.0	13.8	4.9	6.3
Nonphysician medical professional (nurse, paramedic, etc.)	7.0	14.4	33.3	14.3	14.7
Employer provides care through this doctor or practice	6.1	6.3	15.6	4.7	6.0

Source: Reprinted from Stewart, D.W., Hickson, G.B., Peachman, C., Koslow, S., and Altemeier, W., Information Search and Decision Making in the Selection of Family Health Care, *Journal of Health Care Marketing*, Vol. 9, No. 2, pp. 29–39, with permission of American Marketing Association, © 1989.

criterion might be the way a particular doctor's office feels when you walk in for an appointment. A new magazine called *Health Pages* compares 20 managed care plans in the St. Louis, Missouri area on several criteria such as the rate at which they perform childhood immunizations, PAP smears, Caesarian sections, eye exams for diabetes, and mammograms.[6]

The number of criteria used to evaluate alternatives can also vary. As to be expected, fewer criteria are used for simple products like toothpaste or laundry soap.[7] An evoked set of alternatives representing those that meet the consumer's evaluative criteria are determined.[8] In forming the evoked set, the consumer selects a subset of possibilities from which to make the final choice.

Research has found that, when evaluating alternatives, the consumer typically has a set of attributes that are important, and will use each attribute to evaluate the alternatives. In this type of model, developed originally by Fishbein, the consumer selects the alternatives that have the highest evaluation of desired attributes.[9] An example of this process is shown in Exhibit 4–2. Based on the calculations shown

---

Exhibit 4–2 Fishbein Choice Model

$$\text{Attitude} = \sum_{i=1}^{n} \text{Belief} * \text{Importance}$$

1. Rate the importance of each factor on a scale of '1' (very unimportant) to '5' (very important) in choosing a doctor:

Hours for appointments	5
Range of services	3
Office location	7

2. Please rate each group listed below on a scale of '1' (doesn't meet my needs) to '5' (does meet my needs) on each dimension:

	Hours for appointments	Range of services	Office location
Group Health	7	8	2
Johnson Medical	5	6	9
Sutter Clinic	8	4	6

Based on these ratings, the Fishbein model would calculate a consumer rating for each group as follows:

Group Health	5*7 (hours) + 3*8 (services) + 7*2 (location)	=	73
Johnson Medical	5*5 + 3*6 + 7*9	=	104
Sutter Clinic	5*8 + 3*4 + 7*7	=	101

The consumer is most favorably disposed to Johnson and would choose that group.

in this exhibit, the consumer would have the most favorable attitude toward the Johnson Clinic. This outcome is determined by multiplying the importance of the three attributes used to compare the clinics (hours for appointments, range of services, and office location) by the belief held by the consumer regarding how much each clinic meets their needs regarding these attributes.

Purchase

At this stage the consumer makes the *purchase*, selecting one brand or alternative over the others. The decision at this stage may involve final determinations as to when to purchase, or in the case of certain products, how much to purchase.

Post-Purchase Evaluation

Be aware that the consumer's decision-making process does not end at the stage of purchase decision. Upon choosing a particular product or service, the consumer spends some time evaluating that choice. Favorable evaluations might ultimately lead the consumer to repurchase or endorse the product or service.[10]

The importance of the *post-purchase evaluation* has led many health care organizations to measure the satisfaction of their patients or their referral sources. Satisfaction is measured, then, as a confirmation or disconfirmation of the consumer's expectations regarding the performance of the chosen product or service. Consumers can use data obtained from customer satisfaction measurement surveys as part of their internal search information when making subsequent purchase decisions. UniHealth America, an HMO in California, uses a telemarketing firm to check the satisfaction of emergency room visits to any of its 10 hospitals. Physician referrals are made, if requested, along with an assessment of patient satisfaction.[11]

Measuring Post-Purchase Satisfaction

By measuring consumer post-purchase satisfaction, a health care organization can focus management attention on areas of service that need improvement. In the post-purchase evaluation, the organization should measure two elements: (1) it should rate how important a particular aspect of the service encounter was in terms of overall consumer satisfaction, and (2) the organization should measure whether consumer (or patient) expectations were confirmed or disconfirmed. For example, a consumer post-evaluation satisfaction survey might contain the following questions.

A. How important were the following factors in your overall satisfaction?

	Very important				Very unimportant
Quality of food	1	2	3	4	5
Admitting process	1	2	3	4	5
Nursing attentiveness	1	2	3	4	5

B. Please indicate how well each of the following aspects of your hospital stay met your expectations?

	Much better than expected		About as I expected		Must worse than expected
Quality of food	1	2	3	4	5
Admitting process	1	2	3	4	5
Nursing attentiveness	1	2	3	4	5

The outcomes of these post-purchase evaluations will determine the direction for management action, as shown in Figure 4–2. Areas that hold low importance, yet exceed expectations, may present opportunities for management to shift resources into more essential aspects of the service encounter. Areas of high importance in which expectations are exceeded present opportunities to leverage with important markets. A promotional program should reinforce the fact that the organization is meeting customer needs. Status quo areas are those of low importance, where expectations are minimally met but not exceeded.

Dimensions of the service encounter requiring management attention and action are those factors rated as very important by customers where their expectations were not met. In such instances, the service firm must determine whether the problem is perceptual or actual. Let's assume that the results of the survey in the example above reveal that the admitting process requires management attention. The management must first consider the operational factors: Were staffing levels appropriate, given existing resources and customer demand? Was all possible preadmitting information gathered by phone or mail prior to the patient arrival at the facility? If the answer is yes—that operations are functioning normally and that staffing is appropriate—the problem may be perceptual. Consumer expectations must be brought in line with reality. When admitting a new patient, the admitting clerk should explain to the customer how much time the process usually takes. If excessive delays should occur, customers should be informed that these are unusual, and perhaps should be offered a certificate for dessert and coffee in the cafeteria until the backlog is processed.

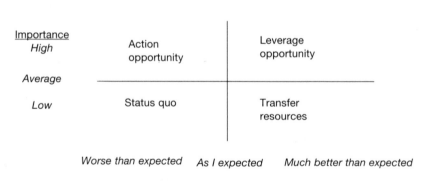

Figure 4–2 Action Opportunities from Post-Purchase Evaluation

Cognitive Dissonance. When a consumer is choosing between two or more relatively equal alternatives, a choice will occasionally lead to the creation of *cognitive dissonance*, a mental state of anxiety brought on because the consumer is unsure of the chosen alternative.[12] For example, an employee might suffer great cognitive dissonance in choosing between two managed care plans. Using as an example the California coalition report in Exhibit 4–1, the consumer (i.e., the employee) can see that the two plans were rated favorably. Now, when the consumer enrolls in one of these plans for the next calendar year, the consumer wonders whether he or she made the right choice, or whether the alternative health plan would have been better. Often when dissonance occurs, consumers will again engage in search behavior to reduce the dissonance. One of two outcomes can result. In some cases, consumers will try to reinforce the correctness of their own decisions; in other cases, they will denigrate the alternatives not chosen. For health care organizations, this aspect of post-purchase evaluation signals the need to communicate with the buyer or user of a service shortly after the encounter has occurred or the contract has been signed. Post-purchase communication in the form of a letter, newsletter, or phone call can reinforce the consumer's belief that the correct choice was made by choosing ABC HMO.

Alternative Decision-Making Sequences

Not every situation in which the consumer is required to make a choice involves the sequence of steps shown in Figure 4–1. There are several alternative decision situations that modify the model previously described. Decision making varies as a function of how involved the consumer is with the decision. Exhibit 4-3 shows the matrix that represents the degree of involvement and the extent of decision making.

In this model, **involvement** refers to the level of the consumer's personal investment in the purchase.[13] High involvement product purchases tend to be those that represent risk (selection of a surgeon), significant cost (choice of a health plan), or social implications (the clubs or associations joined). Low involvement product purchases are not very important to the consumer or represent little risk or cost. The matrix also shows a second dimension of search that refers to the degree of effort the consumer expends in moving from internal to external search and the extensiveness of that external search.

Routine Decision Making

The **routine decision-making** situation involves repetitive purchasing. In these instances, there is often little difference between competing market alternatives. As can be seen in Exhibit 4–3, routine decision making can involve both high and

Exhibit 4–3 Consumer Decision Making and Involvement

Decision making/involvement	High	Low
extended	complex (health insurance plan selection)	variety seeking (over-the-counter pharmaceuticals)
routine	brand loyalty (primary care physician)	inertia (Band-Aid selection)

Source: Adapted from *Consumer Behavior and Marketing Action*, 3rd ed., by H. Assael, p.152, with permission of South-Western College Publishing, © 1987.

low involvement. In the case of high involvement, the consumer engages in little extended decision making in frequently choosing to use his primary care physician. The consumer has developed loyalty to the provider. In product marketing, this situation is referred to as **brand loyalty** in which the consumer regularly chooses the same product or service to fulfill a recognized need.

Complex Decision Making

Complex decision making involves situations in which there is high involvement and extended search. This scenario might well arise in health care situations. A consumer facing major surgery might decide to consult with a couple of physicians for their recommendations. The patient might also research any available data on mortality and morbidity statistics as they apply to particular hospitals and doctors. The individual might also ask friends or family for their insights as to places to go for treatment. Obviously in such situations, risk is high and extended search becomes warranted.

Limited Decision Making

Limited decision making involves extended search in low involvement situations. In traditional product marketing, this occurs when the consumer seeks variety or engages in impulse purchasing. In health care, this situation often occurs when consumers buy over-the-counter pharmaceutical products. The consumer is not particularly tied to one brand and sees little real risk in choosing an alternative. After using one particular cold remedy, an individual might decide to explore alternatives to seek a more effective brand.

PSYCHOLOGICAL INFLUENCES ON DECISION MAKING

There are a variety of personal, psychological factors that affect a consumer's decision-making process. To market effectively to consumers it is useful to understand these elements: motivation, attitudes, lifestyles, learning, and perception.

Motivation

Motivation encompasses the goals or needs that propel a consumer to action. At any point in time, an individual can have multiple needs that result in some course of action.

One of the more well-known models regarding motivation is Maslow's Hierarchy of Needs shown in Figure 4–3.[14] Maslow developed this framework to help explain individual behavior and the differences among individuals regarding their behavior. According to Maslow, the differences in behavior might best be explained by understanding where an individual is in terms of this hierarchy. The needs at the lower end of the pyramid (e.g., physiological, safety) are the most basic. As a consumer begins to satisfy these needs, higher-order needs such as self-esteem or self-actualization begin to be addressed.

For a marketer, this framework is particularly useful in considering the positioning of products or services. A smoke detector can be positioned as meeting safety needs. Many health care plans highlight their ability to meet the safety needs of a family's loved ones. Wellness programs and smoking cessation clinics might be best positioned as responding to needs of self-esteem or self-actualization, rather than safety.

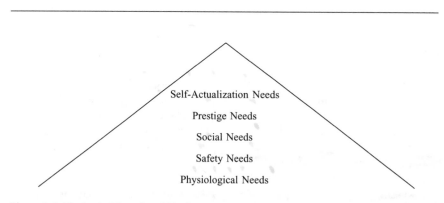

Figure 4–3 Maslow's Hierarchy of Needs

Attitudes

Attitudes and values both affect a consumer's decision-making process. **Attitudes** represent a consumer's enduring cognitive evaluations, feelings, or action tendencies toward some person, object, or idea.[15] As discussed in the alternative evaluation stage, the Fishbein model of attitude formation (shown in Exhibit 4–2) has attitudes being formed as a function of the importance of the attributes and the evaluation that the person or object contains some amount of that particular characteristic.

Since attitudes are predispositions to act in a certain way, marketers have often focused on the measurement of attitudes. Measuring consumer attitudes toward a product or service is not necessarily a measure of purchase intention. A consumer may have a favorable attitude toward the Mayo Clinic but may not seek treatment there for a variety of reasons, such as travel inconvenience, the proximity of other favorably evaluated clinics, or insurance restrictions.

While attitudes represent customers' predispositions, attitudes can be changed to some degree with varying marketing strategies.[16] Because attitudes are comprised of attributes, changing attitudes involves trying to shift the way consumers evaluate certain aspects of these attributes. One approach involves trying to shift consumers' evaluations of how much a particular brand of product or service possesses a particular attribute. For example, if pediatric coverage and availability was deemed important by HMO subscribers, the HMO would tout the availability of its large staff of pediatric clinicians ready to meet subscriber needs. A second tactic involves changing the level of importance attached to a particular attribute. That same HMO might decide that its linkage with an academic medical center is a valuable component of its program. The market positioning might tout the backup expertise available in the rare instances when needed. A third strategy to change attitudes would involve helping consumers to develop an appreciation for other attributes to consider when evaluating alternatives.

Lifestyle

Lifestyle is an important aspect affecting a consumer's decision-making process. **Lifestyle** is the manner in which people live as demonstrated by how they spend their time, what they think, and the interests they have.[17] In the 1980s, for example, the term "yuppies" was popularized to express a group of young, urban professionals who were characterized by a certain upscale, ambitious, and materialistic lifestyle and behavior. BMW automobiles, Chardonnay wine, and Burberry raincoats were some of the hallmarks of a "yuppie" lifestyle.

In marketing, lifestyle profiles of consumers are often developed through the use of AIO statements.[18] AIO refers to attitudes, interests, and opinions. A sample of AIO statements that might be used to define a health-conscious consumer are shown in Exhibit 4–4. These types of questions used in lifestyle analysis have also been referred to as psychographics.

VALS

One of the most commercially popular forms of lifestyle analysis is the VALS2™ system. VALS stands for Value And Life Styles, a program developed by SRI International, a Menlo Park, California research and development company.[19] This classification scheme categorizes consumers into one of eight different basic lifestyle groups: actualizers, fulfilleds, believers, achievers, strivers, experiencers, makers, and strugglers. Figure 4–4 shows a breakdown of these profiles. These profiles define people based on their self-orientation and their resources. Resources are defined not just in financial terms, but refers to the full range of psychological, physical, demographic, and material means or capacities consumers have to draw upon. Resources include education, income, self-confidence, health, and eagerness to buy. Self-orientation can take three primary directions:

- *Principle-oriented.* These people are guided in their choices by their beliefs and principles rather than by feelings, events, or desires.
- *Status-oriented.* These individuals are heavily influenced by the actions, approval, and opinions of others.
- *Action-oriented.* These people desire social or physical activity, variety, and risk taking.

VALS2™ has proven especially useful for understanding consumer preferences in media, electronics, travel and lodging, recreational activities, automotive purchases, home furnishings, and clothing.

Exhibit 4–4 Sample AIO Statements

1. I enjoy exercising whenever I get the chance.
2. It is important to watch your caloric intake.
3. In recent years too much attention has been paid to cholesterol levels.
4. When I exercise daily I feel better.
5. Most of the stories on holistic medicine make me suspicious about the benefits.
6. I get nervous when my physician isn't fit.
7. I'm not sure exercising regularly really helps.
8. I like to read stories about nutrition and fitness.

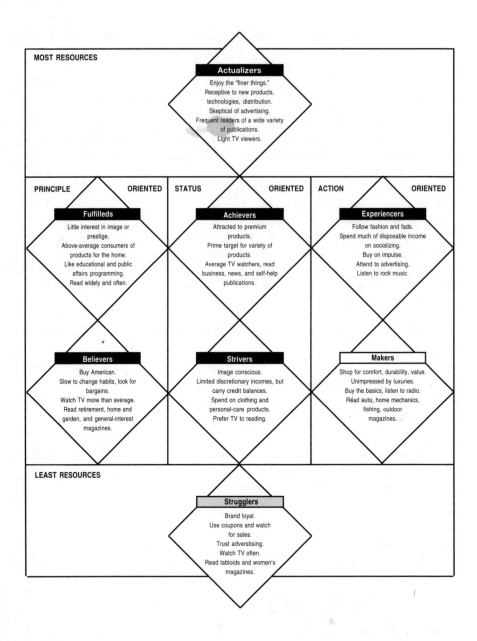

PRIZM

A similar lifestyle program called PRIZM (Potential Rating Index by Zip Market) is commercially marketed by Claritas PRIZM of New York, a marketing consulting firm. This program examines census data and consumer lifestyle by zip code to develop a geodemographic profile. The company has developed approximately 40 different lifestyle profiles of neighborhoods that can be applied to any zip code. A marketer can then target specific appeals to certain areas, and use more targeted media in each area. Unlike the VALS2™ approach, PRIZM is not based on attitudes. The foundation of PRIZM is demographics combined with consumption and media data. The PRIZM method is discussed in greater detail in Chapter 6 with a description of some neighborhood profiles.

Learning

Learning involves the changes in a person's behavior as a result of past experiences. Learning occurs as a result of a drive, stimulus, cues, responses, and reinforcement. The drive is a threat that motivates the individual. The stimulus is the object or factor that can reduce the drive. Related to stimuli are the cues, which are aspects calling attention to the stimuli. Response is the act of satisfying the drive. And finally, there is reinforcement, which is the reward.

Marketers can use learning theory as the foundation for a marketing plan to help the consumer enter the decision-making stage of problem recognition. A consumer has a drive or need for safety. The stimulus might be an advertisement touting the complete services and easy accessibility of Good Samaritan's integrated health care system. The cue might occur when a consumer drives by several facilities and sees the Good Samaritan name on the buildings. The response is the consumer's purchase of the Samaritan health plan, with appropriate reinforcement following in the form of satisfied use.

Learning theory also includes two other aspects that are useful in marketing. Learning facilitates generalizations among stimuli. *Generalizations* are the extensions of past reinforced behavior to other stimuli. A female patient who has had a positive experience in the birthing center of a hospital might generalize that positive level of care to other clinical programs in the same facility.

A second aspect of learning is referred to as *discrimination*, the ability to determine differences between stimuli. A consumer who has had an unsatisfactory experience during one inpatient stay might, from this past reinforcement, be able to discriminate better when having a similar experience (stimulus) with another provider.

Perception

A final psychological aspect affecting decision making is **perception**, the process by which individuals organize, select, and interpret information.[20] Consumers tend to change and reorganize information so that it is consistent with their past experiences and knowledge.

On any given day, consumers are exposed to a vast array of advertisements and messages. Not all of these messages are attended to or processed, because the perception process is selective. The process of selectivity can occur at several stages of the communication process.

Selective exposure is when the consumer only pays attention to a particular set of advertisements. As discussed earlier in terms of dissonance, an individual who recently selected a particular health plan may only pay attention to advertisements for that plan to help them reinforce their choice. *Selective comprehension* is the interpreting of information in a way that is consistent with past attitudes, beliefs, and knowledge. This aspect of perception is important for marketers to understand. A message sent by the advertiser may be perceived in a very different fashion by the intended audience. A hospital, for example, may decide to use an advertisement with humor as the primary appeal. To the intended audience, this message might imply that the hospital is not serious enough about the issue to have faith in this facility as a place for care. Later, in Chapter 11, pretesting will be discussed as one way to overcome or assess this potential problem.

A third aspect of selective perception is that of *selective retention*. Consumers only retain a fraction of the material to which they are exposed. In advertising, the recognition of selective retention has given rise to media strategies that use repetition to reinforce past advertisements. Selective retention is a concern for marketers as consumers move through the stages of internal and external search. An interesting dictum regarding the problem of selective retention, which remains as true today as it was when first published over 100 years ago, is shown in Exhibit 4–5.

Perceived Risk

Within the area of perception is the concept of *perceived risk*, which can be defined as the concerns or anxieties a consumer anticipates regarding a product or service purchase. Purchases represent risk.[21] Several types of perceived risks have been identified in marketing, which are relevant in the health care decision process. Financial, performance, and physical risks are obvious concerns. For certain services, such as mental health or sexual dysfunction clinics, there may also be perceived social risks. For the marketer of such services, strategies must be developed to reduce the perceived risk. A mental health clinic might underscore for patients that mental health is not a problem to hide; or in a different strategy, the clinic might stress its procedures for confidentiality.

Exhibit 4–5 Hints to Advertisers

The first time a man looks at an advertisement, he does not see it.
The second time he does not notice it.
The third time he is conscious of its existence.
The fourth time he faintly remembers having seen it before.
The fifth time he reads it.
The sixth time he turns up his nose at it.
The seventh time he reads it through and says, "Oh, bother!"
The eighth time he says, "Here's that confounded thing again!"
The ninth time he wonders if it amounts to anything.
The tenth time he thinks he will ask his neighbor if he has tried it.
The eleventh time he wonders how the advertiser makes it pay.
The twelfth time he thinks perhaps it may be worth something.
The thirteenth time he thinks it must be a good thing.
The fourteenth time he remembers he has wanted such a thing for a long time.
The fifteenth time he is tantalized because he cannot afford to buy it.
The sixteenth time he thinks he will buy it someday.
The seventeenth time he makes a memorandum of it.
The eighteenth time he swears at his poverty.
The nineteenth time he counts his money very carefully.
The twentieth time he sees it, he buys the article, or instructs his wife to do so.

Source: Thomas Smith, *Hints to Intending Advertisers*, London, 1885.

Behavioral researchers have found that there are certain characteristics that affect the degree to which a person reacts to perceived risk. A greater willingness to accept risk has been found among those who have higher self-confidence, higher self-esteem, lower anxiety and lower familiarity with the problem.[22]

SOCIOCULTURAL INFLUENCES ON DECISION MAKING

Sociocultural factors in addition to psychological influences can also affect consumer decision making. These sociocultural elements include family life cycle, social class, reference groups, and culture.

Family Life Cycle

Consumers' decision making and purchase behavior change over the course of their lives. The **family life cycle** describes the stages the typical consumer passes through from childhood through death of a spouse.[23] The stages of the traditional family life cycle are represented in Exhibit 4–6. In each stage, different conditions lead to a focus on different types of purchases.[24] For example, even though single individuals are represented in several stages (bachelor stage, empty nest I, solitary survivor, and retired) the focus of purchases varies dramatically. For marketers, consideration of just marital status would be too restrictive with regard to the implication for purchases.

Modified Life Cycle

The typical family structure of the past seems less and less applicable to today's market.[25] Many consumers remain single by choice throughout their entire lives, and growing numbers of married couples enter into divorce. The traditional life cycle depiction is becoming less relevant, a modernized view of the family life cycle, or *modified life cycle*, reflects these ever more common variations of the life cycle. In this revised version (as seen in Figure 4–5), singles are comprised of people who are single, separated, divorced, and widowed.[26]

Family Decision Making

Within the traditional family life cycle, historical decision-making patterns have emerged. Early in the formation of the family unit there is a tendency for a large amount of shared decision making as the household is established. Over time, however, *family decision making* has become specialized into either husband- or wife-dominant. Men have traditionally dominated decisions to purchase automobiles, life insurance, and investments. Women dominated decisions to buy appliances and home furnishings. In health care, women often were the primary decision makers regarding selecting the source of care. As the household structure changes, however, and women work outside the home in growing numbers, the traditional patterns of decision making are changing. As the woman's income rises relative to her spouse, her influence in decision making has also increased. For example, women have been found to now influence 80 percent of all new car purchases.[27] Regarding health care, the number of women in the work force has also affected the health care decision-making situation. In the past, the man often chose the health plan, since he was working outside the home in a setting that offered insurance. That is no longer the case. Increasingly, both spouses may be offered health plan options at their respective work sites.

There are also two other decision-making patterns that emerge in families. One involves *syncratic decisions* in which the husband and wife participate jointly. The other form includes *autonomous decisions*, those decisions of lesser importance that the husband or the wife decide independently.

Exhibit 4–6 The Traditional Family Life Cycle

Stage	Characteristics
1. Bachelor stage; young single people not living at home	Few financial burdens. Fashion opinion leaders. Recreation oriented. Buy: Basic kitchen equipment, basic furniture, cars, equipment for the mating game, vacations.
2. Newly married couples; young, no children	Better off financially than they will be in the near future. Highest purchase rate and highest average purchase of durables. Buy: Cars, refrigerators, stoves, sensible and durable furniture, vacations.
3. Full nest I; youngest child under six	Home purchasing at peak. Liquid assets low. Dissatisfied with financial position and amount of money saved. Interested in new products. Like advertised products. Buy: Washers, dryers, TV, baby food, chest rubs and cough medicine, vitamins, dolls, wagons, sleds, skates.
4. Full nest II; youngest child six or over six	Financial position better. Some wives work. Less influenced by advertising. Buy larger-sized packages, multiple-unit deals. Buy: Many foods, cleaning materials, bicycles, music lessons, pianos.
5. Full nest III; older married couples with dependent children	Financial position still better. More wives work. Some children get jobs. Hard to influence with advertising. High average purchase of durables. Buy: New, more tasteful furniture, auto travel, nonnecessary appliances, boats, dental services, magazines.
6. Empty nest I; older married couples, no children living with them, head in labor force	Home ownership at peak. Most satisfied with financial position and money saved. Interested in travel, recreation, self-education. Make gifts and contributions. Not interested in new products. Buy: Vacations, luxuries, home improvements.
7. Empty nest II; older married couples, no children living at home, head retired	Drastic cut in income. Keep home. Buy: Medical appliances, medical care, products which aid health, sleep, and digestion.
8. Solitary survivor, in labor force	Income still good but likely to sell home.
9. Solitary survivor, retired	Same medical and product needs as other retired group; drastic cut in income. Special need for attention, affection, and security.

Source: Reprinted from Wells, W.D., and Gubar, G., Life Cycle Concept in Marketing Research, *Journal of Marketing Research*, November 1962, p. 362, with permission of American Marketing Association, © 1962.

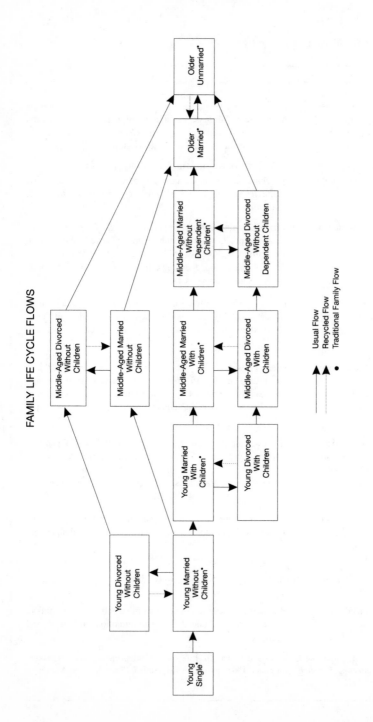

FAMILY LIFE CYCLE FLOWS

Figure 4–5 The Modernized Family Life Cycle. *Source:* Reprinted from Murphy, P.E., and Staples, W.A., A Modernized Family Life Cycle, *Journal of Consumer Research*, Vol. 6, No. 1, pp. 12–22, with permission of The University of Chicago Press, © 1979.

Social Class

A second sociocultural influence on consumer behavior is social class. **Social class** has been defined as relatively stable and homogeneous divisions in society in which individuals, families, or groups share relatively similar interests, values, lifestyles, and behaviors. A combination of factors determine whether an individual belongs to one social class vs. another. Income, education level, source of net worth, and type of housing are but a few of these factors. Exhibit 4–7 shows one such topology of social class.

This listing summarizes the characteristics of seven social classes in the United States. Although there are many differences within social classes, there is far greater variation between social classes in terms of behaviors and lifestyles. The percentages represented for each social class are approximations of their distribution in society. To marketers, the issue of social class is valuable in that it shows that more than income relates to a consumer's lifestyle or behavior.[28] People of lower social class tend to shop closer to home. In terms of the consumer behavior

---

Exhibit 4–7 Social Class Distinctions

<u>Upper Americans</u>
Upper-Upper (0.3%)—The "capital S society" world of inherited wealth, aristocratic names

Lower-Upper (1.2%)—The newer social elite, drawn from current professional, corporate leadership

Upper-Middle (12.5%)—The rest of college graduate managers and professionals; lifestyle centers on private clubs, causes, and the arts

<u>Middle Americans</u>
Middle Class (32%)—Average pay white–collar workers and their blue–collar friends; live on "the better side of town," try to "do the proper things"

Working Class (38%)—Average pay blue–collar workers; lead "working class lifestyle" whatever the income, school background, and job

<u>Lower Americans</u>
"A lower group of people but not the lowest" (9%)—Working, not on welfare; living standard is just above poverty; behavior judged "crude," "trashy"

"Real Lower-Lower" (7%)—On welfare, visibly poverty-stricken, usually out of work (or have "the dirtiest jobs"); "bums," "common criminals"

Source: Reprinted from Coleman, R.P., The Continuing Significance of Social Class, *Journal of Consumer Research*, Vol. 10, No. 3 pp. 265–280, with permission of the University of Chicago Press, © 1983.

model described initially, lower social class members engage less often in external search of information prior to purchase.

Reference Group

Social class is significant to marketers in that other members of a social class often serve as a consumer's reference group. A **reference group** is one that influences an individual's thoughts or behaviors.[29] There are three forms of a reference group. The reference group to which one belongs is considered the *membership reference group*. The reference group to which one does not wish to belong is considered the *dissociative reference group*. Finally, the reference group to which one aspires to belong is referred to as the *aspirational reference group*. From a promotional strategy perspective, it's important to understand the differing types of reference groups. Showing images of dissociative reference groups to a target market would destroy the value of a promotional campaign.

Reference group influence is most significant when use of the product or service is visible to the group.[30] Products such as designer clothing, cars, or brands of sneakers such as Nike or Reebok are greatly affected by the reference group. Reference group influence also tends to be higher the less necessary a product is. The more commitment a person feels to belonging to a particular group, the greater the influence of that group. The more relevant the particular purchase or behavior is to the functioning of the group, the more pressure or influence is exerted by the reference group. Reference group influence is also strong, the less confidence the individual has in his decision. The example of choosing a health care plan highlights what is often a difficult issue for many consumers. In this case, coworkers also involved in the same decision making may play a major influencing role in the ultimate plan selection.[31]

Declining Middle Class

A major concern within the United States has been the growing evidence of the disappearance of the middle class. Figure 4–6 shows this perspective of the middle class as defined by income. The percentage of people who are considered affluent or working class has grown dramatically from 1950 to 1992. Today, 40 percent of that working class exists below the poverty level. For marketing, and potentially for health care marketers, this shift in population class is having a dramatic effect on buying. In recent years, many major brands that once appealed to the middle class (as shown in Table 4–2) have significantly lost their presence and share in the marketplace. The major growth has occurred at either the low end or the high end. So too, for medical organizations, this shift to the extremes in terms of social class may raise similar questions about the group to whom the organization is positioned.

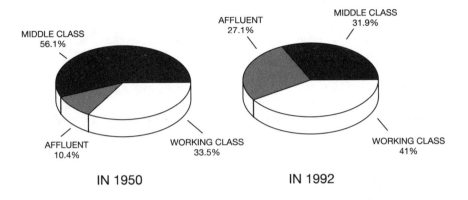

Figure 4–6 Declining Middle Class. *Source:* Statistical Abstract of the United States, 1994 (Washington, D.C.: U.S. Department of Commerce, 114th Edition), p. 465; Statistical Abstract of the United States, 1950 (Washington, D.C.: U.S. Department of Commerce, (71st edition), p. 271.

Culture

Culture, as defined in an earlier chapter, refers to the values, attitudes, and ideas that are transmitted from one generation to another within a group of homogeneous individuals. These values, such as achievement or success, might well influence decision making. American society places a strong value of success in work. Many products and advertisements are directed at ways of demonstrating the fulfillment of this cultural value.

In the United States there has been a growing recognition of subcultures and their different purchasing behaviors, values, and attitudes that affect their decision making. As marketers become more skilled in the management of data bases, they will be able to target particular subcultures more effectively through use of micro marketing strategies. Ads, products, and communication strategies can all be tailored to reflect different subcultural norms.

Table 4–2 Disappearing Middle Brand

Lower End	Middle Brand	Premium
Hyundai	Chevrolet	Lexus
Wal-Mart	Sears	Nordstrom's
Days Inn	Holiday Inn	Four Seasons

Hispanic Subculture

One of the fastest-growing subcultures in the United States is among Hispanics, people of Latin American origin. Predominant in states in the northeast, southeast, and far west regions of the United States, Hispanics will represent significant proportions of the population in many major metropolitan areas. Many distinct media have been established to target this group. It is essential to recognize the differences in certain subcultures. For example, within some segments of the Hispanic population, gynecological examinations are considered only for the promiscuous.[32]

African-American Subculture

Presently 11 percent of the population in the United States is African-American. The income levels of this group on average have been below the average for Caucasians and Hispanics (as was shown in Figure 3–3). Another factor that this group has had to overcome has been historic problems of racism and segregation and their impact on the education of successive generations. Marketers are increasingly recognizing the growing influence and buying power of this particular subculture as historic boundaries and limitations have been removed.

INDUSTRIAL BUYER BEHAVIOR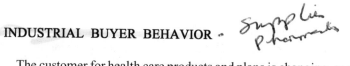

The customer for health care products and plans is changing, as witnessed in the 1990s during the national debate about health care reform. Historically, a health care organization considered its customers to be physicians and patients. With the burgeoning growth of managed care in the United States beginning in the late 1970s, many health care organizations and providers now face a more formidable and complex customer—employers. Employers represent all types of businesses, from a large company that purchases health care for its employees through an occupational medicine program, to an HMO that contracts for inpatient services, to a nursing home that might purchase the services of a physician to monitor the health status of its residents.

In the 1990s, especially, small companies have banded together to form group purchasing coalitions whose purpose is to buy health care coverage for their members at affordable prices. In Detroit, Michigan a purchasing organization has formed between MUST (Management and Unions Serving Together) and the AFL-CIO of metropolitan Detroit. This buying entity negotiates on behalf of union locals representing 125,000 covered lives. Similar coalitions have been established such as the one in Kansas City, Missouri, with 56 companies belonging to the Mid-America Coalition of Health Care.[33]

In any case, marketing to large corporations, small companies, and other business organizations requires an understanding of organizational buyer behavior and how it differs from the individual consumer behavior described earlier. Understanding these differences fosters the development of a more effective marketing strategy relative to the four Ps of the marketing mix.

Organizational Differences

Organizations differ from consumers in terms of the buying process along several distinct characteristics.

Number of Organizations

Compared to consumers, the industrial, or organizational, market is smaller. While a hospital serves hundreds of thousands of consumers in any given year, that same hospital may only deal with two or three managed health care plans in its respective market.

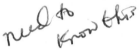

Demand Variations

A second major aspect of organizational buying is the variation in demand. One aspect of industrial demand, referred to as **derived demand**, is the demand for one product or service (such as the managed health care plan) that is derived from the demand for another service or product (consumer need for health care services). In marketing to organizations, providers need to understand who the organization's customers are.[34] To market effectively to a managed care plan, a medical group should know what services the managed care plan's subscribers expect to receive from a medical group that they would select for care.

Another dimension of industrial demand is the tendency to be price inelastic. Demand is considered price inelastic when price cuts or price hikes have little effect on total level of demand. Since industrial demand is derived demand, there is less opportunity for health care organizations to influence or stimulate primary demand in the industrial market than there is in the consumer market.

If the price of Tylenol drops, it is unlikely that a hospital, for example, would order a significantly larger amount of the product. If the price reduction is short-term, there may be some loading up on inventory, but only to a point, since Tylenol does not account for a significant proportion of the cost of treating a particular patient. Similarly, the price of Tylenol would have to rise substantially before a hospital might decide to shift to another product. In this example, the demand is price inelastic. Among individual consumers, demand would probably be far more elastic. A coupon offering a 50 percent price reduction on a large bottle of Tylenol would, no doubt, stimulate significant demand. On the other hand, a doubling of the Tylenol's price would likely lead to a dramatic reduction in demand.

Greater Total Sales Volume

Another characteristic of organizational buying is that its total sales volume is greater than that of the consumer market. For example, a consumer purchase of a particular pharmaceutical product represents the sale of one unit sold in the retail market. That sale on the industrial side represents multiple sales from the purchase of raw materials and other goods to support the production of the product.

Geographical Concentration

Industrial markets are often characterized by greater geographical concentration than consumer markets. In the Cincinnati metropolitan area, for example, CIGNA Companies, a national insurance company headquartered in Bloomfield, Connecticut, can market to a half-dozen hospitals within a five-to-ten-mile radius of the downtown area. Many consumers in the Cincinnati metropolitan area, however, actually reside beyond the state of Ohio in neighboring Kentucky.

Professional Buying

Organizations differ from consumers in that their buying function is usually a structured, formal decision-making process. Many large companies, for example, have purchasing departments that institutionalize the buying process. Other businesses or organizations have a contract negotiation department to deal with the "buying" of health care services from providers or facilities.

Often in these settings, individual providers are judged by defined, well-established buying criteria. To a large degree, these buying characteristics are similar to the evaluative criteria used by consumers in the alternative evaluation stage of the decision process.

Buying Center

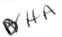

The major difference between the industrial vs. consumer market is the **buying center**, a group of people involved in the decision to purchase a product or service. The buying center allows for many perspectives and broad expertise to be brought to bear on the purchase. For a company selecting a health care plan, the buying center might be comprised of the firm's medical director, financial officer, human resources director, union representative, and possibly, the employee assistance representative.

The buying center makes organizational marketing more complex for the organization offering a service. The firm making a presentation to a buying center has to deal with many views and must gauge the relative influence each party has in the buying process. To market effectively to the buying center, four questions must be answered:

1. Which individuals in the buying center are responsible for our particular product or service?
2. What is the relative influence of each member of this group?
3. What are each member's decision criteria?
4. How does each member of the group perceive our firm, our products, and our salespeople?[35]

Negotiation Variations

Industrial buying also differs from consumer buying in terms of two aspects of the negotiation process, frequency and complexity. Organizational purchases are made less frequently than consumer purchases. A consumer buys primary care medical services several times during the year. A managed care plan, however, most likely will negotiate a contract with a medical group annually. Marketing to organizations, then, requires a detailed knowledge of the timing of their purchase cycle.

Organizational buying is also more complex than consumer purchasing—many details of a contract must be negotiated before agreement is reached. A manufacturer, for example, might negotiate with an occupational medicine clinic regarding the services to be performed on site, the handling of workers' compensation claims, and the contract's payment terms.

With the growing emphasis on managed care, health care organizations are now sharing risk with vendors. In risk-sharing arrangements, the supplier will receive greater reward if the buyer meets their objectives. In health care, risk sharing is increasing between suppliers and buyers and between providers and buyers. For example, Group Health of Puget Sound in Seattle, Washington is a large HMO. In persuing their goal to control the cost of care, Group Health signed a capitated agreement with Owens and Minor, a large distributor of hospital and physician supplies and equipment. Group Health pays the supplier a set fee per subscriber per month for medical-surgical products. The more products Group Health uses, the less Owens makes. The supplier now tries to ensure proper training and inventory control as both the buyer and supplier now have the same incentive.[36]

Vendor Solicitation

An additional difference between consumer and industrial behavior relates to the solicitation of vendors. When a business organization identifies a need for a product or service, it solicits vendors to submit bids or make presentations for supplying the product or service. When individual customers identify a need, they actively identify solutions to address the need.

Close Buyer-Seller Relationships

With most consumer purchases, the seller rarely develops a significant relationship with the individual. Industrial buying is just the opposite. Since there are fewer customers and the negotiations are often complex, the vendor develops a detailed knowledge of the customer.

The Industrial Buying Process

Similar to consumer behavior, industrial buying can be divided into three basic types of purchasing situations: new task, modified rebuy, and straight rebuy.[37]

New Task Buying

In the new task buying situation, organizations face a new situation in which a purchase is required. In this buying situation, a company gathers information from various vendors who can meet the need. This situation is like an extended problem-solving scenario for the consumer and is often very time-consuming.[38] Employers are often approaching health care as a new task buying problem, and so need to collect quantifiable information. In Cincinnati, four companies (Kroger, Cincinnati Bell, GE Aircraft Engines, and Proctor and Gamble) have asked 14 hospitals to collaborate on patient outcomes measurement. The companies hired Iameter, Inc. to collect and analyze hospital data to provide severity-adjusted outcome information.[39]

Modified Rebuy

In the modified rebuy situation, the buyer seeks to modify or alter the purchase. Changes can be made to the price or to product specifications. A company might reopen negotiations with an insurance company, asking it to provide a managed care plan in addition to the indemnity product offered to employees. In the modified rebuy scenario, the existing vendor protects against losing the customer.

Straight Rebuy

Straight rebuy involves making repeated purchases of a product that has generated a positive experience and good past evaluations. Straight rebuy decisions are usually programmed purchases that involve little complexity. Basic industrial supplies are often purchased in a straight rebuy mode. A medical group might purchase checks or office supplies through a straight rebuy sequence. Straight rebuys rarely involve buying centers and usually do not require negotiation for the purchase.

The Buying Center

The buying center was identified as a major difference between industrial and consumer buying behavior. As described earlier, there are many participants in the buying center and these participants can assume one of several roles within it.[40]

Users. These are the people who will use the product. They may include an individual such as an employee representative, who provides the user perspective regarding the particular health plan, judging it for convenience and patient responsiveness.

Influencers. Influencers are individuals both inside and outside the organization who affect the final decision. The chief financial officer in a hospital is often a major influencer, regarding the specific financial details of managed care contracts that are signed. A company might hire a benefits consultant to review alternative health insurance products.

Gatekeepers. Gatekeepers are the individuals who control the flow of information into the buying organization. Many pharmaceutical companies must develop strategies for dealing with the physician's gatekeeper, who is often the secretary.

Deciders. This is the person who has the authority to make the final choice between vendors. The management level at which decision authority rests depends on the cost of the purchase or the risk to the organization. In most hospitals, the director of purchasing would be considered the decider for a capital equipment purchase such as a wheel chair. Yet, in the use of infusion pump equipment, the decider would more likely be a clinician involved in the treatment regimen using this specialized equipment.

Buyers. Those responsible for dealing directly with the suppliers are the buyers, often called purchasing agents. Purchasing agents often are solely responsible for managing straight rebuy situations, without consulting with the buying center.

CONCLUSIONS

Understanding how the customer behaves is at the core of effective marketing strategy. Consumer decision making involves a series of steps and is affected by a variety of internal and external factors. Industrial buying behavior is a formal process in which the decision-maker role is complicated by the type of purchase and composition of the buying center. As health care rapidly moves to a managed care environment, this aspect of decision making will require greater understanding in order to develop effective marketing strategy.

KEY TERMS

Consumer Decision-Making Process	Lifestyle
Evaluative Criteria	Learning
Involvement	Perception
Routine Decision Making	Family Life Cycle
Brand Loyalty	Social Class
Complex Decision Making	Reference Group
Limited Decision Making	Derived Demand
Motivation	Buying Center
Attitudes	

CHAPTER SUMMARY

1. Buyer behavior that results in purchase is a multistage process involving problem recognition, search, evaluation, purchase, and post-purchase evaluation.

2. Post-purchase evaluation is a critical component of buyer behavior. Organizations should assess whether customer expectations are confirmed or disconfirmed by their interactions with the service or use of the product.

3. Consumer decision making depends to a large degree on the amount of consumer involvement in the purchase. The level of involvement is related to the degree of risk and the extent of search behavior.

4. The consumer decision-making process is affected by several influences: motivation, attitudes, lifestyles, learning, and perception.

5. Perception is an important aspect of buyer behavior and must be considered in marketing strategy. Perception affects what people see, understand, and retain.

6. Individual behavior is related to the stage a person is in his or her life cycle. As the composition of the typical family has changed, so have the traditional stages of the life cycle been modified.

7. Within the United States, there are several distinct social classes, each of which reflects norms of behavior, attitudes, and values.

8. Culture is recognized as the transmission of attitudes, values, and norms from one generation to the next. Within the United States there is the growing emergence of several distinct subcultures that influence buying behavior.

9. *Organizational buying behavior is characterized by, among other things, the number of companies, demand variations, sales volume, professionalism of the buyer, and geographic concentration.*

10. *A major defining characteristic of organizational buying behavior is the buying center, which involves many individuals at different levels and positions within the firm.*

11. *There are three variations of industrial buying: new task, modified rebuy, and straight rebuy.*

CHAPTER PROBLEMS

1. For several years, Annie Brouck's employer has offered a traditional indemnity plan for health care coverage for herself, her husband Jim, and their children, Tess and Tasha. Recently, the cost of the monthly premium for this insurance coverage increased dramatically. Annie's employer has decided to offer an HMO in addition to this traditional insurance plan. Describe the steps Annie might follow in deciding whether to choose this plan.

2. In recent years, there has been a growing attempt to measure the performance of health care providers. The federal government has published morbidity statistics. Other organizations, such as the California Cooperative–HEDIS Reporting Initiative (shown in Exhibit 4–1), show information on the performance of HMOs in preventive care as further information for consumers to consider. Explain how these data may affect the consumer decision-making process.

3. In terms of decision-making sequences, how would you explain and describe: (a) the 25-year-old, healthy worker who sees the same physician for minor medical needs; (b) the retired individual who calls the state medical society and seeks a second opinion prior to open-heart surgery; and (c) the consumer who sees a new brand of headache remedy on the shelf and decides to try it?

4. On what level of Maslow's Hierarchy of Needs would you place each of the following decisions: (a) buying health insurance, (b) going skiing, (c) following a low-fat diet?

5. The Select Care HMO has decided to offer the first managed care product in a small community of 25,000 people in West Virginia. Prepaid health care is a concept that is new to this region. In conducting a consumer survey prior to the introduction of the plan, Select Care finds that attitudes toward HMOs are very negative. Some people believe they will be denied care if they join an HMO, while others feel this form of health care delivery is a socialistic approach to medicine. What options are open to Select Care in trying to change these attitudes?

6. The United States is experiencing a decline of the middle class. What does this trend imply for the future of organizations such as: (a) the U.S. Public Health Service, which operates many inner-city health clinics for the economically disadvantaged, and (b) the Scripps Clinic, a large multispecialty group practice in southern California? For years, the Scripps Clinic was seen as an exclusive medical provider known not only for treatment but for its research.

7. A medical group has decided to develop an industrial medicine program for employers. This program would help in the treatment of on-the-job injuries, workers' compensation requirements, health education, and toxicology analysis. The group has hired a new salesperson to approach a major furniture manufacturer in the community about the program. In preparing for her first call, the salesperson makes a list of the possible members of the buying center. Prepare the list.

NOTES

1. A description of this model was developed extensively in J.F. Engel, R.D. Blackwell, and P.W. Miniard, *Consumer Behavior*, 7th ed. (New York, N.Y.: The Dryden Press, 1993).

2. J.F. Engel, R.D. Blackwell, and P. Miniard, *Consumer Behavior*, 7th ed. (New York, N.Y.: The Dryden Press, 1993).

3. For external search approaches, see J.E. Urban, P. Dickson, and W.L. Wilkie, Buyer Uncertainty and Information Search, *Journal of Consumer Research* 16, no. 2 (1989):208–215.

4. See S.E. Beatty and S.M. Smith, External Search Effort: An Investigation Across Several Product Categories, *Journal of Consumer Research* 14, no. 1 (1987):83–95.

5. J.D. Johnson and H. Meischke, Cancer Information: Women's Source and Content Preferences, *Journal of Health Care Marketing* 11, no. 1 (1991):37–44.

6. Consumer Magazine Rates St. Louis Area Health Care, *Business & Health* 12, no.1 (1994):10.

7. A useful discussion of evoked set formation is found in J.E. Brisoux and M. Laroche, Evoked Set Formation and Composition: An Empirical Investigation under Routinized Response Behavior Situation, in *Advances in Consumer Research*, Vol. 8, ed. K.B. Monroe (Ann Arbor, Mich.: Association for Consumer Research, 1981), 357–361.

8. J.A. Howard, *Consumer Behavior in Marketing Strategy* (Englewood Cliffs, N.J.: Prentice Hall, 1989), 176–177.

9. M. Fishbein, An Investigation of the Relationships between Beliefs about an Object and the Attitude toward That Object, *Human Relations* 16, no. 3 (1963):233–240.

10. For additional discussion of past-purchase behavior and feelings, see M.C. Gilly and B.D. Gelb, Post Purchase Consumer Process and the Complaining Consumer, *Journal of Consumer Research* 9, no. 3 (1982):323–328.

11. CA Hospitals Boost Referrals with Outside Program, *Physician Relations Advisor* 3, no. 3 (1994):42–43.

12. L. Festinger, *A Theory of Cognitive Dissonance* (Stanford, Calif.: Stanford University Press, 1957), 260.

13. C. Costley, Meta Analysis of Involvement Research, in *Advances in Consumer Research*, Vol.15, ed. M. Houston (Provo, Utah: Association for Consumer Research, 1988), 554–562.

14. A.H. Maslow, *Motivation and Personality* (New York, N.Y.: Harper, 1954), 80–106.

15. D. Krech, R.S. Crutchfield, and E.L. Ballachey, *Individual and Society* (New York, N.Y.: McGraw-Hill Publishing Co., 1962).

16. R. Lutz, Changing Brand Attitudes Through Modification of Cognitive Structure, *Journal of Consumer Research* 1, no. 4 (1975):49–59.

17. H. Assael, *Consumer Behavior and Marketing Action*, 3rd ed. (Boston, Mass.: Kent Publishing, 1990), 275.

18. See J.T. Plummer, The Concept and Application of Lifestyle Segmentation, *Journal of Marketing* 38, no. 1 (1974):33–37.

19. For further explanation and detail on VALS, see *The VALS2™ Segmentation System* (Menlo Park, Calif.: SRI International, 1989).

20. For a review of the consumer perception process and marketing implications, see J.R. Bettman, *An Information Theory of Consumer Choice* (Reading, Mass.: Addison-Wesley Publishing Co., Inc., 1979).

21. J. Taylor, The Role of Risk in Consumer Behavior, *Journal of Marketing* 38, no. 2 (1974): 54–60.

22. J.C. Mowen, *Consumer Behavior* (New York, N.Y.: Macmillan Publishing Co., Inc., 1993).

23. W.D. Wells and G. Gubar, Life Cycle Concept in Marketing Research, *Journal of Marketing Research* 3, no. 4 (1966):355–363.

24. J. Wagner and S. Hanna, The Effectiveness of Family Life Cycle Variables in Consumer Expenditure Research, *Journal of Consumer Research* 10, no. 3 (1983):281–291.

25. P.E. Murphy and W.A. Staples, A Modernized Family Life Cycle, *Journal of Consumer Research* 6, no. 1 (1979):12–22.

26. *Ibid.*, 17.

27. For a discussion of the purchasing roles of husbands and wives, see S.C. Bennett and E.W. Stuart, In Search of Association Between Personal Values and Household Decision Processes: An Exploratory Analysis, in *AMA Educators Conference Proceedings* (Chicago, Ill.: American Marketing Association, 1989), 259–264; and E.W. Stuart and S.C. Bennett, Perception of Marital Roles in Decision Processes: A 1980s Update, in *AMA Educators Conference Proceedings* (Chicago, Ill.: American Marketing Association, 1988), 77.

28. R.P. Coleman, The Continuing Significance of Social Class, *Journal of Consumer Research* 10, no. 3 (1983):183–194.

29. D. Brinberg and L. Plimpton, Self Monitoring and Product Conspicuousness on Reference Group Influence, in *Advances in Consumer Research*, Vol.13, ed. R. Lutz (Provo, Utah: Association for Consumer Research, 1986), 297–300; and W.O. Bearden and M.J. Etzel, Reference Group Influence on Product and Brand Choice, *Journal of Consumer Research* 9, no. 2 (1982):183–194.

30. Bearden and Etzel, Reference Group Influence, 183–194.

31. *Ibid.*, 188–192.

32. M.C. Jaklevic, Programs and Compaigns Reach Out to Members of Ethnic Communities, *Modern Healthcare* 24, no. 1 (1994):32.

33. D. Wise, Detroit Sponsors Group Buying Effort, *Business & Health* 13, no. 1 (1995):47–50.

34. W.S. Bishop, J.L. Graham, and M.H. Jones, Volatility of Derived Demand in Industrial Markets and Its Management Implications, *Journal of Marketing* 50, no. 1 (Fall 1984):95–103.

35. T. Bonoma, Major Sales: Who Really Does the Buying? *Harvard Business Review* 60, no. 3 (1982):111–119.

36. L. Scott, Hospitals Feel Vendors' Cost Cuts, *Modern Healthcare* 24, no. 46 (1994):62.

37. P.J. Robinson, C.W. Farris, and Y. Wind, *Industrial Buying and Creative Marketing* (Newton, Mass.: Allyn & Bacon, Inc., 1967).

38. P. Doyle, A.G. Woodside, and P. Mitchell, Organizational Buying Behavior in New Task and Rebuy Situations, *Industrial Marketing Management* 8, no. 2 (1979):7–11.

39. F. Cerne, Cincinnati: Major Employers Call the Shots on Health Care Delivery, *Hospitals and Health Networks* 67, no. 24 (1993):44–45.

40. F. Webster, Jr., and Y. Wind, *Organizational Buying Behavior* (Englewood Cliffs, N.J.: Prentice Hall, 1972).

5

MARKETING RESEARCH

LEARNING OBJECTIVES

After reading this chapter you should be able to:

- Understand the nature of the marketing research process

- Know the difference between primary and secondary data

- Recognize the range of alternative sampling methodologies

- Understand the value of alternative data collection methodologies

- Appreciate the necessity of a marketing information system

THE MARKETING RESEARCH PROCESS

Marketing research is a multistep process that involves the systematic gathering of consumer information, or data, that will help an organization identify specific issues of concern to consumers. Organizations use these data to design marketing strategies that will address consumer needs. Conducting marketing research involves a five-stage process, which is displayed in Figure 5–1. Following these five steps will ensure that the data finally collected will help in managerial decision making. The five steps to marketing research include: (1) problem recognition, (2) identification of research objectives, (3) research design, (4) data collection, and (5) analysis and evaluation of results.

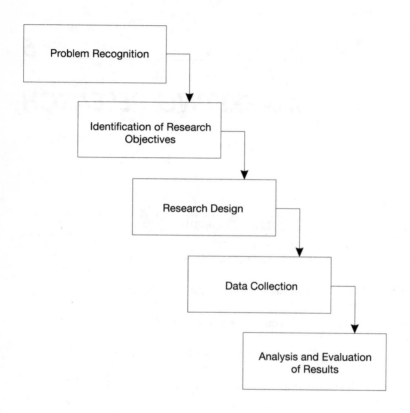

Figure 5–1 The Key Steps to Marketing Research

PROBLEM RECOGNITION

The first stage of the marketing research process, problem recognition, involves the definition of the problem. In order to collect the appropriate information to answer an organization's question, a clear definition of what should be researched is important. Clearly specified, problem definition leads to better articulation of the research objectives.

An HMO, for example, might find that acceptance of its plan among corporate health benefit officers is less than expected. Now, the problem might be defined as one of understanding the competitive position of this plan when compared to competing HMOs. A second way to define this problem might be to understand health benefit officers' attitudes toward prepaid health care plans. Or, a third definition of the problem might be to assess the image of this particular HMO among corporate health benefit officers. In each instance, the type of information and possibly the methodology used to collect the data might vary.

Because the problem recognition stage is critical to the resultant research process, all important members of the organization should be included in this phase of the research. Involvement of both management and clinical personnel is essential to obtain an accurate assessment of the problem definition.

IDENTIFICATION OF RESEARCH OBJECTIVES

Determining the research objectives is the second stage of the market research process. Research objectives can take one of four forms. One common research objective is exploratory, when an organization needs to determine the cause of the problem. For example, an HMO might conduct exploratory research to determine what is causing membership attrition. A second common research objective is descriptive. These marketing research efforts attempt to identify new issues or markets. For example, a study might be conducted to describe the needs of referral physicians in dealing with a physician relations department at an academic medical center. A third common objective of marketing research is to test hypotheses. A marketing director at a hospital, for example, might want to determine what impact doubling the advertising budget for a women's mammography screening program will have on demand for appointments. A final research objective is predictive, in which an organization tries to forecast demand for a service. A study might be conducted to predict the demand for an occupational medicine program in which routine lab work is performed at the company site.

It is important to recognize that the individuals involved in problem definition and in the subsequent stage of specifying the research objectives are often different from those individuals who actually conduct the research. Those involved in the first two stages of the research are the people affected by the issue. Implementation of the actual research process is usually done by marketing research staff or by outside organizations skilled in the methodology of market research.

RESEARCH DESIGN

After the research objectives have been specified, it is necessary to create the research design. This step is of critical importance. The research design is the plan for the entire study. This plan will specify the data needed, and the methods that will be used to collect them and to analyze and interpret the results. The data needs could consist of either primary data or secondary data.

Primary Data

Primary data are information collected to address a specific research question. There are many alternative methods that are used to acquire primary data. These methods consist of qualitative and quantitative data-gathering forms. Qualitative information is information that is not quantified. Quantitative data consist of empirical information. To collect either form of data, companies can either observe individuals or ask individuals questions. There are many alternative methods that must be decided upon in conducting marketing research. A number of these will be discussed later in this chapter.

The major advantage of primary data is that the information is collected for the particular problem or issue under investigation, which usually means that the data are current. Another major advantage is that primary data collection allows the organization to maintain confidentiality about the problem and the resulting information collected. Primary data, however, have some disadvantages. The collection of primary data can entail significant cost, and can require an extended period of time to accomplish.

Secondary Data

Secondary data are data that were collected previously for another purpose.[1] These data could be collected either within the organization or by outside agencies. A hospital might collect patient information for admissions and then use this information to help develop a profile of who is using the facility. While not originally collected for other purposes, admissions information can be a useful source of secondary data to address other questions that the organization might have.

Useful secondary data are collected by the federal and state governments, as well as by many commercial organizations. Exhibit 5–1 lists various types of secondary data. The *Statistical Abstract of the United States* publishes information such as fertility rates, births, and marital status on various segments of the population. Much of these data, for example, might be incorporated into the planning for a women's health program.

There are many commercial firms that provide valuable secondary data sources, including one such as Urban Decision Systems, Inc., which offers a useful way to examine a variety of census data.[2] This company can provide both a historical and a forecasted census analysis to a hospital that is considering opening a clinic in a particular location. This analysis can be done on a variety of parameters, including a one-mile and two-mile radius around the intended location. Table 5–1 provides a sample analysis of a proposed clinic site. As the data in this table indicate, a significant decline in the number of households with an income level between

Exhibit 5–1 Selected Secondary Data

Statistical Abstract of the United States
U.S. Bureau of Census, Department of Commerce, Washington, D.C. 20230

This guide provides a general overview of statistics collected by the federal government and other public and private organizations. Some of the topics covered include geography and environment, labor force, communications, population, employment and earnings, business enterprises, vital statistics, transportation, energy, manufacturers, foreign commerce and aid, standard metro-area statistics, and more.

Social Indicators
Government Printing Office, Washington, D.C. 20402

Triennial. Charts and tables on population; the family; housing; social security and welfare; health and nutrition; public safety; education and training; work, income, wealth, and expenses; culture, leisure, and the use of time; social mobility; and participation. International data are provided for comparison. Extensive technical notes accompany each section. Includes references for further reading and a subject index.

Standard & Poor's Industry Surveys
Standard & Poor Corp., New York, N.Y.

Separate pamphlets for 33 industries, updated quarterly and annually. This is a valuable source for basic data on 33 industries, with financial comparisons of the leading companies in each industry. For each industry there is a "Basic Analysis" (about 40 pages) revised annually, and a short "Current Analysis" (about eight pages) published three times per year. Received with this is a four-page monthly on "Trends and Projections," which includes tables of economic and industry indicators, and a monthly "Earnings Supplement," giving concise, up-to-date revenue, income, and profitability data on more than 100 leading companies in 33 major industries.

Standard Rate & Data Service
Skokie, Ill.

SRDS publications (11 for the U.S. and eight to cover foreign countries) give data on advertising rates, specifications and circulation for individual magazines, newspapers, and other media.

The U.S. services are for business publications (monthly); community publications (semiannual); consumer magazines and farm publications (monthly); co-op source directory (semiannual); direct-mail lists (quarterly); newspapers (monthly) and newspaper circulation analysis; print media production (quarterly); spot radio (monthly); spot radio small markets (semiannual); and spot television (monthly). The international editions include all media in one volume and are in the language of the country. There are monthlies for Canada and Britain; bimonthlies for Italy and West Germany; quarterlies for France and Mexico; and semiannuals for Austria and Switzerland.

Three of the monthlies—the ones for newspapers, spot radio, and spot television—contain useful market estimates. At the beginning of each state's section are estimates by county, city, and metropolitan statistical area (MSA), for population, households, consumer spendable income (by income categories), total and per household retail sales, retail sales for seven store

continues

Exhibit 5–1 continued

groups, passenger car registration, farm population, and gross farm income. The "Market Data Summary" at the front shows rankings of these various statistics and areas of dominant influence; also population by age and sex.

Handbook of Labor Statistics
U.S. Bureau of Labor Statistics, Washington, D.C.

Annual. The best one-volume source for U.S. labor statistics, ranging 10 to 20 years; essentially the same statistics as can be found currently in the *Monthly Labor Review.* For complete historical data see its *Handbook of Labor Statistics, 1975: Reference Edition,* issued as *BLS Bulletin 1865.* The Bureau of Labor Statistics publishes many other statistical bulletins on specific topics. For a subject list of Department of Labor Publications see *Publications of the U.S. Department of Labor: Subject Listing.*

Statistics of Income
U.S. Internal Revenue Service, Washington, D.C.

Annual. This series is actually published as several separate annuals, the most important of which are: (1) *Corporation Income Tax Returns,* which covers balance sheet and income statement statistics for corporations, and includes statistics for corporations, ranked by major industry and by size of total assets; (2) annual statistics in *Partnership Returns* and *Sole Proprietorship Returns;* (3) *Individual Income Tax Returns.* These are usually published first as short preliminary reports, and then as detailed final reports. Unfortunately, the statistics are often several years old. The 1991 information was first available in 1995.

$40,000 and $49,000 (from 13.6% in 1989 to 9.3% in 1994) was projected at this proposed clinic site. Yet, a significant increase is projected in the $60,000-$74,999 income group. This shift in income might suggest the need to develop a clinic that provides services more tailored to an upscale consumer.

In health care a growing amount of syndicated secondary market research is becoming available. **Syndicated marketing research** is commercial secondary data that regularly provides information on a particular question or problem area. These data provide benchmark information to hospital managers. The major limitation to syndicated information is that these same data can be purchased by competitors in the identical market.

There are several syndicated marketing research databases available. National Research Corporation (NRC) *Healthcare Market Guide* is based on an annual survey of 100,000 households in the top 100 markets in the United States. Individual reports are provided to a variety of purchasers including any hospital or clinic within the top 100 markets. National, state, and regional summaries are also part of the report.

The *Healthcare Market Guide* provides a review of several syndicated secondary research bases available to health care marketers.

Table 5–1 Establishing a Satellite Clinic: Sample Census Data

INCOME: 1980-89-94   URBAN DECISION SYSTEMS, INC.
MINNEAPOLIS, MN: LYNDALE AV & 53RD ST   10/26/89
1.0 MILE RING

	1980 Census		*1989 Est.*		*1994 Proj.*	
POPULATION	21,646		19,991		19,175	
In Group Quarters	304		346		359	
PER CAPITA INCOME	$10,570		$19,360		$24,078	
AGGREGATE INCOME ($ MIL)	228.8		387.0		461.7	
HOUSEHOLDS	8,214	%	8,364	%	8,358	%
By Income						
Less than $ 5,000	416	5.1	141	1.7	89	1.1
$ 5,000–$ 9,999	869	10.6	577	6.9	449	5.4
$ 10,000–$14,999	943	11.5	703	8.4	756	9.0
$ 15,000–$19,999	941	11.5	633	7.6	514	6.2
$ 20,000–$24,999	923	11.2	602	7.2	524	6.3
$ 25,000–$29,999	1,084	13.2	545	6.5	515	6.2
$ 30,000–$34,999	919	11.2	537	6.4	447	5.3
$ 35,000–$39,999	602	7.3	478	5.7	451	5.4
$ 40,000–$49,999	696	8.5	1,136	13.6	778	9.3
$ 50,000–$59,999	385	4.7	1,012	12.1	930	11.1
$ 60,000–$74,999	235	2.9	866	10.4	1,194	14.3
$ 75,000–$99,999	127	1.5	643	7.7	866	10.4
$100,000+	74	0.9	492	5.9	845	10.1
Median Household Income	$25,085		$39,652		$45,583	
Average Household Income	$27,600		$46,275		$55,238	
FAMILIES	5,867	%	5,522	%	5,246	%
By Income						
Less than $ 5,000	79	1.3	24	0.4	15	0.3
$ 5,000–$ 9,999	386	6.6	135	2.5	81	1.5
$ 10,000–$14,999	497	8.5	246	4.5	192	3.7
$ 15,000–$19,999	615	10.5	295	5.3	197	3.8
$ 20,000–$24,999	706	12.0	276	5.0	240	4.6
$ 25,000–$29,999	922	15.7	312	5.6	215	4.1
$ 30,000–$34,999	803	13.7	348	6.3	242	4.6
$ 35,000–$39,999	512	8.7	328	5.9	276	5.3
$ 40,000–$49,999	591	10.1	919	16.6	517	9.8
$ 50,000–$59,999	354	6.0	868	15.7	749	14.3
$ 60,000–$74,999	216	3.7	735	13.3	1,016	19.4
$ 75,000–$99,999	117	2.0	579	10.5	726	13.8
$100,000+	68	1.2	457	8.3	781	14.9
Median Family Income	$28,536		$48,665		$58,669	
Average Family Income	$31,549		$55,433		$67,994	

Source: 1980 Census, Jan. 1, 1989 UDS Estimates. Courtesy of Urban Decision Systems, Los Angeles, California.

1. The *Primary Health Care Decision Maker Profile* provides information on customers including their demographics, economic status, and level of usage of alternative services.
2. The *Quality Image Profile* includes information on which hospitals within the market are perceived as the industry leaders in overall quality and in a variety of factors, such as best physicians, best nurses, and most personalized care. A sample of this report is presented in Table 5–2. A total of 1,203 households are included in these data. As can be seen in Table 5–2, 37 percent think the Texas Medical Center facilities are best for overall quality. Sixty percent, however, of those households that do not have a personal physician think this same facility is the best. The problem for the Texas Medical Center is that this market segment (no physician) is small: It represents only 72 households of the total sample of 1,203 households.
3. The *Hospital Product Line Preference Report* indicates the preferences of consumers for a variety of medical and health care services ranging from cancer treatment and heart care to physical therapy and geriatric care.
4. The *Physician Relationships Report* makes it possible to identify which households in each of the top 100 markets have physicians in both primary care and certain specialty areas. Furthermore, the likelihood that their patients will switch care is also examined.

On-line Databases

The advent of computer technology has greatly eased the search of secondary data sources. There are some 5,000 on-line databases available to anyone with a computer and modem. *Disclosure Database* is one on-line source that provides data on more than 12,000 publicly traded companies, while *County and City Data Book* provides on-line information on social and economic statistics from the U.S. Census Bureau and 15 other federal agencies.

These are but a few of the commercial services available. Each one demonstrates that, for many organizations, the research plan might include purchase of secondary data as opposed to the collection of primary research information.

With many of the secondary data sources just discussed, there are several advantages. Much available secondary data are relatively inexpensive to collect. This suggests that, regardless of the issues being investigated, it is helpful to begin with a search of existing noncommercial secondary data sources. An additional advantage is that, unlike primary data collection efforts, secondary data can usually be acquired in a timely manner. Also, secondary data can often be more objective, since they are typically collected by a third party.

A major limitation to secondary data is that the available information may not be exactly what is needed to address an organization's research needs. Often, there is also a question with the timeliness or currency of the information. And, since the

Table 5-2 The NCR Health Care Market Guide: Quality

QUALITY PROFILE—HOUSTON, TX

HOSPITAL/FACILITY RECOMMENDED OR GO TO FOR:
BEST OVERALL QUALITY

	Total area house-holds (000)	NRC Fusion Super Groups									Service Utilization			Physician Association		
		Single achievers	Starting a family	Full house	Baby boom families	Single again	Couple cluster	Golden years	Old & alone	Less fortunate	No usage	Light usage (1–4)	Heavy usage (5+)	No Phys	Primary Phys Only	Both Prim/Spec Phys
TOTAL AREA HOUSEHOLDS (000)	1,203	179	217	128	162	124	113	112	59	110	331	601	271	72	893	228
	100.0	14.9	18.0	10.6	13.5	10.3	9.4	9.3	4.9	9.1	27.5	50.0	22.5	6.0	74.2	19.0
	100.0	100.0	100.0	100.0	100.0	100.0	100.0	100.0	100.0	100.0	100.0	100.0	100.0	100.0	100.0	100.0
DON'T KNOW/ NO IMAGE PERCEPTION HOUSEHOLDS	779	117	138	68	104	82	71	75	41	84	284	386	110	62	590	121
	100.0	15.0	17.7	8.7	13.4	10.5	9.1	9.6	5.3	10.8	36.5	49.6	14.1	8.0	75.7	15.5
	64.8	65.4	63.6	53.1	64.2	66.1	62.8	67.0	69.5	76.4	85.8	64.2	40.6	86.1	66.1	53.1
HOUSEHOLDS WITH IMAGE PERCEPTION	424	62	79	61	58	41	42	37	18	26	47	215	162	10	303	107
	100.0	14.6	18.6	14.4	13.7	9.7	9.9	8.7	4.2	6.1	11.1	50.7	38.2	2.4	71.5	25.2
	35.2	34.6	36.4	47.7	35.8	33.1	37.2	33.0	30.5	23.6	14.2	35.8	59.8	13.9	33.9	46.9

Table 5-2 continued

PRIMARY DECISION MAKER HOSPITAL IMAGERY FOR:
BEST OVERALL QUALITY

	Total area house-holds	NRC Fusion Super Groups										Service Utilization			Physician Association		
		Single achievers	Starting a family	Full house	Baby boom families	Single again	Couple cluster	Golden years	Old & alone	Less fortunate	No usage	Light usage (1–4)	Heavy usage (5+)	No Phys	Primary Phys Only	Both Prim/Spec Phys
TOTAL TEXAS MEDICAL CENTER FACILITIES	158	28	32	22	23	17	14	13	4	4	10	83	65	6	116	35
	100.0	17.7	20.3	13.9	14.6	10.8	8.9	8.2	2.5	2.5	6.3	52.5	41.1	3.8	73.4	22.2
	37.3	45.2	40.5	36.1	39.7	41.5	33.3	35.1	22.2	15.4	21.3	38.6	40.1	60.0	38.3	32.7
ST. LUKE'S EPISCOPAL HOSPITAL	54	7	5	7	14	7	7	2	3	1	5	28	21	1	36	16
	100.0	13.0	9.3	13.0	25.9	13.0	13.0	3.7	5.6	1.9	9.3	51.9	38.9	1.9	66.7	29.6
	12.7	11.3	6.3	11.5	24.1	17.1	16.7	5.4	16.7	3.8	10.6	13.0	13.0	10.0	11.9	15.0
HERMANN HOSPITAL	36	6	7	5	3	2	4	5	1	3	1	18	16	5	24	7
	100.0	16.7	19.4	13.9	8.3	5.6	11.1	13.9	2.8	8.3	2.8	50.0	44.4	13.9	66.7	19.4
	8.5	9.7	8.9	8.2	5.2	4.9	9.5	13.5	5.6	11.5	2.1	8.4	9.9	50.0	7.9	6.5
UNIVERSITY OF TEXAS ANDERSON HOSPITAL	25	3	3	3	3	6	1	5		1	1	12	12		19	6
	100.0	12.0	12.0	12.0	12.0	24.0	4.0	20.0		4.0	4.0	48.0	48.0		76.0	24.0
	5.9	4.8	3.8	4.9	5.2	14.6	2.4	13.5		3.8	2.1	5.6	7.4		6.3	5.6
TEXAS MEDICAL CENTER	24	10	9	1	1	1	1	1			2	16	6		19	4
	100.0	41.7	37.5	4.2	4.2	4.2	4.2	4.2			8.3	66.7	25.0		79.2	16.7
	5.7	16.1	11.4	1.6	1.7	2.4	2.4	2.7			4.3	7.4	3.7		6.3	3.7

Source: Reprinted from The NRC Healthcare Market Guide II with permission of the National Research Corporation, © 1989.

health care organization did not monitor or participate in the research plan, there may be underlying questions about the reliability of the information.

DATA COLLECTION

There are a variety of research methods that can be employed to collect primary data. These many methods can be classified into: (1) observational, (2) experimental, and (3) survey research.

Observational Research

Using the **observational research** method, consumers are either observed by another individual or through a mechanical device such as a camera. The most well-known commercial observational method may well be the A.C. Nielsen Company's recording of people's television viewing habits. A mechanical device is attached to the television set, which then records when the television is on and the station that is being viewed. The information is sent, via telephone lines, to the Nielsen Company each evening. From these data, television show ratings are then produced.

The limitation of this information is that it requires viewers to press a button whenever they watch television. It is questionable whether this process is always followed. Eventually, A.C. Nielsen plans to have a system that does not require the viewer to activate the system when watching a television show.

Observational data have also been gathered with hidden cameras in supermarkets. These cameras will track the eye movements of individuals as they scan a supermarket shelf. These eye-tracking studies can then facilitate package design.

Occasionally, organizations will use trained individuals to observe patterns of behavior. For example, a hospital might place a trained observer in its waiting area to observe the admitting process. Observers might track individual patients from their initial encounter in admitting up to their examination in the emergency room. The Cleveland Clinic Foundation developed a "professional shopper" program to improve the organization's ability to identify and monitor areas of patient concern. Trained researchers were used as simulated patients and they conducted observational market research. Information from this effort was used to make changes in employee training and policies.[3]

Observational data are useful in observing what people do, however, they cannot address why people behave in certain ways.

Experimental Research

A second form of data collection is an **experiment**, where factors are manipulated to determine a causal relationship. Experiments are common in fields such as psychology in which specific variables can be measured and controlled to assess the impact of one factor on another. Marketing experiments are often conducted in academic settings. The advantage of experimental research is that it can measure the actual effects of one variable, such as the effect that the size of an advertisement has on message retention. The major limitation to this method is whether the results can be generalized in the real world. As a result of this concern of real-world transferability, experimental research has had less relevance in health care marketing.[4]

Because of experimental limitations, a more common form of experimental research in marketing is the **quasi-experimental design**, in which the data gathering is set up similar to a laboratory experiment, although lacking in control over all variables.

A common example of a quasi-experimental design is a test market. A hospital designs a study to test two alternative media strategies regarding calls to a physician referral line. Two cities are found that have similar characteristics—size of the population, number of competing hospitals, specialty physician population, and telephone ownership. In the first city, the referral line is promoted through a campaign of billboards and limited newspaper advertising. In the second city, television might be the primary communication vehicle with a similar level of advertising support. Responses to the referral line are then assessed across the two cities. While modeled after an experimental design, this in-the-field test cannot control for every variable. There maybe other factors, such as a competitor's response in a particular market, which could affect the tests differentially. Yet, in spite of this lack of controls, this quasi-experimental design may present a truer measure of an issue than a pure laboratory experiment.

Survey Research

A third common method for acquiring primary data is through **survey research**. Survey research can be obtained through one of four common forms: (1) telephone interviews, (2) personal interviews, (3) focus groups, and (4) mail. Table 5–3 lists some of the trade-offs to consider in the use of the four survey research methods discussed in the following pages.

Telephone Interviews

Telephone interviews are a quick way to acquire information. Using multiple interviewers in a telephone interview bank, data can be acquired in a short time frame. When the questionnaire is short, trained interviewers can usually be successful in obtaining a high completion rate from respondents. Telephone interviewing also allows for the targeting of responses. Using qualifying questions, a telephone interviewer can target the profile of respondent desired.

Table 5-3 Alternative Marketing Research Methodologies

Approach Criteria	Personal Interview	Telephone Survey	Mail Survey	Focus Groups
Economy	Most expensive.	Avoids interviewer travel, relatively expensive. Trained interviewers needed.	Potentially lowest costs (if response rate sufficient).	Relatively expensive.
Interviewer bias	High likelihood of bias. Trust. Appearance.	Less than personal interviewer. No face-to-face contact. Suspicion of phone call.	Interviewer bias eliminated. Anonymity provided.	Need trained moderator.
Flexibility	Most flexible method. Responses can be probed. Assistance can be provided in completing forms. Observations can be made.	Cannot make observations. Probing possible to a degree.	Least flexible method.	Very flexible.
Sampling and respondent cooperation	Most complete sample possible, with sufficient call-back strategy.	Limited to people with telephone. No answers. Refusals are common.	Mailing list problem. Nonresponse a major problem.	Need close selection.

Source: Reprinted from *Health Care Marketing Plans: From Strategy to Action*, 2nd ed., by S.G. Hillestad and E.N. Berkowitz, p.100, Aspen Publishers, Inc., © 1991.

The speed advantage of telephone data gathering has been demonstrated at the Cleveland Clinic. In late May 1987, a surgical resident was reported to have AIDS. Publicity was heightened by several news stories. The resident's death occurred five days after the newspaper stories first appeared. The Clinic used overnight telephone polling services to get next-morning market assessment of any public concerns or issues to which the Clinic had to respond.[5]

Computer technology has greatly improved the telephone interviewing process. At many commercial marketing research firms, the phone survey is done by computer. Questions can be randomly reordered on the computer display screen, eliminating potential interviewer bias. Data can be directly entered as the questions are asked to increase the speed of analysis. This direct transmission can also help eliminate the possibilities for errors and missing data. Technology has also helped in the development of computer programs that make calls to unlisted numbers through such procedures as random digit dialing. In this method, calls are made to a randomly drawn sequence of numbers within a particular exchange area. In recent years the use of Wide Area Telephone Systems (WATS) has helped reduce the cost of telephone surveys conducted over broad geographic areas.

Most readers of this text can speak to the limitations of telephone surveys. Many consumers find them intrusive. It is easy for the respondent to terminate the interview by disconnecting. Telephone surveys are also limited regarding the type of questions that respondents can be asked. Many individuals hesitate to answer confidential questions since they are unsure of the caller's identity. Health care organizations can minimize this problem by sending out a pre-survey letter to inform consumers of the incoming call. The prenotification can often increase the survey's response rate.

Personal Interviews

A second way to survey individuals is through personal interviews. Personal interviews can take two forms: One method consists of one-to-one interviewing between interviewer and respondent; the second form is the group method referred to as "focus groups" (see below).

An individual interview is a valuable way to collect data when the respondent must be probed regarding his or her answers. Complicated questions or questions that do not lend themselves to simple dichotomous responses often require personal interviews. This method also has the highest completion rate since the interviewer has the opportunity to develop some rapport with the respondent. Personal interviews are the preferred method when the survey requires the presentation of visual cues or a product demonstration.

Personal interviews have some limitations, with cost being a major factor. Personal interviews require trained interviewers. And, there are often costs related to the interviewer's travel time. The potential for bias is great as the respondents often have concerns about how they appear or what they say to the researcher. A trained interviewer, however, can often effectively minimize the amount of social desirability. Sensitive questions, such as those regarding health issues, can be difficult.

Focus Groups

Another method of conducting survey research is the focus group, a version of the personal interview conducted with a group of consumers simultaneously. **Focus groups** are interviews typically conducted with eight to 10 people and a trained moderator following an interview guide. Focus groups have become a more common, useful approach for acquiring health care information.[6]

Focus groups are often used in two aspects of the research process. First, focus groups can be conducted to develop hypotheses. For example, if a manufacturer of hypodermic needles that have long been the preferred brand among nurses finds that sales to hospitals have declined in recent years, this manufacturer might not understand why sales have dropped. To determine some of the possible reasons for such a decline in sales, the company might conduct focus groups and then investigate these reasons in a larger study. A second common use of focus groups is to gain insight into the results of quantitative studies. An HMO might conduct a study to determine the image of competing plans in their market among households with young children. The study might report that 40 percent of the respondents do not think this particular HMO is good for young families. Focus groups might then be conducted among people with young children to try to gain insight into why this perception is held.

The typical arrangement for a focus group consists of a group of people who are recruited to discuss a particular topic. Exhibit 5–2 shows a portion of the focus group guide that was used in a study to examine physicians' and women's attitudes toward breast cancer screening. The focus group moderator is a trained professional who uses this guide to generate discussion among the group's members. As can be seen in reading these questions, the focus group guide provides an expansive question to the participants to generate discussion. The moderator is there to facilitate the flow of discussion among participants. Focus groups are often used early in the research process when the researcher is not sure of the correct or exact questions to ask in a survey. An analysis of the focus group response can reveal issues that the researcher should explore quantitatively to determine how extensive they are in the general population.

Data from focus groups consist of transcripts of the discussions and often, videotapes. At Texas Children's Hospital in Houston, focus groups of patients' concerns are shown to department managers.[7] The analysis of the focus group consists of looking for major themes or issues that emerged in the discussion. Typically, a company will conduct several focus groups using the same question

Exhibit 5–2 Sample Focus Group Questions

1. Today, it seems that we can hardly pick up a magazine or read a newspaper without hearing about cancer and what might cause it. Are there any forms of cancer that you think women should be particularly concerned about? Are there any things that you are doing to check for this potential health problem?

   PROBE: What do you see as the real risks of women getting breast cancer?

   PROBE: Do you think there is some age when getting breast cancer is most likely? Do you think there is some age when getting breast cancer is no longer very likely?

2. Based on what you've read or people whom you've talked to, what types of tests do you think can be done to check for whether a woman has breast cancer?

3. When women are in their childbearing years, they often feel that their gynecologist or obstetrician is responsible for looking after women's problems such as breast, uterine, or cervical cancer. Do you think so? How does this change as the woman gets older?

4. Now, I'd like to focus our discussion in the little time left to the problem of breast cancer, specifically. Most of us tend to rely on our physician to inform us of the health care tests we need, and when we need them. When it comes to the area of breast cancer, what does your doctor say to you, or suggest to you?

5. There are many alternative methods which have been suggested for the detection of breast cancer. Specifically, some experts have suggested self-exams, thermography (give description), ultrasound (give description), and mammography (give description). Based on what you've heard, read, or experienced, what do you think about each of these different testing methods? (NOTE: Proceed through list individually. First, let me get your reactions to self exams . . .)

   PROBE: Probe on effectiveness, fear, frequency at which test should be conducted.

guide. In this way, the analysis can examine consistent themes that emerge from the multiple groups. Research has demonstrated that when focus group themes are consistent across multiple groups, a larger-scale survey tends to validate these themes.

The major benefit to a focus group is the synergy that often occurs from a group discussion. Also, there are many questions that cannot be fully explored in a more formal survey. Focus groups are often used to examine the reasons why a particular behavior or response occurred in a population. A limitation of focus groups is that they, by design, consist of a limited number of participants. There is no statistical exactness or estimation that can be applied to a focus group since the data are qualitative in origin. As with any method in which an individual is involved in collecting the data, there is always the potential for bias, especially with a moderator who is not well trained.

Mail Surveys

Mail surveys are the fourth common form of survey research. Mail surveys have the advantage of being a relatively inexpensive way to collect data. Typically, costs involve the reproduction of the survey and postage to send and return it. A major advantage of mail surveys is that they provide anonymity to the respondent. Mail is also an inexpensive, efficient way to contact individuals who are dispersed over a large geographical area. In health care, mail surveys have often been used to collect patient satisfaction data. Another advantage to mail surveys is the elimination of interviewer bias.

While mail surveys have these distinct advantages, there are several major disadvantages. The major limitation pertains to response rate and who returns the form. SunHealth Alliance, a hospital consulting firm in Charlotte, North Carolina, surveyed 85 percent of its hospitals and got only a 13 percent response rate to its mail surveys (and an 85 percent response rate to its telephone surveys). While there are several strategies that can be used to improve response rates, as indicated in Exhibit 5–3, no real controls can be enforced to ensure that the person targeted for the survey did, in fact, complete the survey. There is also the concern that the people who complied and returned the survey may, in fact, be different from those who did not respond. While mail surveys provide the advantage of eliminating interviewer bias, they do not allow for any probing of respondents. Completion rates are affected by question format. Too many open-ended questions requiring respondents to explain their answers in great depth often result in lower return rates.

Designing a Sample

When conducting a study, a basic issue to determine is who should be surveyed. Most marketing research involves a **sample**, which is a collection of data from only a portion of a target population. A **census** is when data are collected from all members of the target population. The sampling process involves six steps.

Step One

Initially, it is essential to define the population. The *population* is the description of all people or elements of interest to researchers and from which a sample will be selected. For example, an academic medical center might define the population as "all pediatricians in the state who referred to a tertiary care facility within the past two-year period."

Step Two

The second step is to specify the *sampling frame*, which is the means of representing the sample population. The sampling frame may be a telephone directory or the medical society mailing list. A perfect sampling frame is one in which every element of the population is represented only once.

Exhibit 5–3 Factors Found To Influence Response Rates

1. Prenotification of respondents
2. Incentives (included with survey is best)
3. Cover letter
4. Stamped response return envelope
5. Follow-up contact
6. Survey length (under four pages)

Note: For a detailed discussion, see F.J. Yammarino, S.J. Skinner, and T.L. Childers, Understanding Mail Survey Response Behavior, *Public Opinion Quarterly*, Vol. 55 (1991): pp. 613–619.

Step Three

The third step involves specifying the sampling unit. The *sampling unit* contains the elements of the population to be sampled. For example, if a survey was going to include clinical directors of comprehensive cancer programs, and there was no such directory, the sampling unit might have to be hospitals. The sampling unit is also partially dependent upon the overall design of the project. If, for example, the survey is to be conducted by telephone, the sampling unit will necessarily be telephone numbers. A mail survey requires a sampling unit of addresses.

Step Four

Selection of the sampling method is the fourth step. The *sampling method* is the way the sampling units are to be selected. Any sampling method is dependent on five choices:

1. probability vs. nonprobability
2. single unit vs. cluster of units
3. stratified vs. unstratified
4. equal unit vs. unequal probability
5. single stage vs. multistage

These five choices, when combined, provide a possibility of 32 different sampling schemes.

Probability vs. Nonprobability Sampling. A *probability sampling* is one in which the sampling units are selected by chance—for each unit, there is a known chance of being selected. The advantage of a probability sample is that an objective measure of the sample's reliability can be made. An additional advantage is that probability sampling often does not require much detailed information about the population to be surveyed.

A major disadvantage to probability sampling is that a listing of the universe population, or at least a good estimate, is needed. In much research, in fact, one may not want to take a probability sample. For example, in an exploratory study, one might want to sample just the successful HMO salespeople to determine what they are doing to win accounts, rather than sampling all HMO salespeople.

There are two basic forms of probability sampling: Simple random sampling is a process that requires that each unit's chance of being chosen is known and equal. Simple random samples have the advantage of being easy to understand, and the data analysis techniques are simple. The major disadvantage to simple random samples is that they require a list and number of every item in the universe. Additionally, when there are large variations in the data, it's possible to gather highly misleading samples. Figure 5–2 shows some data for household expenditures on medical care during the past year. Two simple random samples could lead to dramatic differences in the inferences drawn regarding health care expenditures, as shown in the bottom half of the figure.

Systematic sampling is similar to the simple random sampling process. This approach involves picking a random starting point, and then taking every "Kth" unit in the frame. If, for example, a hospital wanted a sample of 500 patients from a total universe of 100,000, the "Kth" unit would be 200, and then every 200th unit in the frame would be included in the sample.

The advantage of systematic sampling is that, unlike simple random sampling, a designated number does not need to be assigned to every item in the universe. In fact, this approach does not even require a list if units are being sampled over time such as is common to patient satisfaction surveys (e.g., the hospital in the above example surveying every 200th patient). There is some difficulty with this approach, however, when trying to measure sampling error. A well-designed probability sample often does not require large numbers to estimate the results confidently. Table 5–4 shows the sample sizes needed in order for the researcher to be 95 percent and 90 percent confident in the results for defined populations. It is important to realize that as the population becomes more finely specified, the size of the sample increases relative to each characteristic.

A *nonprobability sample* is one in which the chance selection procedures are not used. Nonprobability samples have the advantage of offering better selection of respondents. This factor is particularly true in exploratory research. The major disadvantage, as with all nonprobability samples, is that no mathematical calculation of sampling error is possible. Selection is often based on the judgment of the

Household	Medicine Expenditure
1	$ 60
2	2,700
3	500
4	1,200
5	180
6	800
7	4,200
8	120
9	900
10	1,400
11	1,100
12	3,000
13	4,500
14	650
15	1,300
16	900

Total = $23,510

Average/Household = $1,469.38
Standard Deviation = $1,344

Sample A	
Household	Expenditure
1	$ 60
14	650
9	900
5	180
8	120
Total Expenditure =	$1,910
Average/Household =	$382
Estimate of total Universe =	$6,112

Sample B	
Household	Expenditure
7	$4,200
12	3,000
15	1,300
2	2,700
10	1,400
Total Expenditure =	$12,600
Average/Household =	$2,520
Estimate of total Universe =	$40,320

Figure 5–2 Variations in Simple Random Samples

Table 5–4 Sizes of Samples To Be Confident of Accuracy

Population	Sample size that will provide 95% confidence level	Sample size that will provide 90% confidence level
Infinity	384	271
100,000	384	271
50,000	381	269
10,000	370	263
5,000	357	257
3,000	341	248
2,000	322	238
1,000	278	213
500	217	176
100	80	73

Note: Error margin held constant at +/–5 percentage points

Source: Adapted from *PACE Manual* with permission of Phi Delta Kappa, © 1984.

researcher, which could limit the ability to generalize the results. There are several variations of a nonprobability sample.

A convenience sample is a nonprobability sample where the only criterion for inclusion is the convenience of the unit to the researcher. The advantage of this approach is obvious—it is fast and uncomplicated. The major problem of this method is that the sampling error cannot be determined.

Purposive samples are a nonprobability approach in which units are selected from the universe population on the basis of some form of "expert" judgment. The problems with this method are similar to convenience samples. There is also no way to measure the expertise of the judge in reducing sampling errors.

Of all the nonprobability samples, quota samples involve the most systematic approach to obtaining a representative sample. In a quota sample, the characteristics believed to relate to a representative sample of the population are identified. Then, the proportion of the universe population having the characteristic of interest is estimated. The sample is then allocated among those cells. For example, if it was estimated that women were responsible for the selection of the primary care provider in 80 percent of all families, then 80 percent of households included in the quota sample would contain females.

The quota sample is the most attractive of all nonprobability sampling approaches in trying to control reliability. This method also requires the researcher to focus on relevant population subgroups and minimizes the possibility of unusual samples. Its major disadvantage is that it is hard to use more than a limited number of control characteristics on which to develop a quota sample.

In deciding between probability or nonprobability samples, researchers must consider what kind of error tolerance is needed in the results. Highly accurate estimates of the population values would require a probability sample. A related concern is whether nonsampling errors are likely to be large. If the population is relatively homogeneous on the variables of interest, a nonprobability sample might be sufficient.

Single Unit vs. Cluster Sampling. Single unit vs. cluster sampling is the second variation to sampling methods. In *single unit sampling*, each sampling unit is selected individually. In *cluster sampling*, units are selected in groups. For example, if the unit to be sampled is a household, single unit sampling would require that each household be selected separately. One form of cluster sampling would be to change the sampling unit to city blocks. Then, every household on the particular block selected would be included in the sample.

With cluster sampling, the population to be sampled is divided into mutually exclusive and exhaustive subsets. A random sample of these subsets is then selected. A *one-stage cluster sample* is one in which all the population elements in the selected subsets are included in the sample. If, however, a sample of elements are selected from within each subset, this is referred to as a *two-stage cluster sample*. Since a sample of subgroups is chosen with a cluster sample, it is desirable that each subgroup be a small-scale model of the population. In cluster sampling, the subgroups formed should be as heterogenous as possible.

The choice between single unit and cluster sampling is an economic issue between cost and value. Cluster sampling usually costs less per sampling unit than does single unit sampling, yet for similar sample sizes, the sampling error will be greater with a cluster sample than with a single unit sample. This greater sampling error occurs because there is less variability within a cluster than for a population as a whole. Since single unit sampling uses the population as a whole, this method of sampling reduces sampling error.

Stratified vs. Unstratified Sampling. This is a third sampling variation. A *stratified sample* is a probability sample that involves dividing the population into mutually exclusive and exhaustive subsets and randomly sampling elements from each group. In an unstratified sample, the population is not divided into subsets. This approach is similar to cluster sampling in that both divide the population into mutually exclusive and exhaustive subsets. The difference is that, with stratified sampling, a sample of elements is chosen from each subgroup, while with cluster sampling, a sample of the subgroups are selected. In stratified sampling, each element of the population must be divided into only one subset.

A stratified sample is a common approach in health care research. Consider an HMO that wants to survey member satisfaction. If surveys are administered at the clinic site, it is likely that heavy users of the HMO might be oversampled relative to the total membership, since heavy users are receiving more care. To protect against this oversampling, the HMO might divide its members' strata based upon the amount of their utilization. User groups might be divided into heavy, medium, light, and nonclinic users. Members from each group would be sampled based on the proportion of the membership base that each group represents. If the HMO wants to survey users' satisfaction, the sample proportions would be drawn to represent the heavy users as a proportion of their use relative to the other strata. The strata are drawn so that each individual group is as homogeneous as possible. This type of sample is referred to as a proportionate stratified sample.

Not all stratified samples are proportionate. When some strata have greater variability, more units might be sampled. For example, to determine the average income of physicians across specialties, it might be necessary to disproportionately sample within a specialty, such as neurosurgery, in which the range is broader than a specialty, such as pediatrics, where the income range is narrower.

Equal Unit Probability vs. Unequal Unit Probability. This is the fourth method for selecting sampling units. The only instance in which there is equal unit probability of selection in the sample is when there is no difference in variance among the strata.

Single Stage vs. Multistage Sampling. The final consideration when choosing a sampling method pertains to the number of stages in the sampling process. The researcher must choose between *single stage* or *multistage sampling.* If a perfect sampling frame exists that lists each unit of the population from which the sample is to be drawn, then only a single stage sampling process is needed. Without a perfect sampling frame, a multistage process is often required. Another advantage to multistage sampling is that it often provides a better estimate of the population variance.

Step Five

The fifth step in the sampling process is determination of the sample size. Table 5–4, discussed earlier, shows the required sample sizes for certain populations. Yet more detailed sampling size determinations are possible with the use of sampling theory.

Step Six

The sixth step is to specify the sampling plan, which involves specifying how to implement the sampling choices made in the first five steps.

Questionnaire Design

Questionnaires must be designed to collect survey information. There are several elements that must be considered. Foremost in designing any survey instrument is the requirement for clarity of meaning to the terms that are used. All well-designed survey instruments utilize a pretest in which the survey is administered to a small group of people similar to those who will ultimately participate in the survey. Difficulties with questionnaire design, its wording, and its completeness can all be revealed in a pretest. If the survey requires major revision, this revision can be followed with an additional pretest. Exhibit 5–4 lists the six questions that should be asked about each word in a good survey question.

In addition to pretesting, there are other factors to consider when designing questionnaires. Questions should be written as simply as possible. They should use terms and language with which the audience is familiar. Abbreviations should be avoided. Sending a survey to consumers in which they are asked to indicate their interest or need in referrals to a physiatrist may be meaningless, since a technical specialty designation may be unknown or confusing to the potential respondents.

A second caveat in writing any survey question is to ensure that a certain state of affairs is not presupposed. For example, the following question assumes the patient has contacted the nurse practitioner:

Did you find the nurse practitioner to be helpful?
___Yes ___No

In writing any question, one must ensure that the respondent is capable of giving an accurate answer. The wording of the question must be clear to communicate whether one is seeking a factual answer or an opinion. Some individuals will not respond if they believe a factual answer is required and they are unsure of the correct answer.

Exhibit 5–4 Good Survey Research Questioning Each Word

1. Does it mean what we intend?
2. Does it have any other meaning?
3. If so, does the content make the intended meaning clear?
4. Does the word have more than one pronunciation?
5. Is there any word of similar pronunciation that it might be confused with?
6. Is a single word or phrase suggested?

Question of fact:
     How long did you wait before seeing a doctor? _____

Question of opinion?
     How long do you think you waited before seeing a doctor? _____

With factual questions it is important to remember that memories decay rapidly with time.

Another concern in questionnaire design is to make sure that only one piece of information is asked for at one time. The following question will yield confusion for the respondents and unclear results for the researcher.

Were the billing office and receptionist courteous?
___Yes ___No

Finally, extreme caution should be taken when using adjectives, adverbs, or vaguely defined words. Words such as "several," "most," and "usually" can all have different meanings to different people. For a manager, these definitions complicate actionable results.

Exhibit 5–5 shows a sample patient satisfaction questionnaire that contains many of the questionnaire design problems discussed in this section. Review this survey and critique these items according to the caveats expressed.

Question Formats

There are various question formats that can be used in any survey instrument. Consider the example of a multispecialty clinic that would like to examine the expansion of office hours to include evening appointments. The clinic survey questions could be presented in one of several ways:

1. *Open-ended questions* ask individuals to respond based on their own words. These can take the completely unstructured approach:

What is your opinion of appointment hours?

An alternative would provide more direct response mechanisms.

2. *Multichotomous questions* are those that present the respondent with a fixed alternative. These questions can be phrased in a dichotomous way in which there are two choices presented (Yes, or No):

Would you prefer evening hours by appointment?
___Yes ___No

Exhibit 5–5 Patient Satisfaction Survey

---

1. Do you think our level of tertiary care in nephrology is sufficient?
   ___ yes   ___no

2. Did the telephone receptionist answer your call promptly?
   ___ yes   ___no

3. Rate us on each of the following dimensions:

	Very Good	Good	Outstanding
Caring attitude	1	2	3
Physician's knowledge	1	2	3
Hours of scheduling	1	2	3
Prescription service	1	2	3

4. Is our facility clean and easy to use?
   ___ yes ___ no

5. What is your age?
   ___under 20   ___46 to 55
   ___21 to 30   ___56 to 70
   ___31 to 45   ___over 70

6. How many children do you have?
   ___One child
   ___Two to four
   ___More than four

They can also be phrased through the application of a scale or options list such as the following examples:

(a) Likert scale: Indicates the degree of agreement or disagreement.
     I think evening hours would be more convenient for me.
         (Circle the choice that reflects your view)

Strongly Agree	Agree	Neither Agree/ Disagree	Disagree	Strongly Disagree

(b) semantic differential scale: Uses bipolar adjectives.

Evening hours by
appointment are: Convenient __ __ __ __ __ __ Inconvenient

(c) intention to buy or use scale: Assesses purchase intention beyond attitude.

If evening hours by appointment were offered, I would:

Definitely Use	Probably Use	Not Sure	Probably Not Use	Definitely Not Use
_____	_____	_____	_____	_____

ANALYSIS AND EVALUATION OF RESEARCH

The last stage of the market research process involves the analysis and evaluation of the research results. This analysis might be either qualitative (as in the case of focus groups) or quantitative (using survey methodologies that provide empirical information). In either case, a skilled, unbiased person should conduct the analysis. The quantitative sophistication of marketing analysis has advanced with the use of *multivariate statistical analysis*, which considers the impact of multiple variables on a dependent variable. For example, regression analysis is a multivariate statistical technique that has one dependent variable, such as level of monthly smoking activity, and multiple independent variables, such as age of smoker, gender of smoker, amount of alcohol consumed weekly. The regression analysis can determine how much each variable accounts for smoking consumption, as well as how much the effects of the multiple variables together account for the level of smoking consumption.

Even the most sophisticated analysis, however, is useless if the people within the organization cannot understand the results or translate them into managerial actions. For this reason, it is often helpful to have the analyst prepare mock tables that would appear in the final report. Management personnel can examine whether they would see value in a table that might analyze consumer attitude toward a closed panel HMO by gender, or whether a more important table might provide a breakdown of attitude toward a closed panel HMO by type of health insurance of the individuals surveyed. In this way, the people involved with implementing the changes or dealing with the question being examined can look at what the information might be like. These administrators or managers can then decide whether receiving such data would be helpful, or even worth knowing about. Most importantly, it is essential to have data that would lead to a management action.

Yet it is in this last stage of analysis and evaluation of research results that weaknesses in the problem definition are revealed. Too often, in the presentation of market research, a comment is heard, such as: "interesting, but what can we do with it?" The cause of such frustrations is not so much that the data analysis was poor, or that the questions that led to the information were incorrect, or even that the method of data collection was inappropriate. Rather it is more likely caused by an improperly defined problem and poorly specified research objectives.

Finally, for most health care organizations, it is essential to recognize that the marketplace is dynamic. Competitors are always changing their strategies, customer attitudes might shift as a function of new health care alternatives being offered to them, physician loyalties might change because of new alliances formed between providers. The dynamic nature of the market necessitates a continual monitoring of the marketplace with ongoing market research. Organizations must also manage and coordinate the flow of this information to the decision makers within the company in an organized fashion. The recognition of this requirement has led to the creation of marketing information systems.

MARKETING INFORMATION SYSTEMS

With the onset of more marketing information, individuals are trying to manage the flow of data and information in a more organized fashion. A **marketing information system** (MIS) is "a structured, interacting complex of persons, machines, and procedures designed to generate an orderly flow of pertinent information collected from intra- and extra-firm sources, for use as the bases for decision making in specific responsibility areas of marketing management."[8]

The structure of a hospital's marketing information system might link admissions data with patient and physician referral information. On-line database information and syndicated marketing research information could also be accessed. Key employees would have remote terminal access by modem to the necessary information. Ideally, an effective MIS would be able to construct succinct information reports to the necessary managers on a regular basis.

There are several important ingredients needed to create an organized MIS. Mechanisms must be in place to gather and store the data. Data analysis must be performed, and there must be a way to access the data on a regular or as-needed basis.

The biggest need for an effective MIS is because of the growth in database marketing. **Database marketing** may be defined as "an automated system to identify people—both customers and prospects—by name, and to use quantifiable information about these people to define the best possible purchasers and prospects for a given offer at a given point in time."[9] The objective of database marketing is to target particular customers more effectively. In implementing a database marketing approach, for example, each patient's record, which is entered into the MIS, is assigned a distinct code. Every patient who used the hospital's services would be assigned a database code. In this way, through the MIS support system, targeted mailing could be directed to specific people. Building such an MIS for targeted marketing is the strategy of Mid-Michigan Regional Medical Center in Midland. This provider developed a promotional campaign to encourage consumers to complete a free health assessment quiz. Consumers provided information about lifestyle, family status, and clinical status that could be entered into the MIS for future targeted marketing efforts.[10]

A cardiology department, as another example, might decide in conjunction with nutrition and rehabilitative medicine to offer a health education program called "Healthy Heart." Rather than just advertising broadly in the media, the hospital might access those individuals who utilized related services within the past two years, or whose demographic profile might be relevant for this program.

An effective MIS at Hinsdale Hospital in Illinois was described by Maholtra. This hospital used a support system called the Travenol Market Model, which integrated internal hospital and doctor records with marketing data and hospitalization rates. Using these data, the hospital identified potential high-growth services and geographic locations.[11]

CONCLUSIONS

Fewer areas of marketing are being more rapidly affected by technology than marketing research and information systems. In health care, ongoing market research efforts are needed to understand the customer, in order to market the organization effectively.

KEY TERMS

Marketing Research	Survey Research
Primary Data	Focus Groups
Secondary Data	Sample
Syndicated Marketing Research	Census
Observational Research	Marketing Information System
Experiment	Database Marketing
Quasi-Experimental Design	

CHAPTER SUMMARY

1. Marketing research is a process that involves the collection of primary and secondary data, or a combination of both. These data can be either quantitative or qualitative in form.

2. Secondary data can be obtained from the organization itself, from regulatory agencies, and from commercial firms.

3. The collection of primary market research data can be accomplished through observation, experiments, interviews, and surveys.

4. Mail, telephone, and personal interviews vary in terms of flexibility, cost, and respondent cooperation.

5. An increasingly common qualitative data-gathering method in health care is the focus group, used either to develop hypotheses or to obtain explanations.

6. In conducting market research, organizations can collect data from all members of the target population—referred to as a census—or it can use a subset of the population—referred to as a sample. Designing a sample begins with a definition of the target population.

7. Any sampling method is dependent on five factors: (1) probability, (2) stratification, (3) equal likelihood of selection, (4) number of stages, and (5) level of the unit.

8. In order to develop any survey instrument appropriately, it is essential to pretest the instrument among a group of people similar to those who will receive the final survey.

9. Marketing information systems (MIS) are an approach to organizing an array of data for use in strategic marketing decisions.

10. Organizations are developing database marketing efforts that allow them to identify, profile, and reach individual customers.

CHAPTER PROBLEMS

1. A hospital marketing director has several research projects to undertake this quarter. He must try to determine the appropriate sampling methodology in light of each problem. Provide your recommendation on each issue:

(a) The hospital urology department wants to establish a sexual dysfunction clinic. The department head wants to get an estimate of the number of males aged 35 to 60 in the community suffering some form of sexual dysfunction.

(b) A primary care medical group is trying to determine whether patients are being greeted and serviced appropriately by the billing and admitting departments.

(c) An HMO is trying to determine what concerns physicians have in agreeing to become part of its panel of doctors who will treat the managed care plan's subscribers.

2. A health group wants to identify consumers who: once belonged to an HMO, but left the plan; have at least one child; and live in the primary service area of the town's hospital. Write the questions to target this population and suggest the best method for getting this information.

3. The American Academy of Pediatrics wants to conduct a survey of newly graduated family practitioners to assess why they did not choose pediatrics for their specialization. Provide a definition of the population, suggest a sampling frame, and indicate the appropriate sampling unit.

4. In the previously cited example (Problem 3), suggest the appropriate sampling method in terms of:

(a) probability vs. nonprobability
(b) single unit vs. cluster unit
(c) stratified vs. unstratified
(d) equal unit vs. unequal unit
(e) single stage vs. multistage

5. Listed below are the alternative samples obtained by a health care marketing research firm for its clients. Describe the type of sample each represents.

(a) Ten people sitting in the waiting room are asked to describe the ambiance of the facility and the attitude of the receptionist.

(b) The medical school samples alumni regarding an evaluation of their education. Respondents are selected in an amount equal to the same population of specialties from the graduating class.

(c) The HMO calls every 15th subscriber to assess whether the patient handbook was received, and whether the subscriber has any questions.

6. A nursing home has decided to conduct a short survey to assess whether the family members who are responsible for an elderly resident are satisfied with the care being given. A portion of the survey is listed below.

1. How often do you visit your relative?
___Daily ___3 to 4 times a week ___2 to 3 times a week
___Less than once a week

2. Please rate each aspect of care:

	Excellent	Very good	Good
Nursing quality	1	2	3
Room cleanliness	1	2	3

3. Do you like our newsletters and phone call updates?
    ___Yes ___No

4. Why do you think we are the best nursing home in the area?
    _____.

5. Please tell us your age:
    ___Under 25   ___51 to 65
    ___26 to 35   ___Over 65
    ___35 to 50

Please critique this survey.

NOTES

1. For a useful reference to secondary data sources see, L. McDaniels, *Sources of External Marketing Data*, #580–107 (Cambridge, Mass.: Harvard Business School Press, 1986).

2. This discussion and the following on commercial secondary data is drawn from S.G. Hillestad and E.N. Berkowitz, *Health Care Marketing Plans: From Strategy to Action* (Gaithersburg, Md.: Aspen Publishers, Inc., 1991):65–106.

3. W.R. Gombeski, Jr., C.E. Stone, and F.J. Weaver, Improving Patient Services Through A Professional Shopper Program, *Journal of Health Care Marketing* 6, no. 3 (1986):64–68.

4. P. Cooper and R.D. Hisrich, Marketing Research for Health Services: Understanding Applying Various Techniques, *Journal of Health Care Marketing* 7, no. 1 (1987):54–60.

5. W.R. Gombeski, Jr., J.R. Day, and L. Honacek, Overnight Assessment of Marketing Crises, *Journal of Health Care Marketing* 11, no. 1 (1991):51–54.

6. A useful study of the application of focus group research is presented by E.J. Wargo, Assessing the Potential of an Industrial Medicine Program, *Journal of Health Care Marketing* 7, no. 1 (1987): 79–85.

7. Texas Children's Hospital Films Focus Groups To Improve Service, *Hospital Patient Relations Report* 8, no. 3 (1993):1–2.

8. R.H. Brien and J.E. Stafford, Marketing Information Systems: A New Dimension for Marketing Research, *Journal of Marketing* 32, no. 3 (1968):19–23.

9. S.K. Jones, *Creative Strategy in Direct Marketing* (Lincolnwood, Ill.: NTC Publishing, 1991), 5.

10. L.R. Uttich and G. Dobbins, The Database Difference, *MPR Exchange* 20, no. 3 (1993):4–5.

11. N.K. Maholtra, Decision Support Systems for Health Care Marketing Managers, *Journal of Health Care Marketing* 9, no. 2 (1989):20–28.

$$6$$

MARKET SEGMENTATION

LEARNING OBJECTIVES

After reading this chapter you should be able to:

- Understand alternative market segmentation strategies

- Recognize relevant criteria for selecting market segments

- Identify alternative bases for industrial segmentation

- Appreciate the hierarchy of segmentation alternatives

A basic issue facing most organizations and businesses is deciding which customers to attract to buy their product or use their service. Targeting the market is a major aspect of marketing strategy, as discussed earlier in Chapter 2. A company can decide to target everyone, one market segment, or multiple segments with a different marketing mix strategy.

MASS MARKETING

A mass marketing strategy is an approach in which an organization develops its marketing mix (the four Ps) to appeal to the broadest group, or largest number of people possible. One of the better-known advocates of this approach was Henry Ford, who was cited as saying, "You can have any color car you want, as long as it is black." This is a mass marketing strategy at its ultimate—one color car for the entire car-buying market. The early Model T produced by Ford also did not come with the familiar array of options available to car buyers today.

The underlying rationale of a mass marketing strategy is that everyone in the market wants the same product—delivered, priced, and promoted the same way. Or, if there are differences within the market, they are not usually significant enough to affect demand, nor do they merit being addressed by the organization with a different marketing mix strategy.

A mass marketing strategy has some distinct advantages. Foremost is the cost. A mass marketing strategy for a manufactured product often eliminates retooling costs and can ensure longer production runs. Similarly, a mass marketing strategy makes sense when it is economically infeasible to produce variations in the marketing mix.

The limitations of a mass marketing strategy, however, underscore its limited usefulness. In reality, there are often large differences within a broad consumer market that do affect demand. People have different shopping patterns or work habits, which, for instance, might necessitate different clinic hours for appointments. Differing income levels require differential pricing for certain services or products. A mass marketing strategy can often cause distribution problems. If a product is available at every outlet, no one particular outlet will feel it is worthwhile to push the product. Finally, the major limitation to a mass marketing strategy relates to competitive considerations. A mass marketing strategy that tries to appeal to everyone leaves a company susceptible to having a group, or segment, of its customers won over by another firm that more closely tailors its marketing mix to attract that particular subgroup. It is competition that provides a strong rationale for a market segmentation strategy.

MARKET SEGMENTATION

Market segmentation is the process of grouping into clusters consumers who have similar wants or needs to which an organization can respond by tailoring one or more elements of the marketing mix. While a mass market strategy can be described as bending demand to the will of supply, market segmentation has been described as the bending of supply to the will of demand.[1] Consider the modern automobile industry. Henry Ford would not recognize the production and sales of cars today. Consumers can choose from an array of colors, makes, models, and options. Nike has segmented the market for athletic footwear by the type of athletic activity in which the buyer participates. The Nike line consists of running shoes, weight lifting shoes, basketball shoes, racquetball footwear, tennis, golf, hiking, and even walking footwear. This listing does not even provide a full picture of the colors and variations within each athletic footwear category.

While this view describes a *product* change to respond to individual differences, segmentation can be accomplished with any element of the marketing mix. Individuals in a particular market segment would respond in a like way to one or more elements of the marketing mix. Market segmentation strategies usually fall into one of two categories: (1) concentration strategies, or (2) multisegment strategies.

Concentration Strategy

As described previously in Chapter 2, targeting one segment of the market is referred to as a **concentration strategy**. By focusing on just one market segment, a firm is able to tailor its strategy in an attempt to solidify its position in the marketplace. One advantage of a concentration strategy for the smaller firm is that it may allow the business to target a group that may not be attractive to a larger competitor.

The biggest problem with the concentration strategy is what has been referred to as the **majority fallacy**. Organizations, in deciding to concentrate, will sometimes focus on the largest segment of the market in the belief that it represents the greatest revenue and profit potential. Other competitors may also be attracted to this particular segment for the exact same reasons. As a result of its large size and attractiveness to competitors, the largest segment becomes competitively the most intense, and hence, the least profitable one to target.

An organization that follows a concentration strategy must be able to defend its choice of market segment. The company has no other segments upon which to spread its risk if it is unsuccessful. Another limitation to this strategy is that a firm can develop a reputation that identifies it with just one segment of the market, making it difficult to expand its business to serve other segments. For years, Timex has been known as the manufacturer of reliable, inexpensive watches. It might be very difficult, however, for Timex to market a premium-priced watch.

Niche Strategy

A variation of the concentration strategy is referred to as the niche strategy. A **niche** is a very small, specialized market segment with a highly defined set of needs. A **niche strategy** targets this narrow segment with specialized products or services. For example, a clinic could be established to target only wealthy clientele. A niche within this group might include just senior members of governments or royalty. This niche might have highly specialized needs in terms of travel arrangements, dietary requirements, security precautions, and even accommodations. In 1994, several faculty groups from the Harvard Medical School tried targeting wealthy patients in Europe and the Middle East. With the support of tax incentives from the Irish government, a hospital was established in Ireland to woo patients from these regions. Surgery was to be provided by some of the world's best clinicians. Yet, advanced medical skills and technologies in Europe and the Middle East made it difficult to attract this upscale niche. These wealthy consumers did not feel a need to seek quality care outside their own countries.[2]

Multisegment Strategy

In a multisegment strategy, an organization can pursue several market segments with varying mixes. One approach a company can use is **product differentiation**, a strategy of altering one or more marketing mix elements to respond to various wants and needs of different groups. There are several versions of this strategy. In one version of product differentiation, a company can take the same product, and through different advertising campaigns or pricing, position it differently to two different groups.[3] The Geo Storm automobile might be positioned as an economical car for a young married couple starting out, or as a fun car for the college-aged buyer. A second strategy of product differentiation might involve taking two products and marketing them to two different segments. Kaiser Foundation Health Plan of California can offer its traditional closed-panel HMO model in markets familiar with that type of health plan. In other markets, Kaiser might develop a point-of-service plan that allows members to use an out-of-plan physician for an additional copayment or higher deductible.

Selecting Market Segments

Any company that follows a segmentation strategy must identify which market segments to target. Segments should be selected according to the following criteria.

1. A good market segment should be *identifiable,* that is, easily profiled. The more distinctly a segment can be defined, the more efficiently a company can tailor the marketing mix.
2. *Accessibility* is a second criterion. Can the market segment be reached through either distribution or promotion efforts? Do these consumers shop in a particular store, or can they be targeted through a specialized magazine or newspaper? It is easy to target physicians as a group through an array of publications like the *American Medical News* or *The New England Journal of Medicine.* There is no easy promotional medium, however, to access some physician groups, such as the segment of physicians who refer to academic medical centers for tertiary care problems.
3. A third important criterion for selecting a market segment is whether its members are *inclined,* or likely, to buy the product or service. It may be easy to target a market segment of high-income consumers who live within a

particular zip code. If this market segment is not inclined to purchase the service, it is useless to target the marketing mix to them.

4. A fourth concern is whether members of the market segment are *able* to buy the product or service. This criterion speaks to the economic resources of the market. A medical group might develop a prepaid health plan that is very customer-oriented—appointments are never double-scheduled; physicians stay with patients for as long as needed to answer questions, so that the average appointment interval is one hour; and house calls are made upon request. The cost of the plan, however, might be 10 times that of a competing HMO. While the product is desirable, no one can afford to enroll.

5. A fifth criterion for selecting a market segment is that it should be *profitable* to serve.

6. A group's *desirability* is another criterion by which to judge whom to target. There may be some segments that you do not want to serve because they would be counter to your image or inconsistent with the needs or values of other groups who use your services.

7. A seventh criterion that is relevant when an organization appeals to multiple segments is *consistency*. Are the market segments consistent with each other? Attracting diverse market segments is often difficult because one group may buy or use a product that another group finds irrelevant to its own needs.

8. The final criterion is the *availability* of a market segment. Competitors may already be serving the particular targeted segment, making it hard to shift customers' loyalties.

BASES FOR SEGMENTATION

There are a variety of ways in which a market can be segmented. These can be described as sociodemographic, geographic, psychographic, and by usage.

Sociodemographic Segmentation

There are many common social and demographic variables used for market segmentation. Some of the variables that are especially pertinent to health care marketing in the 1990s include age, gender, and ethnicity, among others.

Age

In health care marketing, age segmentation has particular relevancy. A medical group practice might develop a specific communication strategy geared to the needs of its patients' age group. An internist might publish a brochure in a larger type size. Patients needing to make outside phone calls can use telephones with volume controls. Specialized forms could be developed to help patients remember when to take medications. The group practice might even designate one employee as the senior citizen assistance representative who, for example, could help in the filing of insurance forms.

Age segmentation exists in terms of product. Geriatric medicine is a clinical program geared to the elderly. Based on the environmental analysis presented in Chapter 3, members of older age groups respond well to marketing programs targeted for their market segment. In Springfield, Massachusetts, Baystate Medical Center, a large tertiary hospital, has developed a senior class program that offers tours, lectures, screenings, and other free services. Eighteen thousand senior citizens are members. In 1993, the hospital generated $25 million in gross revenues from this market segment.[4]

Gender

Gender segmentation strategies have been apparent in health care for several years. Studies have found that after age 14, women see physicians 25 percent more often than men, and women also have a 15 percent higher hospitalization rate than men.[5] Since the mid-1980s, a service of growing popularity in many hospitals has been women's health programs, as shown in the advertisement for mammograms in Figure 6–1. Research has shown that women in their 30s and 40s are the key health care decision makers for four generations: their own, their children, their parents, and their grandparents.[6] Other research has demonstrated that women are the primary health care decision makers in 75 percent of all households.[7] Women's health services segment the market based on gender in an attempt to package a bundle of clinical services that are important to women and are provided in a convenient fashion.

Ethnicity

In recent years, greater attention has been paid to cultural and ethnic diversity as a variable to consider in market segmentation. In the United States, the growing presence and importance of the Hispanic market has led many marketers to tailor their marketing strategies to reach this group.[8] Lovelace Health Systems, in Albuquerque, New Mexico, hired a consultant to rewrite signs and forms tailored to this ethnic market segment.[9] Many large metropolitan areas have specialized Spanish-language television shows. St. Francis Hospital, in San Francisco, California, has for many years employed a team of Asian translators to assist in dealing with this patient constituency. The hospital promotes these services through specialized Asian media in the Bay Area. FHP Health Care, a national HMO

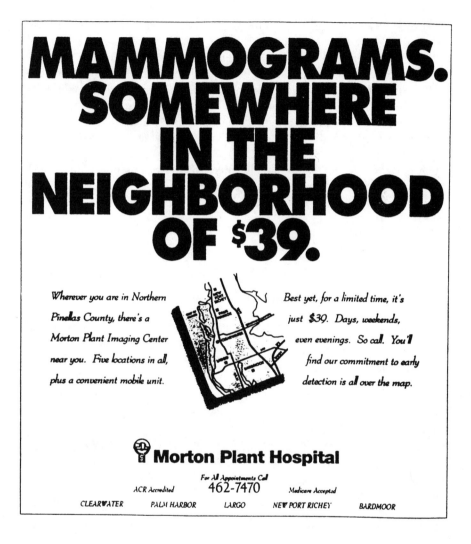

Figure 6–1 Targeting the Women's Marrket. *Source:* Courtesy of Morton Plant HealthCare, Clearwater, Florida.

company based in Fountain Valley, California, has contracted with medical groups who serve Vietnamese and Chinese segments of the population.

In 1993, recognition of cultural and ethnic diversity led the American Medical Association to prepare a monograph on "cultural competence" for physicians. The five key components are:

1. Awareness and acceptance of how cultural differences can affect the delivery of health care.
2. Ability to recognize how one's own culture affects behavior and attitudes.
3. Awareness that misunderstandings and misinterpretations can occur when a provider from one culture interacts with a patient from a different culture.
4. Enough knowledge of each patient's culture to anticipate barriers, plus an awareness that cultures are too complex to understand fully.
5. Ability to adapt and refine one's skills to provide culturally competent care.[10]

Other common sociodemographic variables often used in segmentation strategies include occupation (creating tailored health education programs to particular occupational groups based on the incidence of problems suffered), family status, and education.[11]

Geographic Segmentation

A second major way to segment the market is geographically. Many U.S. manufacturers have found that consumers in different regions of the country have unique preferences for certain food products. Spicier foods, for example, are popular in the Southwest.[12] Japanese-made automobiles have had stronger appeals to consumers on both coasts compared to those in the midwestern parts of the United States.

In health care, geographic segmentation is rarely national; far more often it is regional or local. The major geographic distinctions relevant to health care are urban vs. rural or urban vs. suburban. An urban academic medical center, for example, may pursue a geographic segmentation strategy in attracting patients. In the primary and secondary service areas of the academic medical center, the center may find that it receives few referrals from community physicians. Most of these doctors may admit to their own local hospitals and refer patients to specialists on the staff of these facilities. There may also be a concern among local community physicians that, their patients, once referred to the academic medical center, might become loyal patients of the medical center.

Following a geographic segmentation strategy, then, the academic medical center might open primary care satellites staffed by its own primary care physicians within its primary service area. Outside of the primary and secondary service areas, the medical center may find a stronger referral flow. Physicians in the outlying areas are less concerned about patients going to the academic medical center for routine care, since the medical center is 50 or 100 miles away. In these outlying communities, the academic medical center does not set up primary care satellites. Rather, it establishes a physician relations department to assist with patient referrals from these physicians and to reinforce and encourage their referral pattern. Or, the medical center might set up a referral network. Table 6–1 shows the participants in the Duke Oncology Consortium, which links the Duke University Medical Center cancer program in Durham, North Carolina, with several oncology programs across the South.

For most health care marketing, geographic segmentation allows organizations located in markets with rather heterogeneous factors to tailor a marketing mix on the basis of location.

Psychographic Segmentation

A third major way to segment the market is psychographically, which refers to lifestyle and social class.

Lifestyles

Segmentation by lifestyle is a common approach to segmenting the market. Individuals are grouped based on their behavioral characteristics, attitudes, and opinions. To conduct lifestyle segmentation, marketing researchers profile consumers based on their responses to AIO (attitude, interest, and opinion) statements. An example of some responses to health care–related AIO statements was shown in Chapter 4. Such questions, rated on a scale ranging from "strongly agree" to "strongly disagree" help identify a health-conscious consumer's attitudes, interests, and opinions. A research firm can then match specific demographic characteristics to this profile of a health-conscious consumer in order to more closely profile this market segment.

Table 6–1 Duke Oncology Consortium

	# of New Cancer Patients/Year	# of Beds
Cabarrus Memorial Hospital Concord, N.C.	500	457
Florida Hospital Orlando, Fla.	1,800	1,342
Good Samaritan Medical Center West Palm Beach, Fla.	1,000	341
Lewis Gale Hospital Roanoke, Va.	546	406
Presbyterian Hospital Charlotte, N.C.	2,000	642
St. Joseph's Hospital Asheville, N.C.	1,160	331
Total	**7,006**	**3,519**
Duke University Medical Center Durham, N.C.	3,400	1,125
Grand Total	**10,406**	**4,644**

In Chapter 4, the VALS2™ system of profiling consumers was discussed. This system is a version of psychographic segmentation. The PRIZM system, also described in Chapter 4, is a version of psychographic segmentation that is tied to demographic and geographic segmentation bases. The PRIZM system describes lifestyle profiles of different neighborhoods. A selection of some PRIZM profiles is shown in Table 6–2.

A health care version of psychographic segmentation is being used by Stanford University of Palo Alto, California in conjunction with Consumer Insights, a marketing consulting firm in San Rafael, California. The company uses a 25-question survey and a mathematical algorithm to classify consumers into nine market segments, called Profiles of Attitudes Toward Healthcare (PATH). Segments are given names such as "clinic cynics" and "ready users." Stanford University identified psychographic segments in its market area and is reshaping its advertising strategy to respond to these groups.[13]

Social Class

Social class is included in the Chapter 4 discussion of consumer behavior. It is often used as a basis for psychographic segmentation. Individuals within certain social classes hold similar attitudes and have similar purchasing patterns. Many advertisements are often directed to particular social classes in their appeal for products.

Table 6–2 Selected PRIZM Profiles

	% of U.S. Households
Blue-Blood Estates: America's wealthiest neighborhoods	1.1
Norma Rae–Ville: Lower middle-class mill towns and industrial suburbs, primarily in the South	2.3
Gray Power: Upper middle-class retirement communities	2.9
Single City Blues: Downscale, urban, singles districts	3.3
Towns and Gowns: America's college towns	1.2
Furs and Station Wagons: New money in metropolitan bedroom suburbs	3.2
Heavy Industry: Lower working-class districts in the nation's older industrial cities	2.8

Source: Reprinted from *Clustering of America* by M.J. Weiss, pp. 4–5, with permission of Harper Collins, © 1989.

Usage Segmentation

The last major category for segmentation is grouping people based on product usage or purchase. Of all the bases for segmentation, usage segmentation may be the most valuable. This approach segments the market based on the percentage of a product that consumers buy or a service that they use. Since the ultimate goal of any marketing strategy is to affect a consumer's purchase decision, segmenting based on purchase can relate marketing strategy directly to consumer actions. There are several ways in which this can be done: usage rates, type of usage, brand loyalty, and benefit segmentation.

Usage Rates

One of the more interesting bases for segmentation that are relevant for health care include usage rates. Table 6–3 describes some usage rates for three product categories: colas, beer, and canned hash. Within marketing, a phenomenon called the **heavy half consumer** has been identified, in which a small group of consumers account for a disproportionate amount of a product's sales. Sometimes this is referred to as the 80/20 rule: Eighty percent of a product's sales are accounted for by 20 percent of the people who purchase the product.

While a heavy half segment does not mean that the group always must purchase 80 percent of a product's sales, this segment does account for a disproportionate percentage of the sales relative to its size in the total market.

Table 6–3 The Heavy Half Consumer

	Nonusers	Medium Users	Heavy Users
Colas			
	P-22%	P-39%	P-39%
	C-0%	C-10%	C-90%
Beer			
	P-67%	P-16%	P-17%
	C-0%	C-12%	C-88%
Canned Hash			
	P-68%	P-16%	P-16%
	C-0%	C-14%	C-86%

Note: P=People; C=Total Consumption of product for this group.

Table 6–3 displays data indicating the existence of a heavy half segment across three product categories: colas, beer, and canned hash. Looking at the far right-hand column, one can see that 39 percent of consumers buy 90 percent of all the soft drinks sold. Here is an instance where a small (39%) segment of the market accounts for a disproportionate percent of product consumption. The heavy half segments are more dramatic for beer and canned hash. Seventeen percent of all people account for 88 percent of all beer consumed, and 16 percent consume 86 percent of all the canned hash sold.

A similar case for heavy half segments can be made within health care. Many HMOs, for example, have experienced heavy utilization by a small segment of their subscriber panel. A small percentage of the primary care physicians who refer to a specialty group account for a disproportionate share of all referrals.

Heavy half segmentation has some important marketing implications. Consider the heavy half segment for beer (i.e., the 17 percent that consumes 88 percent of all beer sold). The major marketing objective of a beer company is to maintain its loyalty. No changes in the product or service should be made until it is pretested with these heavy half purchasers. For the medium users (the 16 percent of the market that consumes 12 percent of all beer sold), a brewer's marketing objective is different. The goal here is to increase purchases in this group. A beer brewery may try to convince these individuals that ordering a fine imported beer—as opposed to ordering a glass of fine Chardonnay— will imply they are sophisticated consumers. A company might use a slogan such as, "Come to think of it, I'll have a Heineken!" Finally, there is the third group of nonusers. Sixty-seven percent of consumers do not buy any beer. With a nonuser group, marketing research is necessary to determine why people do not use a product. Typically, there are two subsegments within this population. Some people do not buy beer because they do not like it. For a beer company, little can be done with this segment. Some people, however, do not purchase beer, but they have never tried it. The key here is to determine a legal (for an alcoholic beverage company) way for this segment to sample beer.

Heavy half segments also exist within health care. An HMO can examine their utilization level by subscriber and will, most likely, find the existence of this phenomenon. Twenty or 30 percent of the HMO's subscribers may account for a disproportionate share of all subscriber utilization. Similarly, a specialist whose business is primarily derived from primary care doctors' referrals might experience that 50 or 60 percent of all their referrals are derived from a much smaller percentage of all the doctors who refer to them.

Consider the implications of heavy half segmentation in health care. The strategies and marketing objectives differ in a fee-for-service vs. a managed care model. In a fee-for-service setting, the objectives are similar to the beer company. A specialist who has a heavy half segment of primary care physician referrals wants to maintain the loyalty of that group. No changes will be made regarding how patient referrals are handled unless first checked with the loyal users. The worst strategy would be to change the service in response to a few complaints, only to find that the change is unpopular among the heavy half segment.

With the middle group, marketing strategy must examine ways to increase their referrals. Does this mean improving access? Providing better feedback? Expanding the type of specialties represented in the group? In a particular service area, a specialist might find a large number of physicians who do not refer at all to the medical practice. What must be determined is which physicians don't refer because they are satisfied with their present referral source. Some portion of the physicians who do not refer are in this group because they are unfamiliar with the practice or the physicians within the group. This segment is one to which a very directed promotional strategy effort must be developed.

To increase referrals and attract referrals from physicians who presently do not use the Cleveland Clinic Foundation, this organization has established the Cleveland Clinic CompreCare Affiliate program. Open to physicians who are not affiliated with the Cleveland Clinic Foundation, this program has no cost to participating physicians or minimum referral requirements. Among other benefits, the program provides a monthly newsletter, a toll-free telephone line for scheduling appointments, a guarantee regarding information feedback, and continuing medical education courses. The Foundation has tracked referrals from physicians who participate in the CompreCare program and found a 77 percent increase among those who had not referred prior to the incentive program, and a 34 percent increase among medium referrers (one to six patients a year). The third group included physicians who had been heavy previous referrers.[14]

This heavy half scenario and related objectives change dramatically in a managed care setting. In a managed care model, the objective is to identify the heavy users of health services and to determine how to reduce their demand. For example, an HMO might profile the heavy users to determine whether there are any consistent usage patterns. This might lead to some intervention or more thorough screening prior to appointment scheduling. It also might require shifting certain deductible requirements to minimize excessive use. The middle users are, for most managed care plans, the individuals who follow standard levels of use and requirements. It is the last group, the nonusers among the subscriber pool, which is the financial lifeblood of the managed care plan. For this segment of the market, the managed care plan must develop retention strategies to ensure that these nonusers see value in the product that they purchased.

For traditional marketers, there are some commercial sources available to help them in profiling heavy half users, along with their media habits. Table 6–4 displays a sample from a media usage database published by Simmons Market Research of Chicago, Illinois. This source provides an overview of heavy half users for a wide variety of product categories. This sample page shows the breakdown for female users of cold syrup and the publications that these indivi-

Table 6–4 Media Usage by Usage Segments: Cold Syrups

	All Users				Heavy Users 2 Times a Day or More				Light Users Once a Day or Less Often			
Total U.S. '000	A '000	B % Down	C Across %	D Index	A '000	B % Down	C Across %	D Index	A '000	B % Down	C Across %	D Index
94655	49105	100.0	51.9	100	29371	100.0	31.0	100	19734	100.0	20.8	100

	A '000	B % Down	C Across %	D Index	A '000	B % Down	C Across %	D Index	A '000	B % Down	C Across %	D Index
Newsweek	4025	8.2	53.5	103	2546	8.7	33.9	109	1479	7.5	19.7	94
The N.Y. Times Daily Edition	600	1.2	41.4	80	412	1.4	28.5	92	188	1.0	13.0	62
The N.Y. Times Magazine	730	1.5	45.3	87	506	1.7	31.4	101	224	1.1	13.9	67
Omni	415	0.8	48.4	93	296	1.0	34.5	111	120	0.6	14.0	67
1,001 Home Ideas	1747	3.6	64.3	124	1047	3.6	38.5	124	700	3.5	25.8	124
Organic Gardening	765	1.6	55.7	107	525	1.8	38.2	123	240	1.2	17.5	84
Outdoor Life	883	1.8	52.9	102	472	1.6	28.3	91	411	2.1	24.6	118
Parade Magazine	18790	38.3	51.5	99	11517	39.2	31.5	102	7273	36.9	19.9	96
Parents	2982	6.1	57.6	111	1723	5.9	33.3	107	1258	6.4	24.3	116
People	10010	20.4	53.4	103	5943	20.2	31.7	102	4067	20.6	21.7	104
Playboy	617	1.3	61.6	119	343	1.2	34.3	110	274	1.4	27.4	131
Popular Mechanics	269	0.5	54.3	105	171	0.6	34.5	111	98	0.5	19.8	95
Popular Science	414	0.8	53.5	103	265	0.9	34.2	110	149	0.8	19.3	92
Prevention	2261	4.6	48.7	94	1327	4.5	28.6	92	934	4.7	20.1	96
Psychology Today	976	2.0	57.5	111	558	1.9	32.9	106	418	2.1	24.6	118
Reader's Digest	10780	22.0	52.5	101	6589	22.4	32.1	103	4191	21.2	20.4	98
Redbook	5102	10.4	54.0	104	3084	10.5	32.6	105	2018	10.2	21.4	102
Road & Track	119	0.2	45.9	89	78	0.3	30.1	97	41	0.2	15.8	76
Rolling Stone	1130	2.3	52.4	101	713	2.4	33.1	107	417	2.1	19.3	93
Scientific American	225	0.5	41.4	80	158	0.5	29.1	94	67	0.3	12.3	59

(Total U.S. '000 column values: Newsweek 7521; The N.Y. Times Daily Edition 1448; The N.Y. Times Magazine 1610; Omni 858; 1,001 Home Ideas 2716; Organic Gardening 1373; Outdoor Life 1669; Parade Magazine 36507; Parents 5180; People 18747; Playboy 1001; Popular Mechanics 495; Popular Science 774; Prevention 4647; Psychology Today 1696; Reader's Digest 20546; Redbook 9446; Road & Track 259; Rolling Stone 2157; Scientific American 543)

continues

Table 6-4 continued

	Total U.S. '000	All Users				Heavy Users 2 Times a Day or More				Light Users Once a Day or Less Often			
		A '000	B % Down	C % Across	D Index	A '000	B % Down	C % Across	D Index	A '000	B % Down	C % Across	D Index
Self	2978	1668	3.4	56.0	108	984	3.4	33.0	106	684	3.5	23.0	110
Seventeen	2886	1513	3.1	52.4	101	927	3.2	32.1	104	586	3.0	20.3	97
Shape	1609	858	1.7	53.3	103	616	2.1	38.3	123	242	1.2	15.0	72
Ski	387	223	0.5	57.6	111	107	0.4	27.6	89	116	0.6	30.0	144
Skiing	470	338	0.7	71.9	139	193	0.7	41.1	132	145	0.7	30.9	148
Smithsonian	3134	1578	3.2	50.4	97	1024	3.5	32.7	105	554	2.8	17.7	85
Soap Opera Digest	3950	2316	4.7	58.6	113	1254	4.3	31.7	102	1062	5.4	26.9	129
Southern Living	5281	2933	6.0	55.5	107	1739	5.9	32.9	106	1194	6.1	22.6	108
Sport	200	148	0.3	74.0	143	69	0.2	34.5	111	79	0.4	39.5	189
The Sporting News	329	196	0.4	59.6	115	112	0.4	34.0	110	84	0.4	25.5	122
Sports Afield	391	231	0.5	59.1	114	169	0.6	43.2	139	63	0.3	16.1	77
Sports Illustrated	4030	2205	4.5	54.7	105	1342	4.6	33.3	107	863	4.4	21.4	103
Star	7721	3883	7.9	50.3	97	2380	8.1	30.8	99	1503	7.6	19.5	93
Sunday Magazine Network	22054	11517	23.5	52.2	101	7209	24.5	32.7	105	4308	21.8	19.5	94
Sunset	2198	956	1.9	43.5	84	589	2.0	26.8	86	367	1.9	16.7	80
TV Guide	22342	12686	25.8	56.8	109	7800	26.6	34.9	113	4886	24.8	21.9	105
Tennis	470	303	0.6	64.5	124	167	0.6	35.5	115	135	0.7	28.7	138
Time	9171	4794	9.8	52.3	101	2970	10.1	32.4	104	1823	9.2	19.9	95
Travel & Leisure	1174	631	1.3	53.7	104	448	1.5	38.2	123	183	0.9	15.6	75
True Story	3354	1908	3.9	56.9	110	1108	3.8	33.0	106	800	4.1	23.9	114
USA Today	2168	1266	2.6	58.4	113	762	2.6	35.1	113	504	2.6	23.2	112
USA Weekend	16198	8201	16.7	50.6	98	4958	16.9	30.6	99	3244	16.4	20.0	96
U.S. News & World Report	4705	2407	4.9	51.2	99	1440	4.9	30.6	99	967	4.9	20.6	99

Table 6–4 continued

	Total U.S. '000	All Users				Heavy Users 2 Times a Day or More				Light Users Once a Day or Less Often			
		A '000	B % Down	C Across %	D Index	A '000	B % Down	C Across %	D Index	A '000	B % Down	C Across %	D Index
US	3124	1592	3.2	51.0	98	955	3.3	30.6	99	636	3.2	20.4	98
Vanity Fair	1270	641	1.3	50.5	97	370	1.3	29.1	94	271	1.4	21.3	102
Vogue	4910	2758	5.6	56.2	108	1486	5.1	30.3	98	1272	6.4	25.9	124
Wall Street Journal	1456	839	1.7	57.6	111	537	1.8	36.9	119	302	1.5	20.7	99
The Washington Post Magazine	1237	740	1.5	59.8	115	443	1.5	35.8	115	297	1.5	24.0	115
Weight Watchers	2266	1255	2.6	55.4	107	751	2.6	33.1	107	503	2.5	22.2	106
Woman's Day	13653	7369	15.0	54.0	104	4485	15.3	32.8	106	2883	14.6	21.1	101
Woman's World	5363	2970	6.0	55.4	107	1741	5.9	32.5	105	1229	6.2	22.9	110
Workbench	625	403	0.8	64.5	124	262	0.9	41.9	135	141	0.7	22.6	108
Working Mother	1606	1068	2.2	66.5	128	650	2.2	40.5	130	418	2.1	26.0	125
Working Woman	2615	1519	3.1	58.1	112	863	2.9	33.0	106	656	3.3	25.1	120
Wrk Mother/Wrk Woman (Gross)	4221	2587	5.3	61.3	118	1512	5.1	35.8	115	1074	5.4	25.4	122
Yankee	1122	677	1.4	60.3	116	420	1.4	37.4	121	257	1.3	22.9	110
Read Any Magazine (Msrd)	80579	42215	86.0	52.4	101	25577	87.1	31.7	102	16638	84.3	20.6	99
Daily Newspapers													
Net One Day Reach	57292	29375	59.8	51.3	99	17986	61.2	31.4	101	11389	57.7	19.9	95
Read Only One	47242	24085	49.0	51.0	98	14656	49.9	31.0	100	9429	47.8	20.0	96
Read Two or More	10050	5290	10.8	52.6	101	3330	11.3	33.1	107	1960	9.9	19.5	94
Weekend/Sunday Newspapers													
Net One Day Reach	63490	32386	66.0	51.0	98	19724	67.2	31.1	100	12662	64.2	19.9	96
Read Only One	57010	29073	59.2	51.0	98	17645	60.1	31.0	100	11427	57.9	20.0	96
Read Two or More	6480	3314	6.7	51.1	99	2078	7.1	32.1	103	1235	6.3	19.1	91

Source: Reprinted from *The 1990 Study of Media and Markets*, Vol. P–25, with permission of Simmons Market Research, Chicago, Illinois, © 1990.

duals tend to read. Simmons provides this breakdown for heavy, medium, and light user groups.

Type of Usage

A second segmentation based on usage is type of usage, or how the product is used.[15] Orange juice manufacturers can develop different marketing mix strategies geared to different types of usage segments. Orange juice can be used as a breakfast drink, a mixer for alcoholic beverages, or as an alternative to other beverages. The marketing mix strategies will be tailored specifically for each of these segments. For the breakfast drink market, the product needs to be distributed in grocery stores; advertisements should show it being used in the morning; and the pricing should compare to other morning drinks, such as grapefruit juice. For the alcoholic beverage mix segment, the distribution strategy must shift to liquor stores. The alternative beverage segment might require a packaging change. For instance, orange juice can be packaged in single-serving cans or juice boxes for children's lunches. Vending machine distribution also becomes a major element of this marketing mix strategy.

Johnson & Johnson has used a similar usage segmentation appeal for its Retin-A product. Originally prescribed by dermatologists as an acne medication, Retin-A's usage broadened in 1988 with the publication in the *Journal of the American Medical Association* of a study reporting Retin-A's benefits for improving wrinkles in sun-damaged skin.[16] UpJohn has found a similar usage segment for its product, minoxidil. Long used as a prescription medication for the treatment of hypertension, minoxidil was also found to be effective as a topical ointment for the treatment of some forms of baldness. Known commercially as Rogaine®, this product was subsequently launched to a very different usage segment, as shown in Figure 6–2.

Brand Loyalty

A third usage segment categorizes consumers by their level of brand loyalty or the degree to which they purchase or use the same brand of product or service. Some consumers who repeatedly use the same multispecialty group practice for all their medical care can be described as *hard core loyal*. Some consumers might occasionally use the medical group for some services, and use practitioners outside the group for different clinical needs. These individuals might be termed *split loyalists*. A third group, defined as *switchers*, try different facilities for care. Profiling these segments helps a medical group develop a better understanding of who belongs to a respective target market. This profiling can assist in developing strategies for increasing the loyalties of the *split loyalty* segment. For example, McStravic has suggested targeting loyal hospital users with newsletters, birthday cards, health tips, and update reports to reinforce positive impressions.[17]

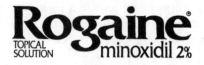

The good news is there's one product that's proven to grow hair...

Rogaine®
TOPICAL SOLUTION minoxidil 2%

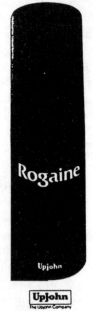

Rogaine is the *only* product that's ever been proven to grow hair. *Rogaine* is made by The Upjohn Company and its active ingredient is minoxidil. *Rogaine* has been available by a doctor's prescription since September of 1988 for male pattern baldness of the crown.

The one and only, according to the Food and Drug Administration (FDA).

You may have read in the news lately about other products that claim to grow hair or prevent hair loss.

A recent ruling by the FDA recognized that only *Rogaine* has been proven to be effective and safe for hair growth. Further, the FDA stated that the ingredients in all other products that say they grow hair or prevent hair loss are "ineffective." It recommended that "these products be eliminated from the . . . market."

Rogaine grows hair for a good percentage of men.

Your doctor will help you determine how good a candidate you are for treatment with *Rogaine*. Each individual responds differently.

In medical tests conducted by doctors on men throughout the United States over a twelve-month period, it was proven that

© 1989 The Upjohn Company   J 2098

Rogaine grew hair. 39% had moderate to dense regrowth, 37% had minimal regrowth, 13% grew soft, downy, colorless hair that was barely visible, and 11% had no regrowth. (In these same medical tests, the men using *Rogaine* evaluated their moderate to dense regrowth at an even higher rate, 48%).

Few of the men in the tests reported side effects. The most common side effect of *Rogaine* was itching of the scalp, which occurred in 5% of the men.

Generally, it takes four months of use before there is evidence of regrowth.

Nearly two million men have started using *Rogaine*. Should you?

More and more doctors are confidently prescribing *Rogaine* for more and more men every day.

If the FDA ruling hasn't convinced you to try it, consider this fact: two million men have tried it already.

It just might work for you.

So call your doctor for an appointment. Or, for more information, a list of doctors near you, and a certificate worth $10 as an incentive to visit your doctor (sorry, this offer is available for men only), call the toll free number below.

1-800-253-7300, ext. 201.

For a summary of product information, see adjoining page.

Upjohn
The Upjohn Company

Figure 6–2 Rogaine® Advertisement. *Source:* The Upjohn Company, Kalamazoo, Michigan, copyright © 1989.

Benefit Segmentation

A final basis for usage segmentation is **benefit segmentation**, the grouping of people based on the benefits sought from the product.[18] To implement this approach, an organization must understand what benefit customers are seeking from the product purchase, and then must analyze the existing brands available on the market. This process can help to identify benefit segments not presently being served. Figure 6–3 displays a benefit segmentation approach for the toothpaste market. Three major benefit segments are identified. One segment prefers decay prevention in their toothpaste, a second wants to improve their cosmetic appearance, while the third group prefers taste. To appeal to each of these segments, there are distinct product ingredients. A fluoride will provide for decay prevention, an abrasive improves the whitening of teeth for cosmetic value, and adding flavoring targets the taste-benefit segment. As Figure 6–3 shows, some major brands have been positioned for each benefit segment. Crest is best known for its decay prevention properties. Ultra Brite has long touted what it will do to brighten a person's smile, and AIM is positioned for taste. An interesting addition to the competition among toothpaste brands has been the appearance of Mentadent by Lever Brothers, an international consumer products company in New York. Mentadent touts its decay prevention *and* tooth whitening properties. The product package shows two separate streams of toothpaste on a person's brush. Clearly, Lever Brothers is trying to appeal to two benefit segments, the decay prevention and cosmetic segments.

A similar benefit segmentation approach has been proposed for the preventive health care market. John and Miaoulis, two academic health care marketing researchers, conducted an exploratory study with 175 consumers. While conducting in-depth interviews, the researchers identified six segments, shown in Table 6–5. This representation suggests important implications for vitamin marketers in targeting the hypochondriac segment where brand preference rather than product utility is the key, since this is a proactive group of purchasers. The self-

Benefits/ingredients	fluoride	abrasive	flavoring
decay prevention	Crest		
	Mentadent		
cosmetic		Ultra Brite	
taste			AIM

Figure 6–3 Benefit Segmentation of the Toothpaste Market

Table 6–5 Preventive Health Care Benefit Segments

Name of Segment	Health Seekers	Followers	Band-Aiders	Do Not Bug Me	Hypochondriacs	Self-Sufficient
Benefits sought	Long life, continued good health.	Want someone else to be concerned about their health, looking for guidance.	Recognition for being hard workers and rarely sick.	Relief from everyday pressures and tensions. Looking for ways to cope with problems.	Tremendous need for recognition, want people to notice them and to assure them that they are okay.	Self-reliance. Home remedies do the job.
Category beliefs	Preventive medical services are the key to a longer and healthier life.	Not sure whether preventive services can deliver what they offer, best to follow the crowd.	Preventive care is for other people who get sick a lot. When your time is up, it's up!	Needs to smoke, eat, etc. to deal with tension. It is just too tough to quit.	Do not wait—see the doctor right away. Must get all possible medical attention to make sure everything is okay.	I can take care of myself. Don't trust doctors and hospitals.
Health services sought	Very broad range of services; nutritional counseling, exercise programs, hypertension tests, dental, etc.	Generally the annual physical; await symptoms before seeking medical services.	Primary treatment oriented; seek only essential preventive services, e.g., vaccinations.	Annual physical.	Any and all.	Home remedies and over-the-counter drugs.
Degree of participation	High, very active, continuous.	Sporadic.	Minimal.	Seldom.	Excessive.	Nonparticipation in institutional medicine.

continues

Table 6-5 continued

Name of Segment	Health Seekers	Followers	Band-Aiders	Do Not Bug Me	Hypochondriacs	Self-Sufficient
Occasions of use	Corresponds to particular health needs at various life stages.	Depends on the degree of persuasiveness of the preventive service.	Following work-inhibiting symptoms, accidents, etc.	To keep employer and/or family off his/her back.	Symptom-of-the-day club members.	Only have remedies.
Personality/lifestyle	Rational, open-minded, appreciates "savings" from preventive services. Plan ahead, body conscious.	Other-directed, highly impressionable by "knowledgeable others."	Family-oriented, set in ways; not impressed by wonders of science.	Easygoing, gregarious on the outside; anxious and very nervous on the inside.	Dependent and lacking self-confidence. Seeks attention from others.	Independent, previous bad experiences with doctors.

Source: Reprinted from John, J., and Miaoulis, G., A Model for Understanding Benefit Segmentation in Preventive Health Care, *Health Care Management Review*, Vol. 17, No. 2, pp. 24–25, Aspen Publishers, Inc., © 1992.

sufficient segment may be a potential target market for health clubs, if these organizations position themselves correctly. Seen as a means to avoid using the medical system, health clubs could attract the self-sufficient market segment.[19]

SEGMENTING BUSINESS MARKETS

For the remainder of the 1990s and beyond, health care organizations will continue directing their marketing strategies and products to employers and business organizations of all sizes. Segmenting of industrial markets requires different perspectives than segmenting of consumer markets. Four broad classifications might be considered for business markets: demographics, operating variables, purchasing approaches, and usage requirements.

Demographics

Business demographics consist of variables such as size of the company (in terms of revenue or number of employees), industry type, and customer location.

Size of Company

Size of company is a particularly relevant variable for health care organization segmentation. For example, small companies have different price sensitivities, as well as clinical needs, for occupational medicine contracts than large companies do. A small company might also require the assistance of a third-party administrator in the analysis of alternative health care plans, or stop-loss insurance as it considers health coverage options for its employees. Focusing on the smaller business segment was the approach of the Group Health Cooperative of Puget Sound, in Seattle, Washington, when it developed its "Options" program. Targeted to companies with less than 500 employees, the program allowed small companies to choose from an array of health care options typically available to larger firms. Through Options, companies could offer employees an open-ended plan with an HMO component. This variation allowed employees a choice of physicians. These smaller firms also could choose deductibles and copayment levels for the indemnity component.[20]

Industry Type

Industry type is a valuable segmentation variable. The federal government provides a classification scheme referred to as the **Standard Industrial Classification (SIC) Code**. The SIC system groups organizations based on their major business activity or the major service or product that firms provide. The SIC system provides a way for health care organizations to identify the SIC codes of the businesses it is trying to target, and possibly to identify or group them according to similar product or clinical needs. While the SIC codes are a useful way to access data collected on company segments, there are some limitations to their usefulness. First, the government assigns each company only one particular SIC designation. For large companies that engage in several business areas, the diversity that exists within the company will be lost by this classification method. Second, the codes are not available for every industry within every geographical area. The federal government will not reveal data when two or fewer organizations exist with a particular classification code within a specific geographic area.

Customer Location

Customer location is a third useful segmentation scheme. A hospital may provide off-site services, such as laboratory or minor emergency care, in locations where its major business customers are located.

Operating Variables

A second manner in which companies might be segmented is by operating variables, which include company technology, product use, and customer capabilities.

Technology

The technology that a company utilizes in its own business often heavily affects its own particular buying needs. For example, a company that is a sophisticated technical service business might employ a large number of highly educated consumers. Its work force's medical needs might involve more psychosocial elements compared to medical interventions required by a firm engaged in the manufacture of steel fire escapes. This latter firm would have a work force that engages in a significant amount of heavy lifting. This work force also would probably have a lower educational level. Prior research in health care has shown that health status is correlated to educational level. Employees of the steel plant might require more health education seminars, such as smoking cessation clinics or dietary intervention, to improve their health status.

Product Use

A second operating variable on which segmentation is based is product use. Companies that use a similar product or service generally have other characteristics in common. For example, an HMO might target companies that offer to their employees the same product or indemnity plan from the HMO's competitor. This analysis provides insight into which factors result or contribute to the buying decision. Identifying a segment of customers who purchase particular health care products or services from a weaker competitor can also provide a target group from which to generate additional revenue.

Customer Capabilities

Analyzing the distinct capabilities or position of companies can result in defined market segments. For example, small companies might have no in-house medical director to assist in analyzing medical plans. Such companies represent a segment receptive to contract management strategies to assist in plan selection. Other companies might not have an in-house physician to assist in job-related injuries. A medical group could provide on-site clinical assistance.

Purchasing Approaches

A third way to segment business markets is to classify companies by the way they make their purchasing decisions.

Purchasing Procedures

Companies differ in terms of the procedures they employ in dealing with sellers. The customer's purchasing process should be a defining consideration in setting up the marketing strategy to target the prospective company. Some businesses approach the health care buying decision through contracts, others mix that approach with a traditional insurance approach. In segmenting by the way companies make purchases, a health care provider might have to develop a range of possible responses, as shown in Figure 6–4. A contractually dominant buyer might be a preferred provider organization (PPO) while a noncontractual buyer is the traditional corporate purchaser. The health care buying market is moving increasingly toward a contractually dominant setting. If buyers selectively purchase, or carve out, coverage of certain clinical areas, strategic business units would have to be established to compete for service-specific contracts.[21]

Purchasing Criteria

Most companies have some purchasing criteria by which they evaluate vendor bids. Some firms have explicit criteria that are published and made available to prospective sellers, while other companies have more subjective criteria. These purchasing criteria are similar to the benefit segmentation described with consumers. Some firms might emphasize the plan's cost as their primary criterion, while

MARKET STRUCTURE

	Bundled dominant	Mixed	Discrete dominant
Noncontractual dominant	Develop broad service and general marketing capabilities.	Offer a midrange of services, but focus on certain specialties. Target marketing efforts to general population and specific target groups.	Offer a narrow range of specialty services. Target marketing efforts. Strongly coordinate marketing and production functions.
Mixed	Develop broad service capability. Target marketing efforts to general population, employers, third parties, and enrollees.	Offer a midrange of services, but focus on certain specialties. Target marketing efforts to general population, target groups, employers, third parties, employees, patients, potential patients, and enrollees.	Offer a narrow range of specialty services. Target marketing efforts to patients and potential patients, employers, and third parties. Strongly coordinate marketing and production functions.
Contractual dominant	Develop broad service capability. Target marketing efforts primarily to employers, third parties, and enrollees.	Offer a midrange of services, but focus on certain specialties. Target market efforts primarily to employers, third parties, patients, potential patients, and enrollees.	Offer a narrow range of specialty services. Target marketing efforts primarily to patients, potential patients, and third parties. Set up strategic business units.

CONTRACTUAL ARRANGEMENT

Figure 6-4 Purchase Procedure Segmentation. *Source:* Product Lines in a Complex Marketplace: Matching Organizational Strategy to Buyer Behavior, *Health Care Management Review*, Vol. 15, No. 2, p. 13, Aspen Publishers, Inc., © 1992.

others consider employee satisfaction relative to the plan's cost. Within purchasing criteria, some employers have established health care performance criteria by which to judge alternative health plans. As a response to some of these concerns, for example, US Healthcare, a publicly traded HMO based in Philadelphia, Pennsylvania, is developing its own report card on its physicians. This information can be made available to subscribers, as well as to prospective customer businesses to show that the provider is assessing its own performance and can demonstrate it to the buyer. Segmenting the market by purchasing criteria allows for a more tailored marketing mix strategy.

In health care, purchasing criteria of growing importance are the service characteristics demanded by the buyer. Company needs vary regarding how they expect or desire their particular account (and those of their employees) to be serviced by a health care organization.

Usage Segmentation

Similar to consumers, companies can also be segmented, based on usage factors, which can include variables such as the volume of purchase, frequency of purchase, or the application. For the most part, these are similar to previously described consumer usage variables. Again, it is crucial to consider that, just like consumers, organizations also can represent a heavy half segment. The same issues and marketing objectives are also relevant in industrial segmentation strategies.

THE HEURISTICS OF SEGMENTATION

Described within this chapter were several possible methods for segmenting the market, whether targeting individuals or companies. Health care marketers should decide what is the most helpful way to segment, as well as determine how these alternative methods relate to each other. Health care marketers need to recognize that, by segmenting, provider organizations are trying to produce a differential response from the market segment as opposed to the mass market. In other words, if segmenting the market and tailoring the marketing mix to particular consumers has no effect on purchase consumption, then there is no value to segmenting. To know that there are large hospitals and small hospitals relative to bed size is to describe segments demographically. If this demographic segmentation scheme, however, cannot be related to a purchase difference, then it is purely descriptive, and irrelevant to marketing strategy. If, however, larger hospitals have different purchasing criteria, and separate purchasing managers, and CEOs who frequently read a particular trade publication more often than CEOs from small hospitals, then marketing segmentation strategy can affect usage and purchases.

Figure 6–5 presents a hierarchy of the various segmentation schemes discussed within this chapter. The best level of market segmentation is represented on the far right-hand side of this figure—actual purchase. It is actual purchase that the marketer wants to affect. As one moves from right to left, each successive segmentation approach is less accurate in terms of predicting how the market segment behaves. From a marketing strategy perspective, it is best to know the consumer at each point on this hierarchy.

For example, it would be valuable to describe the market segments according to their choice of an indemnity plan and a managed care option. It would also help the marketer to know their product preferences regarding health care coverage and their brand preferences. In terms of product design and positioning, knowing the product benefits would be invaluable. To develop effective promotional material, as well as possible product features, lifestyle factors would be useful input. Demographics provide the final descriptive characteristics of the market.

Consider working from right to left within the figure. Only knowing the gender or age range of the market segments would be of limited help in designing an attractive HMO package of services. Some inferences could certainly be made for certain age groups. If, in addition to demographics, a company also had lifestyle and psychographic profiles of customers, it could design a better program. For example, the HMO might decide to offer health club benefits.

If there is a tangible rating of product benefits, then the intended product can be designed to resemble more closely the desired product. Brand name preferences can assist in knowing whether the product can be sold under the medical group's name or whether it should assume a different branding strategy. How likely the consumer is to purchase the described product is the next best way to predict behavior, but actual purchase is the best.

These heuristics also provide the rationale for increasing company use of purchase history to define market segments. In many supermarkets today, custom-

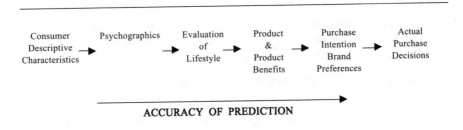

Figure 6–5 Segmentation Heuristics of Purchase

ers are provided with their own ID code, which they may present upon checking out. Consumers receive incentives, such as automatic discounts, if the card is displayed. This also allows for purchase histories to be recorded. These data can be sold to companies to analyze market segments. Customers can be grouped based on who purchased a product during a special promotion. Similar profiling characteristics can be identified to tailor future marketing mix strategies.

CONCLUSIONS

Market segmentation is a common approach used by traditional businesses. Yet, for many years, the health care industry operated close to the dictum of Henry Ford, "You can have health care any way you want, providing it is the one way we deliver it." Segmentation strategies have taken hold, with the realization that the more tailored the marketing strategy is to subgroups within the population, the greater the resulting sales and customers.

KEY TERMS

Market Segmentation
Concentration Strategy
Majority Fallacy
Niche
Niche Strategy

Product Differentiation
Heavy Half Consumer
Benefit Segmentation
Standard Industrial Classification (SIC) Code

CHAPTER SUMMARY

1. *In a mass marketing strategy, the marketing mix is designed to appeal to the broadest market, while in a market segmentation approach, the marketing mix is designed to appeal to subgroups of consumers.*

2. *In following a concentration strategy of targeting only one segment, an organization should not focus only on the largest segment, since competitive intensity can render this segment the least profitable.*

3. *In selecting from multiple market segments, there are several criteria to consider: Segments should be identifiable, accessible, inclined to buy, able to buy, profitable, desirable, consistent, and available.*

4. *Markets can be segmented sociodemographically, geographically, psychographically, and by usage.*

5. *In usage segmentation, it is important to identify the heavy half consumer who purchases a disproportionate share of a product, or who accounts for a disproportionate amount of a service's volume.*

6. As health care moves from a fee-for-service to a managed care environment, the implications are significant in terms of heavy half segmentation. The organization's focus moves from maintaining the heavy half users to keeping the low users and nonusers of the prepaid plan.

7. Business markets can also be segmented by several criteria. The federal government has developed the Standard Industrial Classification (SIC) coding system, which is a common basis for industrial segmentation.

8. As corporations play an increasingly important role in health care purchases, health care organizations may need to segment them by purchase procedures or purchase criteria.

9. There is a heuristic method to segmentation approaches that moves from purely descriptive measures, such as demographics, to actual purchase, such as usage.

10. The ultimate purpose of segmentation is to tailor an organization's marketing mix with the intent of positively affecting consumer behavior. If segmentation does not differentially affect this response, there is little value to segmenting the market on that particular criterion.

CHAPTER PROBLEMS

1. Assume that a multispecialty medical group has decided to segment the market in the community by income level. The group has decided to target a small niche of middle-aged, white-collar professionals who are married, with both spouses working outside the home. How might this medical group tailor its marketing mix to appeal to this segment?

2. A women's health clinic has recognized the need to segment its market. Identify three bases by which this clinic might segment the female market, and identify the manner in which the "product" component of the marketing mix would change in light of the segmentation base used.

3. Examine the benefit segmentation scheme shown in Table 6–5. In what ways might an HMO new to a community try to capture the "follower" segment? How would this strategy differ in trying to attract the "health seekers"?

4. A neurology group practice recently analyzed its level of patient referrals and referral sources. This analysis showed that 60 percent of all referrals came from 35 percent of all the doctors who referred to the group. The remaining referrals came from the other 65 percent of the referral physicians. In examining this referral pattern, it was also revealed that 20 percent of all the primary care

physicians in the group's primary service area had never sent a patient to the group for diagnosis or treatment. As the practice manager of the group, you have been asked by the physicians to develop a marketing strategy to deal with this information.

5. Bethesda Hospital has recently developed an integrated health care system— the hospital and its physicians have formed a new organization, which also is affiliated with a large insurance company. This new structure, called a physician-hospital organization (PHO), offers a prepaid health care plan and competes against other managed care companies. The marketing director of the PHO is planning to approach the employers in the community to encourage them to offer the new health care plan to their employees. Suggest three alternative ways this customer base for the PHO could be segmented, and indicate how each base of segmentation would result in a change in the marketing mix.

NOTES

1. W.R. Smith, Product Differentiation and Market Segmentation as Alternative Marketing Strategies, *Journal of Marketing* 21, no. 1 (1956):3–8.

2. L. Ingrassia, U.S. Overconfidence Leaves This Hospital in Critical Condition, *The Wall Street Journal*, 20 December 1994, A1,A9.

3. P.R. Dickson and J.L. Ginter, Market Segmentation, Product Differentiation, and Marketing Strategy, *Journal of Marketing* 51, no. 2 (1987):1–10.

4. R. Weiss, Market Response Systems: A Community Interface, *Health Progress* 75, no. 61 (1994):68–69.

5. The Health Industry Finally Asks: What Do Women Want? *Business Week* no. 2961 (August 25, 1986):81.

6. J.S. Ghent, Childbirth Education: A Natural Approach To Assessing Healthcare Clients, *Healthcare Marketing Report* 12, no. 5 (1994):14–15.

7. It's a Woman's Market, *Hospitals and Health Networks* 67 (1993):30.

8. J. de Cordoba, More Firms Court Hispanic Consumers, But Find Them a Tough Market To Target, *The Wall Street Journal*, 18 February 1988, 25.

9. M.C. Jaklevic, Programs and Campaigns Reach Out to Members of Ethnic Communities, *Modern Healthcare* 24, no. 31 (1994):32.

10. W. Hearn, Cultural Competence, *American Medical News* 36, no. 40 (1993):13–15.

11. See, for example, W. Power, How Not To Break a Leg: "Arts Medicine" Helps Performers Stay Healthy on the Job, *The Wall Street Journal*, 5 June 1986, 29.

12. L. Carpenter, How To Market to Regions, *American Demographics* 9, no. 11 (1987):11–15.

13. D. Knight, Psychographics Delivers More Than Targeted Ad Pitches, *Healthcare Marketing Report* 11, no. 11 (1993):6–8.

14. Incentive Programs Can Be Used To Boost Business, *Physician's Marketing and Management* 61, no. 1 (1993):6–8.

15. R.K. Srivistava, Usage Situational Influences on Perceptions of Product Markets: Theoretical and Empirical Issues, in *Advances in Consumer Research,* Vol. 8, ed. K. Monroe (Ann Arbor, Mich.: ACR, 1981), 106–111.

16. A. Hagedorn, Johnson and Johnson Says Wrinkle Cream Goes Under Its Skin, *The Wall Street Journal*, 10 August 1989, 19; and From Wrinkle Cream to Cancer Cure, *Business Week* no. 3092 (February 20, 1989):146.

17. R. McStravic, Loyalty of Hospital Patients, *Health Care Management Review* 12, no. 2 (Spring 1987):23–30.

18. R.J. Haley, Benefit Segmentation: A Decision Oriented Research Tool, *Journal of Marketing* 27, no. 3 (1963):30–35.

19. J. John and G. Miaoulis, A Model for Understanding Benefit Segmentation in Preventive Health Care, *Health Care Management Review* 17, no. 2 (Spring 1992):21–32.

20. J.E. Pickens, Group Health "Options" Showing Potential of Market-Responsive HMO/Indemnity Hybrid, *Healthcare Marketing Report* 9, no. 5 (1991):8–10.

21. W.N. Zelamn and C.P. McLaughlin, Product Lines in a Complex Marketplace: Matching Organizational Strategy to Buyer Behavior, *Health Care Management Review* 15, no. 2 (Spring 1990):9–14.

Part III
The Marketing Mix

7

PRODUCT STRATEGY

After reading this chapter you should be able to:

• Learn the range of product and service variations

• Understand the issues of product line formation

• Identify the strategy considerations over the product life cycle

• Know the strategic implications of alternative branding strategies

THE MEANING OF PRODUCTS AND SERVICES

Ultimately for any business, the focus of marketing revolves around the products and services to meet customer needs. Health care business lines involve a range of products and services. The primary distinction between products and services is their degree of tangibility, or the extent to which they can be examined, touched, or experienced before purchase. Products can be divided into two groups: nondurable goods and durable goods. A **nondurable good** is an item that can be consumed in some defined period of time. Examples of nondurable goods include chewing tobacco, food products, and topical dressings for wounds. A **durable good** is a product that lasts over an extended period of time. Items such as automobiles, CT scanners, and computers can all be classified as durable items. A wide range of health care activities involve **services**, which are defined as intangible activities or processes offered to customers to solve problems, and for which the organization is often reimbursed. Open heart surgery, a comprehensive

201

cancer program, and a geriatric medicine clinic are examples of common health care services.

The differences between such items reflect important considerations in any marketing action. Nondurable products are often heavily advertised because consumers frequently purchase such products. Many pharmaceuticals, such as Rogaine®, are heavily advertised directly to the consumer. Retail store displays play a major role in direct marketing to the consumer. For durable products, personal sales often play a major role. General Electric, for example, has an extensive sales force that calls upon hospitals selling the latest G.E. scanning devices. Durable products usually cost more than nondurable items, and are often far more complicated to use. For these products, personal sales are essential to help answer customer questions and to explain the intricacies of the product.

The marketing of services is often more challenging because of their unique elements, given that they are not tangible. Services differ from products on five components, which can be referred to as the five I's.

The Five I's of Services

Service marketing is a challenging and often difficult aspect of marketing. The five characteristics of services that any health care marketer should recognize include: intangibility, inconsistency, inseparability, inventory, and interaction.

Intangibility

Services are intangible in that they cannot be felt, touched, or heard before they are encountered. Cardiac surgery, for example, is intangible. Prior to undergoing such a procedure, a patient cannot see the surgery or examine it as can be done with the purchase of a computer. A major challenge in the marketing of intangible services is to show the tangible benefits from their use.[1] An advertisement for an occupational medicine program, for example, might show a productive worker back on the job; or the hospital birthing center advertisement shows a mother with a contented baby. Because services are intangible, consumer interactions with the processes and the individuals who deliver the service are often the bases by which consumers evaluate the actual service itself.

Inconsistency

Health services are delivered by people—the nurse practitioner, the physician, or the admitting clerk in the group practice. In this regard, service marketing is more difficult than product marketing. In the manufacture of a product, exact standards can be developed by which the production line assembles a car, telephone, or other product within some defined tolerance levels. Deviations in the tolerance can lead to a simple adjustment in the production machines. People-delivered services have inherent variability. The delivery of the service changes with the individual who delivers the service. For example, two surgeons may have noticeably different levels of proficiency at performing a particular procedure. While they perform the same clinical procedure, no one would argue that they are delivering the same service. Similarly, on any given day, the admitting clerks at the hospital may deliver their services differently as a function of their own motivation, morale, or attitude.

For service marketers, the objective in reducing inconsistency is to achieve as much standardization as possible. In McDonald's restaurants, for example, service workers all wear the same uniform to minimize inconsistency. The key, however, to any attempt at reducing inconsistency in people-delivered services is through training.

Inseparability

Services cannot be separated from the individuals who deliver them. The classic example of this characteristic in health care settings is known as the "bedside manner" of the physician. The link between the issues of inseparability and inconsistency underscores the complexity of health care service marketing.

Inventory

Often in the discussion of services, the issue of inventory is ignored. Inventory is a concept that is common to product businesses. In the analysis of costs associated with product businesses, a major concern is the cost of carrying any inventory. Yet, services, too, have inventory. Whenever an employee who delivers the service is not being utilized, but is still being paid, an inventory exists. A hospital emergency room physician who is paid on a contract represents an inventory cost that the hospital carries. As long as the emergency room is not being utilized and the physician has down time, the cost of that inventory is large.

Service businesses can manage the cost of inventory by either managing the service deliverer or by shifting the demand. One strategy for managing the delivery of a service is to employ part-time workers who work at peak time periods. Nurses are frequently paid premium wages for working certain shifts or working overtime to cover unusually busy periods of activity.

Managing the demand for a service is more difficult. It involves shifting demand to nonpeak hours to level out the costs of personnel and overhead. Movie theaters, for example, offer discounted admissions during the afternoon, or matinee, shows. Management's goal is to attract customers throughout the day to defray the costs of building maintenance and the movie rental fees. In health care, accomplishing this strategy requires an understanding of the ebb and flow of customers through the business.

Interaction with Customers

Because services involve processes, an important consideration in marketing a service is the quality of the interaction between the customer and the service provider. One approach that highlights the encounters between a customer and the service is the **customer contact audit**, which is a flow chart of the points of interaction between the customer and the service offering.[2] Figure 7–1 shows a customer contact audit involving a car rental. Each area that is starred (*) represents a point where the customer interacts with the service organization. It is at these points where the consumer evaluates the service's quality. Figure 7–2 shows a similar customer contact audit applied to a primary care visit.

CLASSIFICATION OF PRODUCTS AND SERVICES

Products and services vary in two key ways: in terms of durability and tangibility, as we have just discussed. These variations clearly determine the types of marketing strategy developed for each category. Products and services can also be classified on other levels, in terms of who buys them and how they are delivered.

At the most macro level, products can be classified by the type of users who buy them. **Consumer goods** are products purchased by the ultimate consumer. **Industrial products** are products purchased for use in the manufacture of other products, which will, at some point, be purchased by the ultimate consumer. Both consumer and industrial products have several variations, which are discussed in this chapter. Services can be classified by how they are delivered: primarily by individuals or by machines.

Classifying Consumer Products

A major way to classify consumer products is by the amount of effort and manner of search the consumer uses in purchasing the product.[3] Using this classification scheme, consumer goods fall into three categories: (1) convenience goods, (2) shopping goods, and (3) specialty items. **Convenience goods** are products that the consumer purchases frequently that require little deliberation or search prior to purchase. Cold remedies, analgesics, and chewing gum are all such examples. For marketers of convenience goods, there are two major concerns. Since the consumer engages in little search or deliberation, name recognition and product distribution are critical. Makers of Tylenol, for example, prominently place their brand on eye-level shelves in pharmacies and other stores where medicine is sold.

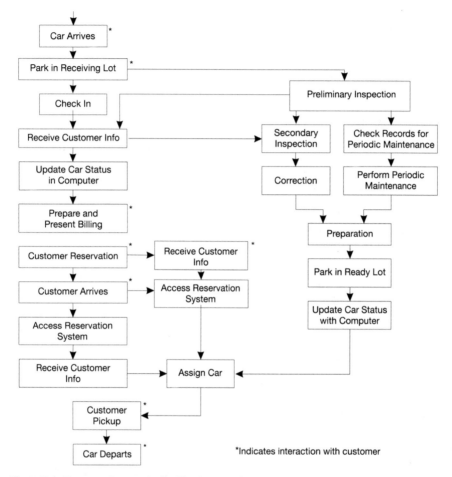

Figure 7–1 Customer Contact Audit: The Car Rental Process. *Source:* Reprinted from *Marketing* by E.N. Berkowitz, R. Kerin, S. Hartley, and C.W. Rudelius, p. 683, with permission of Richard D. Irwin, © 1994.

A second type of consumer product is a **shopping good**. Shopping goods are products in which the consumer engages in a significant amount of search to compare competing brands on selected attributes, such as price, style, or features. Televisions, computers, and cameras are all common examples of shopping goods. Marketers of shopping goods must differentiate their brand from their competitors' on the attributes that are important to their customers. Salespeople often play a major role in helping the consumer learn about alternative brands and ultimately make the purchase.

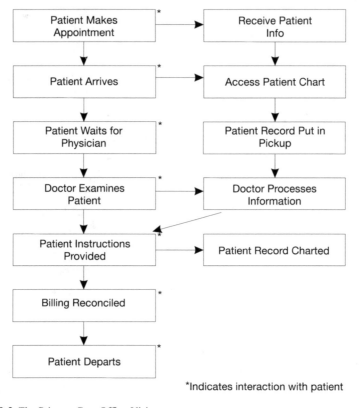

*Indicates interaction with patient

Figure 7–2 The Primary Care Office Visit

A final category of consumer goods includes **specialty items**. Specialty products are those that the consumer specifically seeks out. Often the consumer is very loyal to a particular brand, and will go to great lengths to find that particular item. While specialty items vary from one individual to another, common examples might include a Rolex watch, Joy perfume, or a Sony Discman. Table 7–1 shows a representation of consumer products.

Industrial Goods Classification

Industrial products have two broad levels of classification. **Production goods** are those that are used to become part of a final product. Raw materials fit into this category. A second type of industrial goods is known as **support goods**. These are

Table 7–1 Categorization of Products

Criterion	Convenience Good	Shopping Good	Specialty Item
Degree of Search Effort	little	compares alternatives	seeks specific brand
Price	relatively inexpensive	moderate	usually expensive
Differential Advantage	little on product	often varies by product	identity
Key Marketing Mix Component	distribution	product or price	product (brand)
Customer Loyalty	little	prefer a brand but will substitute	highly loyal
Frequency of Purchase	frequent	infrequent	very infrequent

items used to assist in the producing of other products. Support goods can include buildings, accessory equipment, and supplies. A CT scanner would be considered a support good, as would a desk used in an office, or a paper clip attached to a billing invoice.

Service Classifications

Services can be classified primarily by how they are delivered: whether by people or equipment.[4] Figure 7–3 shows the two major distinctions and examples of each. Services that are primarily equipment-based have fewer problems with inconsistency. Health care services are primarily delivered by professionals and skilled labor.

In the health care industry there is also another common delineator of services. This categorization pertains to the tax status of the organization either as a for-profit or a nonprofit entity. During the 1980s, health care saw a rapid rise in the number of for-profit health care organizations, such as National Medical Enterprises, Hospital Corporation of America, and US Healthcare. The major distinction of these services pertains to the distribution of excess revenues (profits) over expenses. In for-profit businesses, some portion of profit often is directed to shareholders. In nonprofit service organizations, excess revenues are redirected back to the organization to continue the maintenance of the service.

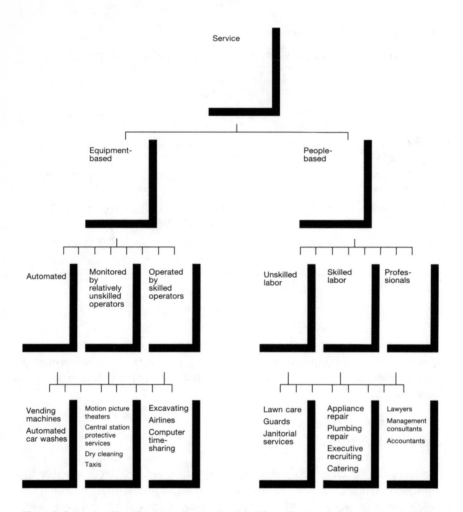

Figure 7–3 Service Classifications. *Source:* Reprinted from Thomas, D.R.E., Strategy Is Different in Service Businesses, *Harvard Business Review,* Vol. 56, No. 4, p. 161, with permission of the President and Fellows of Harvard College, © 1978. All rights reserved.

MANAGING THE PRODUCT

The remaining discussion in this chapter will use the terms "product" and "service" interchangeably. In cases where there are variations in the marketing implications, the differences between products and services will be noted.

Know

Developing the Product Line and Mix

All businesses must decide which products and services to offer. The **product mix** is the entire range of products a firm offers. Figure 7–4 shows a portion of the product line of a large community hospital that provides some tertiary services. This chart shows several distinct **product lines**, which are groups of related services. For example, the product line in Infant and Maternal Health contains the services of obstetrics, pediatrics, gynecology, neonatal care, and an intensive care nursery. In determining the product mix, companies must determine the breadth and depth of the product mix. The **breadth** refers to the number of different product lines in the mix. As can be seen in Figure 7–4, the hospital has a reasonably well-developed product line, consisting of such services as a comprehensive cancer center, sports medicine, and respiratory therapy. **Depth** refers to the number of product items within each product line. Figure 7–5 shows the depth of the product line in the comprehensive cancer center. Significant depth is represented by the number of services offered within this program, which range from invasive procedures such as oncological surgery to supportive assistance with social services.

A real-life example is St. Francis Hospital, in Roslyn, New York, which specializes exclusively in the diagnosis and treatment of heart disease. Although this is a narrow product line, the program has significant depth by including services such as a community outreach program that brings cardiac screening to low-income residents living in medically underserved areas. The hospital operates a cardiac fitness center and offers regional employers a corporate education and screening program. St. Francis also offers an educational outreach program to teach children healthy eating and exercise habits.[5]

Most companies manage multiple product lines and items. In these circumstances, companies must guard against **cannibalization**—when a company's own products steal market share from other products within the company's product line. A hospital, for example, might open a free-standing emergency room only to find that it steals patients from the hospital's main emergency room. The major rationale used to allow for cannibalization is that it is better to offer the product oneself than for a competitor to enter the market with the same product. A company would market the product to appeal to a different market segment that would not have a major impact on other product lines.

The Product Life Cycle

The marketing implications and considerations for any product vary depending on how long the product has been in existence, the number of competitors, and the

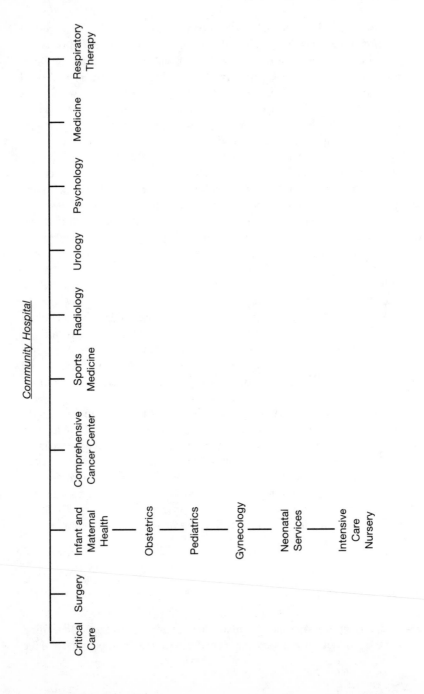

Figure 7-4 Community Hospital Product Mix

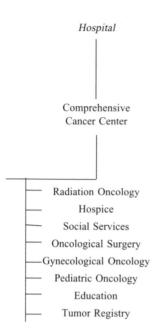

Figure 7–5 Depth in the Product Line

---

level of sales or revenue the product is generating. Central to understanding the marketing of products, then, is the concept of the product life cycle. The **product life cycle** refers to the stages a product goes through as it exists in the market from its first introduction to its final withdrawal.[6] Figure 7–6 shows the four stages of a generalized product life cycle: introduction, growth, maturity, and decline. In this representation the X axis represents time and the Y axis represents gross revenues or sales.

Introduction

The first stage of the product life cycle, introduction, occurs when the product is first rolled out into the marketplace. This might be considered the present market position of subacute care facilities. These organizations, often nursing homes and skilled nursing facilities, are for those patients who no longer need acute care. One thousand such centers were operating in 1994 with a projected tenfold increase by the end of this decade.[7] As seen in Figure 7–6, sales start slowly in the introduction stage and gradually increase. Looking at Figure 7–7, one can see the early stage of the life cycle of ambulatory surgical procedures between 1980 and 1984 before

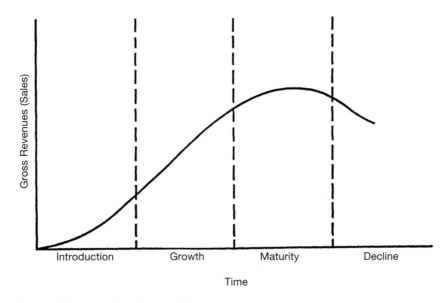

Figure 7–6 The Generalized Product Life Cycle

it began the rapid rise. At this stage of the life cycle there are distinct considerations for each element of the marketing mix.

Product. The key consideration in the introduction stage of a product is quality. Product quality must be at the level that meets customer expectations. A product whose quality suffers at this stage of the life cycle will have a difficult time reaching the growth stage. Early buyers who try the product will become dissatisfied and will discourage prospective buyers. Any repeat purchase probabilities by these early buyers will be quickly eliminated.

In service marketing, the introduction stage of the life cycle is particularly difficult. Since much of the service delivery involves a process and personnel, internal controls become of paramount importance. In introducing an industrial medicine program, for example, an HMO must have procedures in place to provide quick follow-up with the employee assistance professional who processes the paperwork for a company's injured employee. If the system fails, it will be difficult to get that employer to sign a second-year contract for the industrial medicine program.

Price. At this stage of the product life cycle, pricing follows one of two primary strategies. One is a **skimming price** strategy, involving a high initial price rela-

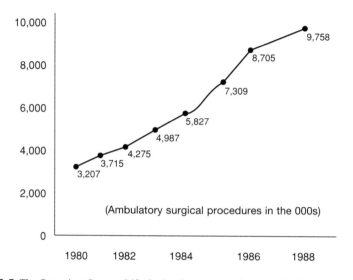

Figure 7-7 The Outpatient Surgery Life Cycle. *Source:* American Hospital Association, Chicago, Illinois, 1989.

tive to competing products or substitutable services. Or, the organization can roll out the new product and price it lower than the competition, using a **penetration price** strategy. There are advantages and disadvantages to each approach.

One advantage to a high initial price is that, for any new product or service, there are often some early buyers who want the product, no matter what the price. These buyers are less price sensitive. Following the skimming strategy allows the organization to achieve a greater margin on these early buyers and to recoup the cost of developing the new product. As competition enters the market, the price subsequently can be reduced. A second major advantage to a high initial price is image. The high price sets off the product as a premium good or a status item. In health care there is some strong logic to this rationale. Since services are intangibles, price is one way consumers can infer the quality of the service, since price is a tangible element. For physicians, the initial pricing of a service sets up their profiles for Medicare and Medicaid reimbursements, as well as for other third-party carriers. As a result, a higher price allows for a more remunerative level of reimbursement from these agencies.

With services, there is another strong reason supporting a skimming strategy. Services require personnel and processes. Often, in spite of an organization's best efforts, there is a shakeout period in which processes for delivering the service must be reworked once actual demand is established. The admitting procedures for a day surgery program, for example, might need to be streamlined. In such cases, when complicated systems or multiple departments are involved in the delivery of the service, a high price acts as a safeguard to discourage too much start-up demand. The organization can use the initial high price as a spigot to control the flow of demand until there is confidence that the systems, personnel, and supporting facilities are in place to meet customer needs.

The disadvantages of a skimming strategy are obvious. If the organization needs to have some economy of scale to deliver the service efficiently, a high price discourages demand. A skimming strategy also may entice competitors to enter the field. A potential competitor watching the premiums being charged by a new HMO may decide it can offer a similar plan at a lower price in the marketplace, and still earn a reasonable return.

The advantage of a penetration strategy is that it keeps the competition out and encourages demand. St. Michael's Medical Center, in Newark, New Jersey, introduced a 20-minute health check for women. The service included an EKG, cholesterol check, blood pressure check, and computerized health test risk appraisal. The introductory price was only $25. After an introductory period, the price was raised to $40.[8] The major limitation of penetration pricing, however, is that setting a low price requires a good understanding of what it costs to produce the product. The organization must understand the per-unit cost to ensure that the low initial price covers the per-unit cost, in addition to providing a return to the company. In a health care business, an accurate per-unit cost of delivery has always been a difficult figure to obtain. In such instances, a low-cost strategy can entail some real financial risks for an organization.

Promotion. Promotion is an essential component to consider in the introduction stage. For a truly new product or service, the company must develop **primary demand**, or purchase interest in this new class of service. A new product requires significant promotional effort to educate the market about a product's capabilities. Glaxo Wellcome PLC, an international pharmaceutical manufacturer, for example, spent significant promotional dollars educating neurologists about a new migraine headache medication. Advertisements in clinical publications, displays at the annual meeting of the American Academy of Neurology, and personal calls in the doctor offices—some of the tactics that were used by Glaxo—are all key promotional components in the introduction stage of the life cycle of the new drug product.

Place. The distribution issues in the introductory stage of the product life cycle are somewhat limited. The key challenge is to obtain some initial exposure for the product.

Growth

In the growth stage of the product life cycle, as shown in Figure 7–6, sales of the product begin to increase rapidly. For example, between 1982 and 1988 there was a 128 percent increase in ambulatory outpatient surgery procedures, as depicted in Figure 7–7. While only 21 percent of all surgical procedures in the United States were done on an outpatient basis in 1984, the number today is closer to 75 percent.[9]

An early sign that one is entering this stage of the life cycle is the appearance of competitors. Once other providers enter the market, the key challenge is to generate **selective demand**, which is preference for the company's product or service. The marketing mix issues regarding the product life cycle also begin to shift.

Product. A key decision for organizations at this stage of the life cycle is whether to expand the product mix. Organizations will often expand the product line by offering a variation of the original product. Sony, for example, offers less expensive versions of its Walkman, which has fewer features and is made from less expensive materials than the original. The purpose of these new variations is to expand the product's appeal to new market segments.

Promotion. While in the introduction stage, the promotional concern was to generate awareness. Now with competitors, the purpose of promotion is to develop product preference. Advertising must create brand awareness. For example, when the first HMO enters a particular community, its major promotional objective is to educate people about this new "managed care" plan. Once other competitors enter the market, each HMO advertises its particular name to generate selective demand.

In the growth stage of the product life cycle, personal sales become more important. Once there is market competition, the competitors battle for middleman support. With the introduction of DAT recorders, for example, each manufacturer's sales force works aggressively to convince retailers to carry its particular brand. So too, in health care, this same personal sales emphasis is occurring with managed care plans. Each plan has a sales force offering its products to large employers. Most health care providers know that employers offer their employees only a limited choice of health plans, just like most retailers carry only a limited number of brands in any particular product category.

Price. The pricing decision in the growth stage depends on the initial price at which the product is offered, and whether the company is broadening its product line. It is difficult to raise the price for a product after its introductory offering. In health care, many HMOs raised their prices after they reviewed utilization rates. Too large a price increase without a substantial change in the product quality, however, can lead to significant buyer dissatisfaction in any business.

Place. A major emphasis of marketing strategy in the growth stage is on the distribution component of the marketing mix—solidifying the loyalty of the middleman. Hospitals, for example, have often faced this dilemma when a competing hospital established a similar medical or surgical service, such as cardiovascular surgery.

Maturity

In this phase of the life cycle, sales begin to slow. An indicator of the mature stage is when the marginal competitors begin to exit the business line. This happens in many communities with an aging population. Selected hospitals in particular communities may leave the pediatric business, for example. In the mature stage of the life cycle, the key objective is to maintain the existing customer base. Some additional growth in sales can occur as the remaining competitors fight for the business of those who have left the market.

Product. There are few major product decisions at this stage of the life cycle. Most companies have a relatively full product line. The key product issue is to develop some new lines that can help reposition the organization to return to the earlier stages of introduction and growth. Kaiser's recent developments in California can be viewed as a strategy to move back up on the growth curve of the life cycle in the face of maturity. Having existed for many years in this market, the Kaiser HMO is a mature product within California. In 1994, Kaiser began offering a point-of-service plan that allows its subscribers a choice—they can receive their health care from a Kaiser provider, or, for the payment of an additional deductible, they can receive care from a non-Kaiser physician.[10]

Price. At the mature stage of the life cycle, pricing becomes far more competitive. Typically, at this stage, there is aggressive price discounting, which contributes to the exit of some marginal competitors.

Promotion. Promotion at this stage involves retention of existing customers. In traditional industries, coupons or promotional games are often used to keep existing customers coming back. McDonald's, for example, offers different promotional products to children as a way to maintain customer loyalty. In the health care setting, such games or promotions would be considered unacceptable. Some institutions, however, have set up senior citizen clubs as a way to tie this population to a particular facility.

Place. The distribution decision at this stage is relatively simple—the profitable channels are maintained and marginal outlets are dropped. At this point, for example, a health care organization may decide to close some free-standing emergency rooms in locations that haven't developed a reasonable return.

Decline SNF

The decline stage of the life cycle is difficult for any organization; it must recognize that the service cannot continue to grow. Services in the decline stage of the product life cycle can consume a disproportionate share of management time and financial resources. There are relatively few options. The most difficult option is to *drop*, or eliminate the service. There may be significant emotional attachment to the service within the organization. A hospital's board of trustees, for instance, might note that from its early days, the hospital always offered pediatric services.

A second option is to *contract* with another party to provide the product or service. In health care, for example, some companies might agree to run a hospital's emergency room or rehabilitation department under a contract.

A final option is to *harvest* the service.[11] This involves paring out the aspects of the service that are truly not profitable and offering a reduced version of the service for loyal customers. In the pediatric example, the hospital could decide to offer a pediatric clinic for primary case consults, but drop its inpatient beds.

Product Life Cycle Issues

The product life cycle is a useful management concept for determining where a service is positioned in the marketplace and what external influences, such as competitors, might affect strategy. Yet, there is no exact way for an organization to determine where a respective service or product is in the life cycle. Nor do all life cycles necessarily have the shape of that shown in Figure 7–6.[12]

Alternative Product Life Cycles

Figure 7–8 displays four other common product life cycles. One life cycle is for a **high learning product** that requires a significant introductory period.[13] These represent rather complicated services for which the immediate benefit might not be seen by the consumer. These types of products often require significant buyer education. A high learning product might include services of a physiatrist. Studies have shown that few people understand what a physiatrist does, including members of the medical profession, who lack the knowledge of this medical specialty's capabilities. Thus, a rehabilitative medicine service staffed by a physiatrist can be viewed in some markets as a high learning product. Significant time must be spent educating potential referral physicians about the value of this service, compared to dealing with orthopedists or physical therapists.

A second variation shown in Figure 7–8 represents the **low learning product** for which the benefits are clearly seen by the consumer.[14] This product has a short introductory period and enters competition rapidly. These products generally are not technologically sophisticated, so that there is lower complexity and a lower cost of entry for the competition. A walk-in medical center can be considered a low learning product. Consumers see these as convenient places for care for minor medical problems. The benefits of reduced waiting time compared to a hospital emergency room, as well as the "no appointment needed" approach, has led to rapid acceptance of this concept.

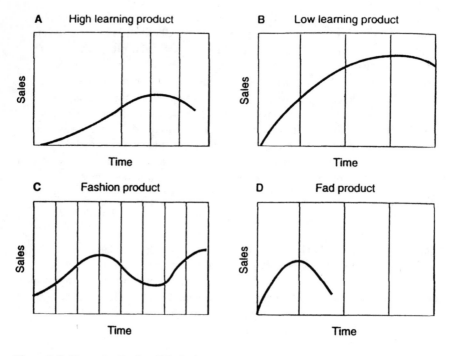

Figure 7–8 Alternative Product Life Cycles

A third life cycle shown in Figure 7–8 represents the fashion product, in which there is a decline and an eventual reemergence of the product. The name of this curve is related to the fashion styles that often disappear only to reemerge years later in modified form. Some fashion magazines were touting bell bottom slacks as the fashion statement of 1993. Yet, bell bottoms were tossed out of most closets at the end of the 1960s. The width of men's ties or the length of hemlines vary in the fashion life cycle.

Figure 7–8 also includes the fad product. There are really only two stages to the fad life cycle: introduction and decline. Pet rocks, wall walkers, and toe socks are all examples of past fads. These items are quickly adopted by consumers for their novelty value, and competitors often enter quickly to capitalize on the sales growth. Yet, as quickly as the sales occurred, the fad can end, once it reaches saturation. The shape of this life cycle can tell the fortunes of many companies. A company fortunate to enter the life cycle early can reap significant financial gain. A competitor entering the fad market too late can find itself with a warehouse full of rocks that no one wants for a pet. In the health care industry, fads occur, often with regard to vitamins and treatment approaches. At one time, for example, bran was cited as a preventative for heart disease. This led to the rapid proliferation of bran additives in many products. After a relatively short time period, however, and the publication of several medical studies questioning the validity of the claim, the bran fad disappeared.

Length of the Life Cycle

It is difficult to affect the length of the product life cycle. In health care, the major factor that moves a service rapidly from introduction to decline is technology. As was seen in Chapter 2, Figure 2–9 shows the impact of new technology on the life cycles of the preceding products over which there has been an improvement. The life cycle of X-rays as an imaging device was fairly long. Yet increased imaging performance became available through the advent of nuclear imaging, which led to X-ray technology becoming mature in terms of performance (and most likely sales). The past 15 years, however, have seen rapid development in imaging technology with the result of shorter product life cycles in terms of the existing technology.

The Life Cycle of Hospitals. In health care management, the life cycle phenomenon is real. Figure 7–9 shows the classic life cycle of inpatient acute-care hospitals in the U.S. from 1965 to 1985. As hospitals reduce beds and convert unused facilities, few would argue that the inpatient side of the hospital business is in the decline stage of the product life cycle.

Product Life Cycle Concerns

While the product life cycle is one of the most common conceptualizations used within marketing, it is not without its limitations. A major criticism is that there is no standard life cycle and that many products defy the life cycle sequence.

A second concern is whether the product life cycle relates to the product class (automobiles), the product form (full-size sedans), or the specific product (Mercury Marquis). The product life cycle treats each product as a new form or a new product class when, in fact, the product may just be a new brand of a product at the growth or maturity stage. This factor may lead to different life cycle strategies.[15] A third concern is that the product life cycle is tied closely to sales. It is often difficult, however, to relate some marketing activities directly to their impact on sales.

Modifying the Product Life Cycle

While it is impossible for marketing managers to alter the external factors, such as demographics or new technology, that affect the product life cycle, there are three strategies they can consider to stretch the life of the product they control.

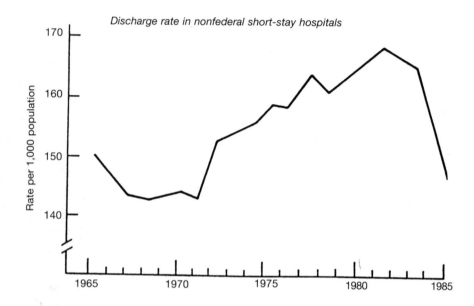

Figure 7–9 The Declining Hospital Life Cycle. *Source:* National Center for Health Statistics, 1985 Summary, *National Hospital Discharge Survey.* Advance data from *Viral and Health Statistics,* No. 127, DHHS Pub No. (PHS) S6–1250, September 25, 1986.

These strategies include product modification, market modification, and repositioning the product.

Product Modification

The strategy of **product modification** involves actually altering the product in some fashion by changing its quality, features, performance, or appearance. A hospital may decide to add more services to its industrial medicine program. A membership at a local health club could become part of the standard package, thereby actually improving the service.

Market Modification

An alternative approach to stretch the life cycle is **market modification,** in which the company tries to increase the use of, or create new uses or new users for, the product.

Increase Use. Promoting more frequent use of a product is common in traditional industries. Brushing your teeth after every meal has long been touted as important by toothpaste manufacturers. There are some strong ethical concerns, however, about promoting the more frequent use of health services. In fact, this aspect of health care advertising was an early concern voiced by opponents of the practice. Physicians believed that the advertising of medical services would lead to unnecessary utilization or demand from consumers for an advertised clinical service that may not be appropriate for all of these consumers.

Create New Uses. This strategy involves identifying new ways to use the product. Arm & Hammer baking soda is an example of a product that has stretched its life cycle very successfully with this strategy. Arm & Hammer baking soda is advertised as a refrigerator deodorizer, toothpaste, cat litter refresher, and also as a baking product. In health care, identifying new uses for medications has become common. A particular drug is often found to be beneficial for the treatment of unrelated problems. As noted earlier, Retin-A is a topical cream originally intended for treatment of severe acne. This product's life has been stretched considerably since put to new use as a topical for early-stage skin cancers, as well as an antiwrinkling preventative for the skin.

Find New Users. Seeking out new target markets is a third way to stretch the life of a product. In the rehabilitative medicine department of the Cleveland Clinic, a seat was developed to assist patients who were wheelchair-bound. This seat (and the process to create it) was originally intended for patients who came to the clinic. To stretch the life cycle of the product, the clinic considered selling the process and technology to other large medical centers for use with their patients.

Repositioning the Product

In offering a service or product, a company must first decide how it wants to position the product in the market. **Product positioning** involves how a product is perceived in the minds of consumers relative to defined attributes and competing products. There are several alternatives a company can consider in the initial product positioning. Target market strategies can include mass market, niche, and growth market strategies.

As noted in Chapter 2, with a mass market strategy, the company tries to attract larger market segments by positioning the product so it appeals to the largest number of customers in the market. A medical group, for example, may offer primary care services at a number of sites in the community, planning to attract the largest volume possible to utilize the service.

Within the mass market strategy, a firm can follow either an undifferentiated or differentiated approach. In using an undifferentiated strategy, the service is positioned to appeal to the larger segments. In a differentiated strategy, services are developed to meet the individual needs of the multiple segments that comprise the total market.

A niche strategy involves selecting a narrow segment or segments of the market. Shouldice Hospital, in Toronto, Canada, received significant attention when it specialized in short-stay hernia repairs. The hospital introduced this service not only within Canada, but also in the United States. The target market was corporate executives who could fly to Canada for treatment, but needed to return to their jobs as soon as possible.

A growth market strategy involves targeting those segments that are going to expand. Prior to the changes in reimbursement, many hospitals targeted oncology as a growing market segment. Demographics, technology, and advances in treatment led many facilities to establish comprehensive cancer programs since this area generated significant revenue by using many services within a hospital's product mix in the diagnosis and treatment of the disease. In the 1980s, however, the government began to change how hospitals were reimbursed for the inpatient care they provided. Historically, hospitals were paid based on the costs incurred during the length of stay for the treatment of a medical problem. This was called cost-based reimbursement. During the 1980s, the government moved to reimbursing hospitals for the treatment of a disease or medical problem at a predetermined rate, regardless of the length of stay or services utilized in the treatment of a condition. Medical problems were categorized into diagnosis-related groups (DRGs). This change in reimbursement meant that an intensive medical service, such as oncology, would no longer be so profitable if it required significant resources. The change to DRGs required the hospital to be efficient, since charges for excessive treatment would no longer be reimbursed by the government.

Assessing Product Position. One way to assess the position of a service in the minds of consumers is through the use of multidimensional scaling (MDS). With this statistical technique, perceptual maps can be developed of a hospital's position relative to competing institutions. In a typical MDS situation, consumers are asked to provide paired similarity ratings of services or hospitals. All possible combinations are provided. Consumers rate desired attributes in order of importance. An MDS map such as that shown in Figure 7–10 then can be developed. These maps help to visualize the service gaps, and also show how the competitive set of alternatives are positioned for consumers.

Branding

When offering any product, a company needs to decide how it will be branded. A **brand** is any name, term, colors, or symbol that distinguishes one seller's product from another.[16] A brand name can be spoken, such as the names Chevrolet, Glaxo, or Crest; or it can be recognized, such as the apple for Apple Computer or the greyhound for the Greyhound Bus Company. A **trade name** is the commercial

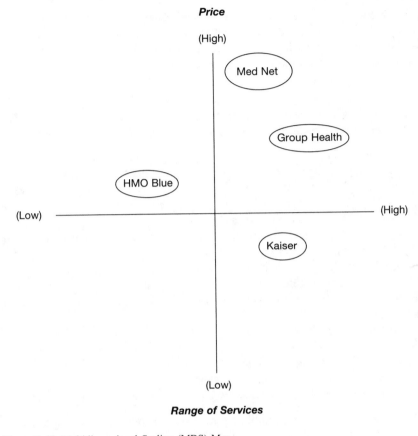

Figure 7-10 Multidimensional Scaling (MDS) Map

name under which a company does business.[17] A **trademark** is a brand name or trade name given legal protection. Services use a service mark in the same way.

To be protected, a trademark must have a distinctive meaning, must be used in interstate commerce, and not be confused with other registered trademarks. Service names cannot be registered unless they describe a particular business, nor can terms that are primarily descriptive, such as "medical services," be registered.[18] In health care, most organizations use their trade name as opposed to a brand name. Yet as more health care organizations produce alternative plans and products, brand names are becoming more common.

Branding is important to consumers because it helps them to identify the product as coming from a particular source. There is a growing recognition of the added value a brand name gives a product through associations made by the consumer. This added value is referred to as **brand equity**.[19] The Mayo Clinic's trade name has significant brand equity. The clinic uses this name on its health newsletter, which is sold by subscription to consumers.

Branding Strategies

There are several strategies a company can use in branding a product or service. These are referred to as multiproduct, multibrand, reseller, or mixed strategies.

Multiproduct Strategy. In using a **multiproduct branding strategy**, the company places one brand name on all the products in its line. This strategy is common to companies such as Honda, which puts its name on its cars, lawn mowers, motorcycles, and home generators. This is also common strategy for health care organizations. A hospital puts its name on the outpatient surgery center, its walk-in emergency centers, and its industrial medicine program. The rationale for this approach is the use of brand equity. Knowing the brand name, consumers have confidence that the new product should work as well as other items in the line. Honda cars are reliable; therefore, so are Honda lawn mowers. Using a well-known name should lead to reduced promotional expenses in any new product introduction.

The risks for a multiproduct strategy, however, are significant. Because the organization uses one name for all items in the line, each new product puts the brand equity at risk. Companies that follow this strategy must ensure that the new product meets the quality standards for which the company is known. Otherwise, a failure in one item may negatively affect other similarly branded products.

Multibrand Strategy. In a **multibrand strategy** the company places a different name on each item. This approach is followed by Proctor and Gamble, which manufactures four different laundry detergents (Tide, Cheer, Ivory Snow, and Oxydol) and toothpastes such as Crest and Gleam. Companies follow this strategy when they are manufacturing products that appeal to different market segments. For example, a specialty health clinic, which has historically been known for sophisticated, high-technology care, may enter the primary care market by opening satellite clinics. Establishing those satellites under a different brand name may by advisable because the historical image of the group is so strong in one particular aspect of care. Extending to primary care may seem inconsistent, or consumers may think the new clinics will not be price competitive. The downside to a multibrand strategy is that each brand must establish consumer recognition. Promotional costs thus tend to be higher and the introductory period of the life cycle may take longer.

Reseller and Mixed Strategies. In a **reseller strategy**, one company sells its product under the name of another company. Sears Roebuck sells Craftsman tools and Kenmore appliances. Sears has no manufacturing facilities—these products are made by other companies and sold under the Sears name. Companies use this strategy when the reseller appeals to a strong segment of the market, or, if the reseller's market segments are different from the manufacturer's. In a mixed strategy, a company offers a product under the name of the reseller and under its own brand name. Michelin makes tires that are sold under its own name and that are also marketed under the Sears name.

Product Acceptance

In offering any new product or service to the market, a major concern is gaining initial product acceptance. A key component is the product's first buyers. If a product cannot obtain initial buyer interest, it will never reach the growth stage of the life cycle.

The Diffusion of Innovation

Consumers differ in the amount of time they require before adopting a new product. The rate at which a product is adopted by the market is called the **diffusion of innovation**. Research in rural sociology and marketing has shown that consumers can be classified in one of five categories, based on the time at which they adopt a product.[20] Shown in Figure 7–11, these categories include: innovators, early adopters, early majority, late majority, and laggards. The characteristics of these groups also differ.

Innovators. These consumers are the first to adopt a new product. Innovators tend to be risk takers who are highly educated and who use multiple information sources.

Early Adopters. These are people who are leaders in their social setting. They tend to be respected by their peers and are turned to for information by slower adopting groups. Early adopters act as opinion leaders and are above average in education.

Early and Late Majority. These two groups represent the bulk of the population. The early majority are deliberate decision makers who have many informal social contacts. The late majority are far more skeptical of new products and are below average in social and economic status.

Laggard. This group represents the last people to adopt. They have a strong fear of debt and are price conscious. Their sources of information are primarily family and close friends. This group tends to be tradition-bound.[21]

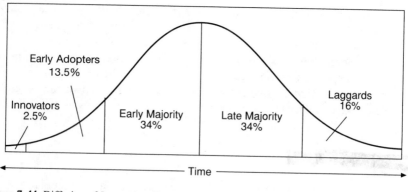

Figure 7–11 Diffusion of Innovation Curve

Most companies develop profiles of the innovators and early adopters. This strategy has been closely followed by health care company sales forces who try to identify which nurse or physician groups might be the most likely to adopt and have the greatest influence on their hospital staffs. Companies send these groups information on new products or invite them to conferences where new product announcements are made. Lyons has suggested four tips for identifying physician opinion leaders:

1. Be a detective. Question physicians to identify the roles colleagues play. Whom would they call to determine what is going on?
2. Find the power brokers, both formal and informal leaders.
3. Focus on the dominant, longstanding referral patterns and potential threats. Reviewing patterns can help identify who has the power.
4. Identify the main leader who assumes the role of motivator.[22]

Factors Affecting Adoption

There are several factors that determine the speed at which a new product is adopted by consumers. These are: relative advantage, compatibility, complexity, divisibility, and communicability.[23]

Relative Advantage. This dimension refers to the perceived benefit or advantage that a new product has over existing products, or over substitutable goods in the market. The more the product has a noticeable and valued relative advantage, the quicker it will be adopted. Health care providers quickly recognized the benefits of arthroscopic surgery on recovery time for simple knee operations. In a short period of time, the hospital lengths of stay for these procedures dropped as surgeons adopted this new invasive technique.

Compatibility. A product that is compatible with existing values or customs will be adopted quicker than one that is not. Among older consumers, the early adoption of microwave ovens was rather slow. The manner in which foods are cooked in microwaves was inconsistent with long-used methods and recipes.

Complexity. A product's complexity will affect its rate of adoption. More complex products are accepted at a slower rate.

Divisibility. A product's divisibility is the degree to which the product can be tried on a limited basis. In consumer product marketing, divisibility can be offered through the use of samples. In health care services this is more difficult to achieve. Many hospitals have offered educational seminars as a way to help consumers experience the hospital staff and the non-technical components of the service.

Communicability. The easier a product's benefits can be communicated, the quicker the rate of adoption. Showing the lower health care costs for an employee enrolled in a health education workshop would be the best form of communication to generate corporate interest in enrolling employees in a new health plan.

CONCLUSIONS

The product component of the marketing mix is the element around which other strategic decisions are made. An organization must initially determine the breadth and depth of its product or service mix. Compared to products, services have some unique elements which, by their very nature, make their marketing more challenging. In either instance, it is essential to recognize the life cycle position of a product or service and the range of strategic options available at each stage. Complicating the life cycle analysis is the reality that the life cycle has various forms. Regardless of the form, however, the health care organization must make decisions regarding product positioning and branding. As the health care marketplace becomes increasingly competitive, the challenge for all organizations will be to facilitate the diffusion of their new market entries.

KEY TERMS

Nondurable Good

Durable Good

Services

Customer Contact Audit

Consumer Goods

Industrial Products

Convenience Goods

Shopping Goods

Specialty Items

Production Goods

Support Goods

Product Mix

Product Lines

Breadth

Depth

Cannibalization

Product Life Cycle
Skimming Price
Penetration Price
Primary Demand
Selective Demand
High Learning Product
Low Learning Product
Product Modification
Market Modification

Product Positioning
Brand
Trade Name
Trademark
Brand Equity
Multiproduct Branding
Multibrand
Diffusion of Innovation

CHAPTER SUMMARY

1. Products and services differ in terms of tangibility. Services can also be distinguished by five I's; intangibility, inconsistency, inseparability, inventory, and interaction.

2. Consumer goods can be differentiated by the amount of effort and manner of search the consumer uses in purchasing the product. Industrial goods are classified as either production or support goods. Service distinctions depend on whether they are delivered by people or by equipment.

3. When establishing the product element of the marketing mix, a company must decide its product mix, product line, and its breadth and depth.

4. All products and services can be described as having a life cycle consisting of four stages: introduction, growth, maturity, and decline. While there is a generalized product life cycle, variations also exist.

5. The length of the product life cycle is affected by uncontrollable forces such as technology and demographics. An organization can affect its sales in each life cycle stage relative to the competition as a function of the effectiveness of its marketing mix strategy.

6. In the early stages of the product life cycle, a new entrant can price high to skim only the most likely buyers, or penetrate the largest market by pricing low.

7. Organizations can stretch the life cycle in the mature phase through either product or market modification.

8. An organization's brand name, if well known and regarded, can have value or equity in the marketplace. In deciding upon the brand name, a firm can pursue a multiproduct, multibrand, reseller, or mixed strategy.

9. Acceptance of a product is the result of its diffusion through the population. Individuals differ in terms of the rate at which they accept new products.

10. The rate of adoption of a new product is affected by its perceived relative advantage, compatibility, complexity, divisibility, and communicability.

CHAPTER PROBLEMS

1. A large academic medical center was interviewing candidates for the position of marketing director. One interviewee was a vice president of marketing for a large consumer food product firm. During the interview, the interviewee was asked what skills he had for the position. He responded, "I've sold products all my life and have been successful. Marketing a food product is no different than marketing a hotel, airline, or hospital." Explain to this candidate how this view might be naive.

2. How would you array the following organizations in terms of the depth and breadth of their product lines: (a) a solo-practice family practitioner who does not deliver babies, (b) a multispecialty group practice that provides primary care at five satellite locations, (c) an academic medical center, and (d) Shouldice Hospital in Toronto, which specializes in short-stay surgery for hernia repair.

3. Listed below are three different organizations at various stages of the product life cycle. Explain the strategy considerations they might undertake for the specific marketing mix variable listed.

Organization	Life cycle stage	Marketing mix variable
1. Prucare, a managed care plan entering a new metropolitan area	Introduction	Promotion
2. HealthStop, an urgent care clinic offering minor ER treatment	Mature	Product
3. Community Hospital, a 234-bed facility with seven pediatric beds	Decline	Product

4. Explain how the advertising copy for an HMO would look if it were trying to develop primary demand? How would the advertising copy change to develop selective demand?

5. A large community hospital, River Valley, has recently begun to acquire physician practices. At issue is whether to rename each acquired practice to "River Valley Associates" or to leave each name alone. What are the trade-offs River Valley should consider in this decision?

6. In 1993, President Clinton developed a task force to propose the restructuring of health care delivery in the United States. At the core of this proposal were large health care purchasing alliances through which regional groups of individuals and employers could buy insurance for themselves or for their employees. All companies would have been required to pay 80 percent of employee premiums; and employees would have paid 20 percent. Purchase of health insurance by individuals and employers would have been mandatory. Alliances would have offered at least three choices of health plans, one of them fee-for-service. In October 1994, after months of debate, the health care reform bill was declared dead by then Senate Majority Leader George Mitchell. Based on the factors that affect adoption, how would you analyze the demise of the President's health care reform proposal?

NOTES

1. V.A. Zeithaml, A. Parasuraman, and L.L. Berry, Problems and Strategies in Services Marketing, *Journal of Marketing* 49, no. 2 (Spring 1985):33–46.

2. M.J. Bitner, B.H. Bloom, and M.S. Tetreault, The Service Encounter: Diagnosing Favorable and Unfavorable Incidents, *Journal of Marketing* 54, no. 1 (1990):71–84; E. Sheuing, Conducting Customer Service Audits, *Journal of Consumer Marketing* 6, no. 3 (Summer 1989):35–41; and W.E. Sasser, R.P. Olsen, and D.D. Wyckoff, *Management of Service Operations* (Newton, Mass.: Allyn & Bacon, Inc., 1978).

3. This original classification was proposed by M.T. Copeland, Relation of Consumer Buying Habits to Marketing Methods, *Harvard Business Review* 1, no. 3 (1923):282–289.

4. D.R.E. Thomas, Strategy Is Different in Service Businesses, *Harvard Business Review* 56, no. 4 (1978):158–165.

5. R. Weiss, A Hospital That Is All Heart, *Health Progress* 74, no. 9 (1993):60–61.

6. A comprehensive discussion of the product life cycle has been presented by D.R. Rink and J.E. Swan, Product Life Cycle Research: A Literature Review, *Journal of Business Strategy* 5, no. 4 (Spring 1985):218–242.

7. A. Waldman, Subaute Care: Spreading the Word, *Healthcare Marketing Report* 12, no. 8 (1994):6–8.

8. M. Luallin, The 20-Minute Heart Check, *Marketer's Guidepost* (Spring 1994):1,8.

9. HMR Clips, *Healthcare Marketing Report* 12, no. 8 (1994):6–8.

10. A. Waldman, Kaiser Expands Choice with New Co-Op Products, *Healthcare Marketing Report* 12, no. 9 (1994):6–7.

11. L.P. Feldman and A.L. Page, Harvesting: The Misunderstood Exit Strategy, *Journal of Business Strategy* 5, no. 4 (Spring 1985):79–85.

12. See W.E. Cox, Jr., Product Life Cycles as Marketing Models, *Journal of Business* 40, no. 4 (1967):375–384; and J.E. Swan and D.R. Rink, Fitting Marketing Strategy to Various Product Life Cycles, *Business Horizons* 25, no. 1 (1982):72–76.

13. C.R. Wasson, *Dynamic Competitive Strategies and Product Life Cycles* (Austin, Texas: Austin Press, 1978), 53–64.

14. Ibid., 66.

15. N.K. Dhalla and S. Yuspeh, Forget the Product Life Cycle Concept, *Harvard Business Review* 54, no. 1 (1976):102–112.

16. P.D. Bennett, *Dictionary of Marketing Terms* (Chicago, Ill.: American Marketing Association, 1968), 18–19.

17. E.N. Berkowitz, et al., *Marketing*, 4th ed. (Homewood, Ill.: Richard D. Irwin, Inc., 1994), 332.

18. D. Cohen, Trademark Strategy Revisited, *Journal of Marketing* 55, no. 3 (1991):46–59.

19. For a detailed discussion of brand equity, see D.A. Aaker, *Brand Equity* (New York, N.Y.: The Free Press, 1991).

20. This concept was presented by E. Rogers, *Diffusion of Innovations* (New York, N.Y.: Free Press of Glencoe, 1962), 81–86.

21. E.M. Rogers, *Diffusion of Innovations*, 3rd ed. (New York, N.Y.: Free Press, 1982), 246–261.

22. M.F. Lyons, M.D., Trying to Get a Fix on Your Medical Staff? Sometimes, It Pays To Go Underground, *Medical Staff Strategy Report* 3, no. 2 (1994):6–7.

23. These factors are drawn from S.L. Lampert, Word-of-Mouth Activity During the Introduction of a New Food Product, in *Consumer Behavior Theory and Application*, ed. J.U. Farley, et al. (Newton, Mass.: Allyn & Bacon, Inc., 1974), 82; and J.R. Mancuso, Why Not Create Opinion Leaders for New Product Introductions, *Journal of Marketing* 33, no. 3 (1969):20–25.

8

PRICE

After reading this chapter you should be able to:

- Appreciate the many factors that affect pricing decisions

- Recognize the array of alternative pricing strategies available to health care marketers

- Calculate break-even pricing

- Learn the positioning value of price

THE MEANING OF PRICE

In its simplest form, **price** is the level of monetary reimbursement a firm demands for its goods or services. From a marketing viewpoint, the price also represents the economic value that the buyer provides to the producer in exchange for a product or service. A company's main priority is to establish a price that corresponds to the level of value that the consumer perceives in the service being offered. Yet, price is far more than just an economic indicator of a product's worth.

In establishing a price, companies realize that the established price has a perceptual or positioning value for the service.[1] Higher prices often connote better quality. Yet in establishing the price, a company must also consider the competitive dynamics of the marketplace. Price can affect consumer demand, as well as competitor response. As a result, the pricing decision is a major aspect of marketing strategy. In this discussion of price, it is important to recognize that the price of a product or service goes by many names. Companies such as Toro charge

232

a *price* for their lawn mowers, physicians charge *fees* for their services, and universities charge *tuition.*

In the health care industry, the issue of price was rarely a marketing concern. Pricing was based on predetermined reimbursement formulas. Often, in deciding price, the main issue was determining where the reimbursement might be most favorable. Considerations of competition or consumer perception of value were not factored into the strategic discussion of price. The health care environment of the 1990s, however, makes the pricing of services as challenging as product pricing in traditional industries. As health care organizations operate under a managed care model of capitation, bidding for contracts becomes a standard business procedure. In pricing services and products, health care providers must consider not reimbursement, but rather what the buyer will consider a value. Competitive considerations have become a key component of the pricing decision, as the number of competing managed care players in the marketplace continues to increase. Based on coverage and deductibles, the old dictum that the consumer doesn't pay for health care is also no longer valid. A recent study by InterStudy, a Minneapolis-based health care research firm, found that of 262 HMOs surveyed nationwide, the plans with the lowest premiums saw enrollment growth averaging 16 percent in 1993, while the highest-priced HMOs experienced only a .08 percent enrollment increase.[2] Health care providers must consider the response of individual consumers and employers to likely charges and fees.

ESTABLISHING THE PRICE

Establishing the price for a product or service effectively is a multistep process. Organizations must: (1) identify the constraints to their pricing policy; (2) determine their objectives; (3) estimate demand and revenue; (4) determine the cost, volume, and profit relationships; (5) select a pricing strategy; and (6) consider the positioning element to their final price.

Indentifying Constraints

Ideally, one might suggest pricing a product high. Obviously, the higher the price the greater the potential for profit. Yet in any pricing decision, several constraints must be recognized to temper the final price level established.

Demand

A major factor in establishing price is recognizing the demand for the product or service. Products in great demand can command a higher price.

Newness in the Life Cycle

In Chapter 7, the concept of the product life cycle was reviewed. Pricing considerations change over the length of time a product exists in the competitive market.[3] Pricing in the early stages of the life cycle depends on several variables. If the company has a limited capacity to meet demand, or if it needs to recoup investment costs prior to competitors entering the market (for a truly new service), it may select a higher price. If, however, an organization needs to generate volume to achieve an economy of scale, or if it wants to minimize the likelihood of competitive entries, it will establish a lower price level.

Typically, the newer a product is in the life cycle, the higher the price that can be charged. When a company holds a patent on a product—such as is common in the pharmaceutical industry—the greater the likelihood it will price the product high. Health care is a service-driven industry, with little ability to establish proprietary rights to what is being provided. This lack of sole providership has made higher pricing more difficult. Many states, however, have required filing a certificate of need (CON) or a determination of need, for example, when a hospital was establishing a new service that required significant capital expense. Once granted to a hospital, this certificate often served as a form of patent or franchise, since the state regulatory agencies try to cap the number of health care providers offering similar services. The regulators determined that duplication of services would lead to greater health care costs. In terms of competitive strategy, however, one can see that increasing the number of competitors would drive prices down.

Single- vs. Multiple-Product Pricing

Many organizations have more than one product or service in their product line. In pricing these products, a company must evaluate whether the products are complementary, in other words, whether the purchase of one product or service will affect the purchase of another item in the line. Organizations can employ multiple pricing strategies when they have complementary products. These are discussed more fully later in this chapter.

Production Cost

A fourth constraint in the pricing decision is the cost of production. A company must determine whether it has high fixed costs or high variable costs to consider in its pricing decisions. A more detailed discussion of the nature of production costs and the types of production costs is provided later in this chapter.

Channel Length

Pricing decisions cannot be made independent of consideration of the channel of distribution (described in Chapter 9). The producer of a product or service, which is provided through resellers, must determine what the final price will be to the end consumer as the product is marked up through the distribution channel. Each member of the channel provides services and adds to the cost, and thus price, of the service at the next level.

Market Structure

Every pricing decision must reflect, to some degree, the nature of the market structure. As noted in Chapter 3, there are four basic types of market structure: pure monopoly, oligopoly, monopolistic competition, and pure competition.

A pure monopoly involves one seller who sets the price for a unique service. This situation existed historically in the communications industry when AT&T, at one time, was the sole provider of telephone service in the United States. It is still a common form of market structure in the energy industry where one company supplies all of the local or regional demand for electricity or natural gas. There is no direct price competition in such a market. Usually, pure monopoly markets result in government or regulatory price control or review. Even in this type of market structure, however, a company must consider whether there are **substitutable goods**, or other products that can satisfy the same basic needs. For example, when the price of electricity rose in many northeastern states in the 1970s, many consumers switched their home heating source to natural gas or oil.

In an oligopoly—a market structure where a few companies control a majority of industry sales—there is often great awareness of competitors' pricing policies. There tends occasionally to be a price leader who dictates the direction of price levels. In the airline industry, for example, one company will occasionally raise fares and hope the others will follow suit, rather than induce a price war that erodes all sellers' margins.

Monopolistic competition exists in markets where many sellers offer substitutable products. These producers want their offerings to be viewed as unique and different from the competition. This shifts the focus of competition and consumer buying decisions away from price. In recent years, hospitals have focused on advertising their particularly unique services and amenities in an effort to create more of a monopolistic competition in the health care market.

As noted earlier, pure competition involves markets with many small producers and many small buyers—the typical market structure faced by many physicians in their office practices. There is relatively easy entry and exit from these markets, and buyers are supposed to have perfect information. This last characteristic tends not to exist in the real world. In a purely competitive market, price levels would be set by the market.

Pricing Objectives

In determining its pricing strategy, an organization must first specify its pricing objectives. There are several objectives that are relevant to pricing programs.

Profit

A common objective for many organizations is to price in a way to maximize profits. In following this objective, companies will utilize a skimming price strategy, especially in the introduction stage of the product life cycle, as discussed in Chapter 7. This strategy may be workable in the short term. The problem with a skimming strategy, however, is that while short-term profits can be maximized, the high price may encourage competitors to offer a similar service at a lower price and thereby capture share. The original company that tried to maximize profits might end up with a small position in the market.

Sales

A second pricing objective is to maximize sales or volume. In following this objective, companies often employ a penetration pricing strategy, which involves setting a low price (as noted in Chapter 7) relative to the competition or to substitutable services. Sales are maximized. The value of this approach is apparent when the firm must meet some economies of scale. Morton Plant Health System in Clearwater, Florida, for example, lowered the price of mammography services from $55 to $39. The health system decided it could make up the price difference in higher patient volume. Between March and December 1993, 11,651 mammograms were performed, compared to 4,199 in 1992.[4]

Unlike a skimming strategy, this approach discourages competition. Following the sales objective, however, requires a good knowledge of the cost curves. Generating sales that lead to a dollar loss will be a short-lived approach for any company.

Market Share

Many companies set their pricing strategy around the objective of gaining market share. This strategy is common in two different types of market conditions. In the early stages of competition for a new product or service, a market share objective is often important to achieve economies of scale to support the operation's overhead. This condition is true for managed care plans that have slashed premiums.[5] A second condition in which market share is often the objective is in industries that have no real growth. In these instances, the opportunities for increased revenue will only come from increasing market share relative to a competitor. Today, many acute care hospitals are aggressively competing with each other for managed care contracts in order to increase market share.

Image

The image a company wants to project is often tied up with its pricing objectives. One pricing strategy is called **prestige pricing**, in which a high price is established relative to the competition, or to the true cost of producing the service. The reason is to project an image of exclusivity or value. This strategy is common to products that are hard to differentiate in any other tangible way, such as liquor. Alternatively, Wal-Mart stores set their pricing strategy as one not to be undersold. Their image is that of a place where the price-conscious consumer shops.

Stabilization

A fifth pricing objective is to establish a price level that will encourage a similar response from competitors. Although overt agreement among competitors to set prices is illegal, a stabilization pricing objective can result in maintaining margins while encouraging competition on other elements of the marketing mix. This is especially true if the pricing strategy considers attributes important to consumers, such as convenience and quality.

Estimating Demand and Revenue

An essential step in establishing any price level is to estimate the demand for the company's product. A key aspect of this phase of pricing is to prepare a **demand schedule**, or summary of the amounts of a product that are desired at each price level. Understanding consumers' price sensitivity at various levels is where marketing research plays a critical role.[6]

In determining consumer response to price, marketers try to assess the degree of **price elasticity**, or change in demand relative to a change in price, which exists in the marketplace. Consumers are said to be price elastic when the percentage demand for a product exceeds the percentage change in price. A study conducted by the Harvard University School of Public Health found that nearly 30 percent of fee-for-service patients surveyed said they would switch to a managed care plan if it lowered their costs by at least 20 percent. In addition, 1 in 11 consumers said they would switch if it lowered their costs by 30 percent.[7] These data indicate a rather price elastic market.

Consumers are price inelastic when the percentage change in demand does not exceed the percentage change in price. Figure 8–1 shows the price elasticity of consumer demand as the monthly premium for a closed-panel HMO is lowered. Based on the curve, one can see that the demand is relatively price inelastic as the monthly premium is decreased from $200 per family per month to $170 (D2) per family per month. The number of subscribers increases dramatically as the premium begins to drop from $150 to $75 (D4). At this point demand might be considered price elastic. The more that a marketer can position a product so that it is perceived as unique, however, the greater the likelihood that demand will be price inelastic. A company that positions itself as a high-quality provider can charge higher prices. Price elasticity is reduced when the customer perceives higher quality in the service.[8]

Cost and Volume Relationships

In establishing the price for a product, marketers must take into consideration the nature of the organization's costs. There are three cost concepts to consider: fixed costs, variable costs, and total cost. **Fixed costs** are those costs that do not change based on the volume of product or service delivered. For example, a hospital that buys a piece of laboratory equipment would incur a fixed cost for the equipment. Regardless of whether 1 test or 100 are performed with the equipment, the cost of the machinery is fixed. **Variable costs** are those costs that vary with the amount of the service delivered. Nursing personnel salaries are considered a variable cost. For example, if patient volume declines, the number of full-time-

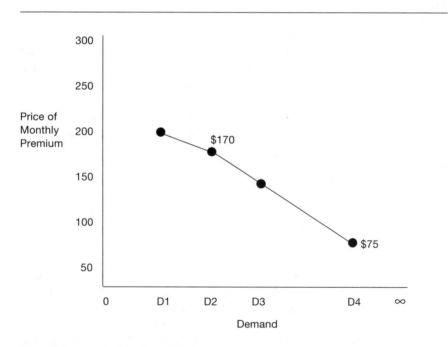

Figure 8–1 Price Elasticity for an HMO

equivalent (FTE) nurses can be reduced. **Total cost** represents the total expense that the firm bears in delivering and marketing its service. Total cost represents the combination of fixed and variable costs. With these concepts in mind, companies can consider the relationship between cost and volume in establishing prices.

Cost-Plus Pricing

One of the simplest approaches to setting price is the cost-plus method, in which the selling price represents the total cost of the service, *plus* some additional amount for profit. While simple in methodology, cost-plus pricing does not consider the differences between fixed and variable costs.

Exhibit 8–1 shows the cost/price relationships that must be recognized. In a high fixed-cost organization, the major consideration is to price for volume. With high variable costs compared to total cost, an organization must price for margin.

Consider the example of the airline industry, in which fixed costs are a high percentage of total costs. Its major concern is to price in such a way to ensure the coverage of fixed costs. As a result, the airline offers significant consumer fare discounts in order to cover fixed costs, if consumers purchase tickets well in advance of their scheduled travel times. This point is shown as T1 in Figure 8–2. As the airline comes closer to covering its fixed costs (T2), prices rise, since the additional revenue generated now contributes to profit. Finally, departure time arrives, and the airplane is ready to leave the gate (T3). Since an empty seat is a wasted seat, it is not long before the airline reduces the fare for a consumer willing to hop on the plane as a last-minute standby.

This same type of pricing as a reflection of production costs is followed by arts organizations. These entities provide subscriber discounts if tickets are purchased several months prior to the performance. Ticket prices rise as the date of the show draws closer. Then, many theater groups will offer significant customer discounts for last-minute rushes for seats as the curtain rises. Similarly, Rick Scott, CEO of Columbia/HCA, a Nashville-based organization that owns over 200 hospitals in the U.S., has discussed the possibility of discounted midnight surgery. Recognizing the high fixed cost of an unused operating room suite, this approach could result in some surgeries being scheduled during off-hours at a lower price. The

---

Exhibit 8–1 Cost/Price Relationships

High Fixed Cost/Total Cost = Volume Sensitive
High Variable Cost/Total Cost = Margin Sensitive

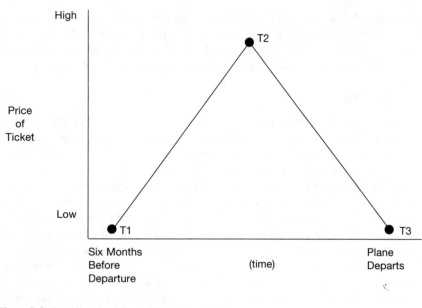

Figure 8–2 Covering Fixed Costs: The Airline Industry

---

target market might be self-paying individuals or those whose insurance coverage carries high deductibles.[9]

Consider this cost-plus scenario: An airline wants to price its tickets at 50 percent above the cost of each flight. The cost of a flight (maintenance, salaries, landing rights, etc.) is $5,000. In addition, the cost of meals, snacks, and beverages is $2 per passenger. If 150 seats on the plane are occupied, the total cost of the flight is over $5,000 (150 × $2 = $5,300). Adding 50 percent profit would yield a total cost of over $5,000 (50 percent × $5,000 = $7,500). Since this cost is based on the assumed volume of 150 passengers, the price per ticket would be $7,500/150 = $50.

If, however, only 100 passengers show up for the flight, total cost does not change very much. As described, the fixed cost represents a higher proportion of total cost. Yet, in this instance, total revenue changes dramatically. With only 100 passengers, the airline's total revenue for the flight is $5,000 ($50 per ticket × 100 passengers). The airline would not cover the total cost of the flight, which is $5,200 [$5,000 + ($2 × 100)].

The opposite of a high fixed cost–to–total cost ratio is the firm whose variable costs are a higher proportion of the total cost of production. With these companies, small increases in margin can result in significant increases in profit.

Break-Even Analysis

An alternative concept that considers the level of sales required at a given price to cover total costs is referred to as **break-even analysis**. Using this price-setting method, a company determines the break-even point needed to cover total costs. This point is derived by the following equation:

$$\text{Break-even point} = \frac{\text{Total Fixed Cost}}{\text{Price} - \text{Variable Cost}}$$

The break-even point is that point of volume where total revenue equals total cost.

Consider the example of the free-standing surgery center shown in Table 8–1. In this case, the average price per procedure is $500. Because of the contractual arrangement with managed care organizations, a 10 percent discount is required. Annual fixed costs total $500,000 and variable costs are $200 per procedure. The volume of procedures now necessary to operate the facility at break-even point is 2,000. Consider what happens if a higher price or lower discount were possible. At a charge of $500 with no discount, the break-even point drops to only 1,667 procedures to cover costs and break even.[10]

At this point it is important for the free-standing surgery center management to recognize the linkage between the break-even point and market share. Identifying

---

Table 8–1 Free-Standing Surgicenter Cost Structure

Factors	Costs ($)
Break-Even Analysis	
Average price per procedure	500
Average discount or allowance (10%)	– 50
Net price per procedure	450
Annual fixed cost (depreciation, interest, utilities, management, etc.)	500,000
Variable cost per procedure	200
Break-Even Computation	
Net price per procedure	450
Variable cost per procedure	–200
Contribution margin per procedure	250 (A)
Fixed cost	500,000 (B)
Break-even number of procedures (B divided by A)	2,000

Source: Reprinted from Pitts, K.B., Pricing and Reimbursement Strategies, *Topics in Health Care Finance*, Vol. 12, No. 2, p. 26, Aspen Publishers, Inc., © 1985.

varying break-even volumes, the organization should consider what percent of the market they can attract, and what discount levels are required by buyers (managed care plans). In this way, an organization can assess the likelihood of generating revenue and the pressures on the ultimate price. For example, if the low price represents a competitive market price—most other competitors discount surgery $75—this constraint must be considered. Yet, if this price level represents a break-even volume of almost 75 percent of all surgery cases, the venture might be considered too risky to enter.

Marginal Cost Pricing

Marginal cost pricing is based on the concept that the price per additional procedure must equal or exceed the cost of an additional procedure. In the previous free-standing surgicenter example, the $200 per procedure variable cost (shown in Table 8–1) equals the marginal cost of each additional procedure.

To understand a marginal cost pricing approach, consider the data shown in Table 8–2, which evaluates the marginal, or variable, cost per procedure. As is common today, assume that the surgery center negotiates with an HMO. This managed care plan guarantees at least 600 procedures, at $325 per procedure. This price exceeds the marginal cost ($200), but it is below the level of the full price with the discount as shown earlier in Table 8–1. Complicate this scenario by assuming that the HMO purchases 100 procedures at the higher price. Table 8–3 shows the

Table 8–2 Free-Standing Surgicenter: Variable Cost Analysis

Expenses	Full cost	Fixed cost	Variable cost
Salaries	$350,000	$140,000	$210,000
Fringe benefits	50,000	20,000	30,000
Supplies	160,000	6,000	154,000
Maintenance and repairs	10,000	8,000	2,000
Utilities	30,000	28,000	2,000
Administrative and general	40,000	38,000	2,000
Housekeeping	20,000	20,000	—
Property taxes	10,000	10,000	—
Depreciation	130,000	130,000	—
Interest	100,000	100,000	—
Total	$900,000	$500,000	$400,000
Number of break-even procedures	2,000	2,000	2,000
Cost per procedure	$ 450	$ 250	$ 200

Source: Reprinted from Pitts, K.B., Pricing and Reimbursement Strategies, *Topics in Health Care Finance,* Vol. 12, No. 2, p. 27, Aspen Publishers, Inc., © 1985.

Table 8–3 Free-Standing Surgicenter: Impact of Volume Increase

	Break-even at 1,000 procedures	Impact of 500 additional procedures	Total income at 1,500 procedures
Revenues			
Current	$900,000	$ -	$ 900,000
Incremental (600 @ $325)	—	195,000	195,000
Lost revenue (100 @ $450)	—	−45,000	−45,000
Total	900,000	150,000	1,050,000
Expenses			
Salaries	350,000	52,500	402,500
Fringe benefits	50,000	7,500	57,500
Supplies	160,000	38,500	198,500
Maintenance and repairs	10,000	500	10,500
Utilities	30,000	500	30,500
Administrative and general	40,000	500	40,500
Housekeeping	20,000	—	20,000
Property taxes	10,000	—	10,000
Depreciation	130,000	—	130,000
Interest	100,000	0	100,000
Total	900,000	100,000	1,000,000
Net Income	$ 0	$ 50,000	$ 50,000

Source: Reprinted from Pitts, K.B., Pricing and Reimbursement Strategies, *Topics in Health Care Finance,* Vol. 12, No. 2, p. 28, Aspen Publishers, Inc., © 1985.

impact of increased volume at reduced price and the profitability of entering into the contract. This marginal cost approach is useful in considering appropriate pricing strategies to attract large-volume purchasers.

Markup Pricing

Markup pricing involves calculating the per-unit cost of producing the service or product and determining the markup percentages needed to cover the cost of selling and profit. This pricing scheme is often used by wholesalers and retailers. The formula for markup pricing is:

$$\text{Price} = \frac{\text{Service Cost}}{(100 - \text{Markup Percent})/100}$$

For example, if a physician pays $6.00 for lab tests and needs a 40 percent markup to cover costs, the price billed to a patient's insurance company for the test would be:

$$\text{Price} = \frac{\$6.00}{(100 - 40)/100} = 10.00$$

Target Pricing

A fourth pricing strategy, **target pricing**, involves setting price to provide a targeted rate of return on investment for a standard level of service delivery or production. For example, a hospital may have an average rate of occupancy of 60 percent. The hospital might compute a target price for services directly paid with the following formula:

$$\text{Price} = \frac{\text{Investment Costs} \times \text{Target Return on Investment (\%)}}{\text{Standard Volume}}$$

Target pricing is common in production firms that are capital-intensive. A major limitation to this method, however, is that price is set with no consideration of market demand, and thus, all the volume needed to generate the target return might not be forthcoming.

Demand-Minus Pricing

A final pricing strategy that is becoming more relevant for health care providers with the advent of managed care is **demand-minus pricing**, which involves determining what price the market is willing to pay and working backwards to compute costs. This pricing concept focuses on a major difference in pricing considerations between financial officers in health care organizations and marketing professionals. Typically, health care prices have been set based on the costs the facility estimated in providing the service. In fact, 20 years ago, hospitals were reimbursed under a procedure called *cost-based reimbursement.* Subsequent reform dictated that hospitals would be paid for services based on diagnosis-related groups (DRGs). This reimbursement mechanism paid a price to treat a disease. Yet, in fact, hospital reimbursement under the DRG system was based on average historical costs.

Under the prevailing managed care models, health care organizations are competing for contracts. Employers and individual consumers who enroll in individual health plans care little about what it costs to provide the service. Rather the determining factor is the buyers' own respective price ceiling, or limit, that they are willing to pay. Past distinctions of inpatient charges, outpatient charges, and the like are irrelevant to the consumer. Health care providers must identify through market research the maximum price a buyer is willing to pay for a bundle of services. The organization must then calculate the markup percentage it needs to cover selling expenses and desired profits. Then, the maximum permissible cost can be computed through the following formula:

$$\text{Maximum Service Cost} = \text{Price} \times [(100 - \text{Markup Percent})/100]$$

Dallas Medical Resource (D.M.R.) is using this pricing strategy with participating hospitals. D.M.R. is a nonprofit corporation comprised of nine major Dallas health care providers and major Texas employers. Employers set prices and the providers decide whether they can meet them. Fina, Inc., a Dallas-based, integrated oil and chemical company, proposed a global price for coronary artery bypass procedures, hip and knee replacements, and neck surgery. The D.M.R.–affiliated hospitals accepted this market price.[11]

Pricing Strategies

There are several types of pricing strategies that firms can use. Many of those discussed in the following pages have not been applied previously to health care, but this is changing as the health care regulatory environment and marketplace evolves. Health care organizations that sell managed care products and services in the marketplace are behaving more like retailers.

Price Lining

One price strategy is **price lining**, in which products in a line are priced within a distinct price range that is significantly different from the prices of substitutes in the next range. The purpose of this strategy is to give the consumer the impression that quality differences exist between the price lines. This pricing strategy works best under conditions where the consumer has little prior experience with the product or service or lacks the expertise to evaluate the service objectively. For many years, for example, Sears Roebuck operated with three distinct price lines of *good, better,* and *best* for its home appliances and household items.

Price lines make it easier for consumers to shop because they can consider the level of product quality they want to buy. For price lining to be effective, however, consumers must perceive a significant difference between the items in each line in terms of quality. When making changes in price lines, marketers must be aware of the fact that a change in one aspect of the line can affect the entire price line.[12]

Odd Pricing

A second pricing strategy has been referred to as **odd pricing**, in which items are priced at just below whole dollar amounts. Perusing the shelves of any supermarket, one will notice the vast array of items marked with a price ending in 5, 7, or 9. Several reasons have been posited for odd pricing. One rationale suggested is that of pluralistic ignorance—one retailer does it because the other competitor is following this strategy. There is no real logic to the approach, however. A second, more plausible, explanation for odd pricing pertains to in-store theft. Odd prices require the cashier to make change for the customer. In so doing, the clerk must record the sale on the cash register and enter the cash drawer in the presence of the customer. If the item were priced at $1.00 or $5.00, the customer might just hand the clerk a bill of the correct amount and leave the store. The cashier could then just not record the sale and pocket the money. A third reason suggested for odd pricing is that it gives the impression that the item has been discounted from a higher price.[13] For example, $4.99 suggests a markdown as opposed to $5.00.

The final explanation for odd pricing is based on a theory of how consumers shop. **Item budget theory** suggests that consumers set out with a predetermined price that they are willing to pay for a particular item. Any item just below this predetermined price will be deemed acceptable. If the item is priced even slightly above that amount, however, it will be considered too expensive. For example, a consumer decides to shop for a new business suit and she decides to pay no more than $400. Seeing a suit priced at $420, the consumer would find the price unacceptable. Priced at $395, however, the suit would fit within the shopper's budgeted amount.

For health care providers, this last explanation of odd pricing based on item budget theory is extremely relevant for pricing health care services in today's marketplace. Through marketing research, providers must determine what is the item budgeted amount that a consumer feels is acceptable for a monthly health plan premium, or for a routine mammogram not covered by insurance.

One-Price vs. Flexible Pricing

With a **one-price policy**, the company charges the same price to all customers who buy the service under the same set of conditions. Discounts may be provided for the timing of the purchase or the level of volume; however, all customers have the opportunity to avail themselves of these discounts. The advantages of this policy are that it instills customer confidence and it is also easy to administer.

A second variation is the **flexible pricing policy**, in which customers will be charged different prices based on their ability to negotiate or on their respective buying power. This strategy is common in the automobile industry where, based on the ability to haggle, a customer might get a lower price than another person purchasing the same car. Recently, because many consumers find this strategy uncomfortable, some automobile dealers have begun promoting one-price policies. Flexible pricing is common in industrial settings where the consumer's buying power can often result in lower prices. The major concern here, however, is to ensure the legality of the pricing policy according to the Robinson-Patman Act, as described in Chapter 3.

Prestige Pricing

A fourth pricing strategy described earlier in this chapter is prestige pricing, in which items are deliberately priced at a high level to connote uniqueness or value. This pricing strategy goes against the typical economic logic of the rational buyer who purchases more as the price declines. The demand curve for prestige pricing is shown in Figure 8–3. As can be seen, at price level P1 demand is D1. Yet as the price rises to P2, demand increases rather than decreases to D2. At some point, however, if the price should increase to too high a level (P3), demand will again decrease to a low level again (D1).

Prestige pricing is a strategy often followed for products or services where it is difficult to distinguish real quality differences or where the perceived risk of purchasing is high.[14] For many years, for example, L'Oreal hair coloring has been promoted on the basis of "It costs more, but I'm worth it." Again, the risk of health care services might provide some logic to prestige pricing, along with the fact that it is hard for the average consumer to discern the quality differences of the service delivered. The only limiting constraint to prestige pricing as discussed at the beginning of this chapter is that the price must not be so high as to generate little demand.

Leader Pricing

Leader pricing is a strategy of attractively pricing an item in the product line and aggressively promoting it to encourage consumers to purchase it and also other items in the line at the same time. This strategy is often implemented by grocery stores. Popular brand-named items are priced low to get consumers into the store, who then complete their grocery shopping by purchasing items priced at more favorable margins for the retailer.

For leader pricing to be successful, the consumer must recognize the promoted price to be a significant value, and the item must be desired.

Bundled Pricing

Bundled pricing involves selling several items or services together for one total price.[15] This strategy has been common in health care for occupational and industrial medicine programs. Companies are offered an array of services, such as health education for employees, pre-employment physicals, job hazard analysis, and toxicology support, for a set price per employee.

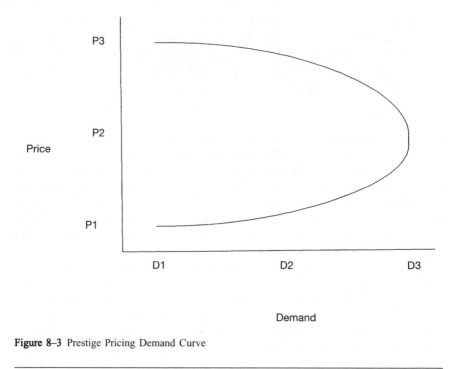

Figure 8–3 Prestige Pricing Demand Curve

For price bundling to be effective, the savings on the bundle must be seen as a real value as opposed to buying the services individually.[16] Fulton described a large metropolitan hospital in the West that bundled its obstetrical services. Services that were bundle-priced included normal delivery, 24-hour, 36-hour, and Caesarian section delivery. Each bundled price included room, recovery, nursery, and hospital-based physician costs.[17]

With "unbundled pricing," a company breaks down the price of the items to be purchased individually. Increasingly in health care, providers are offering customers the opportunity to tailor the product line by offering both pricing strategies.

Going-Rate Pricing

Going-rate pricing is a pricing strategy that involves setting prices relative to the prevailing market price with less consideration for internal costs or margin requirements. This strategy has been common in oligopolistic industries where there are only a few sellers who sell relatively similar items. This situation somewhat describes the hospital competitive environment of the 1970s before many institutions tried to differentiate themselves in terms of the services provided.

Discounts

In many situations, companies often provide discounts, or price reductions, to buyers. There are four common types of discounts: volume, functional, seasonal, or allowances.

Volume or Quantity Discounts. **Volume discounts** are provided to buyers who purchase the service or guarantee to utilize the service at some predetermined level. Legally, volume discounts must be offered equally to all buyers. To offer volume discounts, the seller must be able to demonstrate that there are real cost savings that can be achieved if the service is utilized at some specified volume level.

Functional Discounts. **Functional discounts** on price are offered if the buyer agrees to perform or take over particular functions involved with the product or service. For example, if a manufacturer agreed to provide on-site space for the administration of routine employee exams or for a nurse practitioner to meet with employees, this might be factored into a discount. An employer might also receive a discount if it agrees to distribute all health plan promotional material internally to its employees.

Seasonal Discounts. These are price reductions provided when the product is purchased out of season. The objective of a seasonal discount is to smooth out demand. Hotels offer special discounts on weekends when business traveller use is light. Golf equipment manufacturers will run winter sales to stimulate demand in off-peak times in order to keep the production line operating.

Allowances. Allowances refer to other reductions from the standard price. Occasionally, companies will offer trade-in allowances to customers who bring in an older item for the purchase of a new one. Manufacturers often offer allowances to resellers who agree to use certain promotional material like end-of-aisle displays of the product within their stores.

Positioning Value of Price

Price plays a major strategic role in the positioning of the product, service, or organization. In establishing the price level, companies must consider the competitive environment and the position where they would like their service to be priced relative to the competition. Second, a company must consider how much focus will be placed on price in promoting the service.

Figure 8–4 displays four broad options for price positioning. There are two axes defining these quadrants. The horizontal X axis refers to whether the price to be charged will be high or low relative to the competition. The vertical Y axis refers

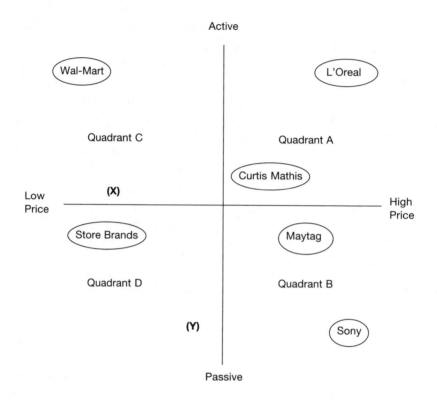

Figure 8–4 Positioning of Price. *Source:* Adapted from Tellis, G.J., Creative Pricing Strategies, *Journal of Medical Practice Management*, Vol. 3, No. 2, pp. 120–124, with permission of Williams & Wilkins, © 1988.

to whether the price will be an active or passive part of the promotional strategy. When price is active, promotional efforts will call attention to the price level. When price is passive, the promotional effort focuses on other attributes of the product or service.

Quadrant A represents situations where prices are high relative to the competition and price is a very active part of the strategy. This approach is useful in situations where it is hard to differentiate the product on tangible dimensions or when promoting a prestige image for the product. Curtis Mathis televisions have been promoted as "The most expensive television set money can buy." L'Oreal hair coloring was mentioned earlier as a prestige-priced item.

Quadrant B involves situations where price is set high but kept a passive element in the marketing mix. Maytag appliances, for example, are premium-priced relative to competitors' products. Maytag, however, does not mention price but focuses instead on the reliability of its product. Maytag advertising often displays their lonely company repairman who is never called for repairs. The implication is that Maytag products never need fixing. Sony audio and video equipment is also priced higher than the competition. Again, Sony focuses on sound and visual quality and advanced technology as its differential advantage.

The third quadrant, C, involves setting a low price and being very aggressive in promoting it. Wal-Mart aggressively promotes its low-price position, which is a common position for many discounters.

The last quadrant, D, unusual for many marketers, entails assigning a low price but not promoting it. In traditional businesses, this is very uncommon. In health care, however, this strategy has been used for services that an organization might be mandated to provide, but for which they did not want significant demand. Many hospitals have often posted notices regarding the availability of free care, if economically necessary. Few institutions, however, would want to promote this option.

CONCLUSIONS

Price is a major aspect of marketing strategy. As the health care industry moves from a reimbursement environment into a retail economy where products and services are offered to consumers, the pricing considerations common to traditional businesses such as Pillsbury and Sony will become more prevalent. The strategic and positioning implications of price cannot be ignored when developing the organization's marketing strategy.

KEY TERMS

Price	Target Pricing
Complementary Products	Demand-Minus Pricing
Substitutable Goods	Price Lining
Prestige Pricing	Odd Pricing
Demand Schedule	Item Budget Theory
Price Elasticity	One-Price Policy
Fixed Costs	Flexible Price Policy
Variable Costs	Leader Pricing
Total Cost	Bundled Pricing
Break-Even Analysis	Going-Rate Pricing
Marginal Cost Pricing	Volume Discounts
Markup Pricing	Functional Discounts

CHAPTER SUMMARY

1. The price an organization establishes has an economic, perceptual, and positioning value to the firm.

2. Multiple factors, such as demand, life cycle, product line, and channel structure, all affect the pricing decision.

3. Organizations can pursue several different pricing objectives that affect their strategy. These are: profit, sales, market share, image, and stabilization.

4. An important consideration in pricing is determining the amount of sales needed in order to break even. This figure is based on the total fixed cost, variable cost, and price charged.

5. In addition to break-even pricing, firms can follow a cost-plus pricing, marginal cost pricing, markup pricing, target pricing, or demand-minus price-setting policy.

6. In establishing prices lines it is essential to have noticeable differences in perceived quality for the distinct lines.

7. Odd pricing is based on item budget theory, which assumes a consumer predetermines the amount to be spent on an item.

8. Prestige pricing is counter-intuitive to the economic logic of a rational buyer. Too high a price, however, will lead to a decline in demand.

9. Bundling, or selling several medical services together at one set price, is becoming a common strategy in health care.

10. There are several ways an organization can reduce the price for a product. Discounts can be based on volume, function, seasonality, or an allowance.

11. Price has an important positioning value depending on how active or passive a role it plays in the promotional strategy, and on the level of the price relative to the competition.

CHAPTER PROBLEMS

1. Explain how a pharmaceutical company's pricing for a nonproprietary drug might change if the objective was: (a) profitability, (b) sales volume, (c) market share.

2. Two medical organizations have recently examined their cost structures. The first group is a radiology practice with a significant investment in diagnostic

imaging equipment. The second group is a single-specialty pediatric practice. The cost analysis reveals the following distribution:

	Radiology Group	Pediatric Group
Fixed Cost	70%	20%
Variable Cost	30%	80%

Explain the implications of these differing cost structures of each medical group in terms of contracting with managed care organizations.

3. An HMO marketing manager reduced the HMO's premium by 10 percent and saw a 20 percent increase in the number of subscribers. He then thought that if the premium was reduced by another 20 percent, he would see a 40 percent increase. What is your analysis of this reasoning?

4. An ophthalmology practice is deciding whether to offer prescription eyeglasses for sale in-house. The new service would require the training and hiring of additional personnel, inventory for glasses and frames, and some minor space alterations. The utilized space in the office would be a charge allocated to the program. The costs for this new service are:

Variable Costs (electricity, labor, supplies)	$80 per completed pair of eyeglasses
Total Fixed Cost	$36,000

How much volume does the group need to break even if they charge $100 per pair of eyeglasses? If they charge $200?

5. Assume that in problem 4 the total market for eyeglasses in this community is 2,400 pair. What are the market share implications of a $100 price? A $200 price?

6. A health club decided recently to offer a yearly membership. Separate fees were to be charged for nutrition counseling, tennis court usage, and aerobic instruction. How might this organization implement: (a) a prestige pricing strategy? (b) a bundled price strategy? (c) price lines?

7. What type of price positioning strategy would you recommend for a medical group that: (a) has customer service features such as weekend appointment hours that distinguish it from the competition, and (b) wants to entice wealthy South Americans to seek treatment in the United States? What is your rationale for each recommendation?

NOTES

1. Several studies consider the perceptual aspect of price. See: J. Jacoby and J.C. Olsen, eds., *Perceived Quality* (Lexington, Mass.: Lexington Books, 1985); V.A. Zeithaml, Consumer Perceptions of Price, Quality, and Value, *Journal of Marketing* 52, no. 3 (1988):2–22; and J. Wind, Getting a Read on Market-Defined Value, *Journal of Pricing Management* (1990):5–14.

2. In Brief, *Business & Health* 12, no. 5 (1994):17.

3. For a discussion of pricing issues over the life cycle, see P.M. Parker, Price Elasticity Over the Adoption Life Cycle, *Journal of Marketing Research* 29, no. 3 (1992):358–367.

4. R.L. Cohen, Retail Strategy Works Wonders for Hospital Mammography Promotion, *Healthcare Marketing Report* 12, no. 8 (1994):12–13.

5. C. Sardinha, HMOs, Hoping To Win Market Share, Slash Premium Hikes to New Lows, *Managed Care Outlook* 7, no. 2 (1994):1–2.

6. For a good review of methods used to measure sensitivity and price see, T.T. Nagel, *The Strategy and Tactics of Pricing* (Englewood Cliffs, N.J.: Prentice Hall, 1987).

7. For Patients, Is Cost More Crucial Than Freedom of Choice? *Medical Economics* 71 (1994):18.

8. Y.K. Shetty, Product Quality and Competitive Strategy, *Business Horizons* 30, no. 3 (1987): 345–52; and K.B. Monroe, Buyer's Subjective Perception of Price, *Journal of Marketing Research* 10, no. 1 (1973):70–80.

9. D. Jones, Election Gives Hospital Giant More Clout, *USA TODAY*, 11 November 1994, B1,B2.

10. This discussion and that of marginal pricing is based on K.B. Pitts, Pricing and Reimbursement Strategies, *Topics in Health Care Financing* 12, no. 1 (Fall 1985):24–31.

11. Dallas Project a Model for Physician-Hospital Collaboration, *Hospital Integrated Strategy Report* 2, no. 1 (1994):8–10.

12. S. Petroshius and K.B. Monroe, Effects of Product-Line Pricing Characteristics on Product Evaluation, *Journal of Consumer Research* 13, no. 4 (1987):511–519.

13. Z.V. Lambert, Perceived Price as Related to Odd and Even Price Endings, *Journal of Retailing* 51, no. 3 (Fall 1975):13–22.

14. G.J. Szybillo and J. Jacoby, Intrinsic versus Extrinsic Cues as Determinants of Perceived Product Quality, *Journal of Applied Psychology* 59, no. 1 (1974):74–78.

15. J. Guiltinan, The Price Bundling of Services: A Normative Framework, *Journal of Marketing* 51, no. 2 (1987):74–85; and D. Paun, When To Bundle or Unbundle Products, *Industrial Marketing Management* 22, no. 2 (1993):29–34.

16. G.J. Tellis, Beyond the Many Faces of Price: An Integration of Pricing Strategies, *Journal of Marketing* 50, no. 4 (1986):146–160.

17. P.R. Fulton, The Forgotten "P"—Pricing Strategies, in *Responding to the Challenge: Health Care Marketing Comes of Age*, ed. P.D. Cooper (Chicago, Ill.: Academy for Health Care Marketing, 1986), 10–12.

DISTRIBUTION

After reading this chapter you should be able to:

- Understand the concept of channel structure and the alternative channels available

- Know the varying levels of distribution intensity and the considerations in implementing each alternative

- Understand the concept of vertical marketing systems and their application in health care

- Describe the nature of channel leadership and the source of channel power

- Recognize the application of retailing in health care strategy

Place, which refers to distribution, is a basic component of the marketing mix. It represents how and where the product is accessed by the consumer. The path a product takes as it travels from the manufacturer to the consumer is referred to as the **channel of distribution**. In both service and product marketing, marketers have several key decisions to make involving the channel of distribution and the place component of the marketing mix, such as: how the product should be distributed, who within the channel should perform specific functions, how much coverage of the market is needed, and ultimately how the channel can be controlled.

ALTERNATIVE CHANNELS OF DISTRIBUTION

All businesses must decide how many other organizations are needed to distribute their product or service. The channels companies use vary in length, with length referring to the number of intermediaries. A *direct* channel is one in which no one stands between the producer of the product and the ultimate consumer. Figure 9–1 shows a direct channel (A). In health care, the most direct channel is between the primary care physician and the patient.

An *indirect* channel may have several intermediaries between the producer and the ultimate consumer. For example, Proctor and Gamble, a consumer products company located in Cincinnati, Ohio, uses the middle channel (B) in Figure 9–1 for the distribution of its many products. So too, an academic medical center that provides sophisticated tertiary services might have an indirect channel with several intermediaries (C), as shown in Figure 9–1. The community hospital, the specialist, and the primary care physician all are involved in early stages of diagnosis, intervention, and care before the patient is referred to the academic medical center. In traditional product marketing, the intermediaries within the

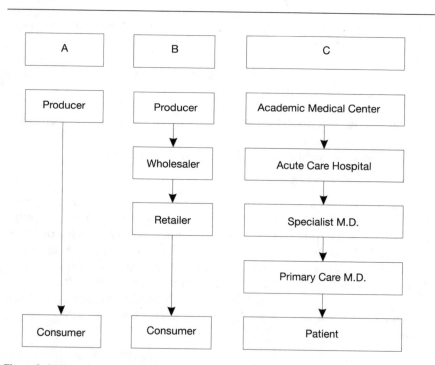

Figure 9–1 Channels of Distribution

channel will vary as to whether they take ownership or title to the goods as they move through the channel. In health care, taking title is not an issue for channel consideration.

Functions in the Channel

A common view that consumers have had of traditional industries is that the middleman, or intermediary, adds cost or little value to the product. In reality, though, most intermediaries perform several valuable functions or **utilities** in the channel of distribution.

Place

A major function of any intermediary is the place value provided to the product or service, by making it more accessible to the consumer. A primary care clinic that offers after-hours care or weekend appointment hours would be offering significant place value to the consumer. Another example is the outreach strategy of U.S. Health Corporation in Columbus, Ohio. The multihospital system operates a medical van that visits two inner-city Columbus high schools to bring prenatal care to pregnant students.[1]

Time

The time utility refers to the fact that many intermediaries store the product until the consumer wants to purchase the item. A department store, for example, may stock some bathing suits for sale throughout the entire year. As a result, a consumer does not need to maintain an inventory in anticipation of future need. Instead, the customer can purchase close to the time the item is required. The value to consumers is that they can use their money for other purposes and the retail store can carry the cost of the inventory. Stores that sell manufacturer overloads or distressed merchandise offer little time value. Since items are not regularly stocked, the customer must purchase them when offered. The store cannot guarantee that the manufacturer overrun of bathing suits available in January will also be available just before the summer months.

In health care organizations, there is a time value provided regarding the ancillary support goods often needed such as durable medical equipment or pharmaceuticals. Any business organization must recognize that the more of each utility it provides, the greater its cost structure. The objective, however, is to provide a level of each utility that the customer values sufficiently enough to pay the additional cost. A primary care group that has its own on-site pharmacy may have a higher cost structure than a group that provides no such convenience.

Possession

A third utility performed in the channel of distribution is that of possession or financing. In traditional businesses, some intermediaries will provide credit, allowing the customer to take the product and pay over time. So too, in health care, some intermediaries vary regarding the provision of possession utility. Many urgent medical care centers that were established in the 1980s as for-profit enterprises required patients to pay for services at the time of delivery. If health insurance was going to reimburse these patients, they had to seek this reimbursement after payment to the urgent care center. Most hospital emergency rooms will, however, bill the patient's insurance company directly, and for the uninsured patient, some will provide services regardless. The patient then works out a repayment schedule with the financial office of the hospital.

Hospitals have begun to recognize the value of this utility. Since 1991, Mastercard and Visa credit cards have been accepted in 5,000 hospitals and in 40,000 physician offices. Many hospitals offer designated health care credit cards under a program by Health Charge Corporation in Skokie, Illinois. This company offers a charge card in the hospital's name, for which the patient can apply upon admission. At discharge, the self-pay portion of the visit is placed on the charge.[2]

Form

The fourth utility provided by some intermediaries is that of form or alteration, in which the intermediary actually changes the product for the customer. Some intermediaries provide customization of the product. In a traditional industry, form utility might be found when a department store alters a suit to better fit an individual. Similarly, form utility might occur at the Rehabilitation Hospital of the Pacific, a 100-bed inpatient acute care rehabilitation facility in Honolulu, Hawaii. This organization has the capabilities to redesign orthotic devices to better conform to the rehabilitation needs of their patients.

Functional Shifting

In spite of criticism often leveled at the middleman, it is important to recognize the concept of **functional shifting**, which involves the movement of different functions such as credit and sorting, between the producer of a product or service and its intermediaries or the customer. The intermediary can be eliminated but then the function has to shift to some other entity in the channel. For example, if the intermediary is eliminated and no longer provides customer credit, then either the customer must assume the credit requirement or the manufacturer must provide the credit.

An extreme form of functional shifting has been described by Trombetta. In the late 1970s, Goodyear established a plant in Lawton, Oklahoma. Area physicians were unwilling to grant any price concessions when approached by the company. Goodyear proceeded to assume the medical functions by setting up its own hospital, medical staff, and labs.[3]

Channel Management

In designing the channel of distribution there are several factors to consider, including determining the degree of distribution required, gaining channel cooperation, and dealing with conflict.

Ultimately, in the deliverance of a service or product, an organization must decide how available the product or service will be to customers. This issue might involve questions of the number of satellite facilities or primary care offices that would be staffed by physicians who participate in a prepaid plan. Secondly, there is always a question of whether any intermediaries who will be involved in the service will cooperate in how the service is delivered. Hospitals, for example, have always been concerned about getting physicians to admit to their hospitals. HMOs often need to convince physicians to join the plan as participating physicians. Both of these situations involve channel cooperation.

Finally, whenever two or more separate entities are involved in the delivery of a service, there is the potential for conflict. Conflict has often existed between hospital administrators and their medical staff. Conflict is now common between administrators of an HMO and the clinicians. Thus, channel management is a major consideration in the establishment of the "place" component of the marketing mix.

INTENSITY OF DISTRIBUTION

For any channel formation, the provider of a product or service must first decide how intensive the distribution should be. This **channel intensity**, as it is called, will then determine how available the product is to the ultimate consumer. In traditional businesses, there are commonly three forms of distribution intensity: intensive, selective, and exclusive. Figure 9–2 shows examples of the three distribution strategies regarding intensity. There are several factors that determine the ultimate selection of any specific strategy.

A major consideration in the selection of an intensity alternative is the consumer and how much effort consumers will expend searching for a particular product or service. The more effort they are willing to expend, the more an organization can

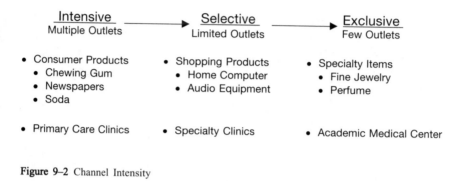

Figure 9–2 Channel Intensity

be selective or exclusive in its intensity. A second consideration is control. The more control the manufacturer wants over the intermediary, the more it would choose the strategy of exclusivity. Retailers, for example, who carry products also carried by their competitors find less reason to be attentive to the demands of the manufacturer, since the manufacturer is not offering them a product that the competition doesn't have. Market coverage is another consideration. The greater the desired coverage, the more the strategy leans toward intensive distribution with more outlets for distributing the service.

Intensive Distribution

This strategy is typical of consumer goods manufacturers. In intensive distribution, the product is available in a large number of outlets. This strategy applies to products such as soda or chewing gum, for which the consumer exerts no effort to find, knowing that there are many available outlets for such products. The traditional view in health care was that patients had their own personal physicians and would accept no substitutes. Increasingly, however, convenience has become a major customer concern, a dimension that affects the amount of effort patients will expend in seeking care from a particular primary care physician.

As a result, many primary care groups increasingly have used intensive distribution efforts by providing multiple satellite facilities and extended hours. Hospitals, too, have not overlooked the growing need to increase intensity of distribution. David Ginsburg, executive vice president for planning and program development at Presbyterian Hospital in Manhattan, commented regarding his organization, "In 1977, Presbyterian had one address, and basically one location. In 1987, we already have twenty different addresses, and we expect in the next century to be even more decentralized."[4]

Exclusive Distribution

The opposite of intensive distribution is exclusive distribution, in which the product or service is offered in a highly restricted number of outlets. Manufacturers of luxury products, which often have high margins, follow this strategy. Rolls Royce, for example, has few auto dealerships in the United States, in the belief that the customer who wants a Rolls Royce will be willing to travel to make the purchase. In the same regard, the manufacturer—by limiting the number of dealerships—can exhibit strong control over these intermediaries. Because a Rolls dealership is exclusive, the manufacturer can place certain demands on it regarding service levels, parts inventory, and sales training. In health care, exclusive distribution has existed for the providers of highly specialized medical services. For example, in Brookline, Massachusetts, the Joselin Clinic at Deaconess Hospital has received international acclaim for diabetic treatment. Patients who want to access this service will not find a satellite of the Joselin Clinic in their community but rather must travel to Brookline.

Selective Distribution

An intermediate intensity strategy is that of selective distribution. As noted in Figure 9–2, this approach involves fewer retailers than the intensive approach, and is particularly attractive to manufacturers of shopping goods. At this distribution level the consumer compares alternatives on selected attributes and compares the value. Intermediaries are restricted to those whom the manufacturer believes will provide the best product support. By providing some selectivity among intermediaries, the manufacturer can require them to meet certain objectives. Nikon, Sony, and Ping are three companies that follow selective distribution. Nikon does not sell its cameras in every outlet where cameras are sold. Rather they use selected outlets that see Nikon cameras as a differential advantage and present them more favorably to customers than Kodak or Minolta cameras. Sony follows a reasonably selective distribution approach for its products. Ping only distributes its golf clubs through golf professionals. While there may be two golf pros in one community, both know that if the customer wants Ping clubs they cannot buy them at the local sporting goods store or golf retailer.

In health care, the use of selective intensity strategies has increased. Historically, the Mayo Clinic in Minnesota and the Ochsner Clinic in Louisiana followed an exclusive intensity approach. If consumers wanted to use the services of either facility they had to travel to Rochester or to New Orleans, respectively. Now, as customer requirements have changed, both facilities have increased their distribution intensity. The Mayo Clinic has opened satellites in Jacksonville, Florida and

Scottsdale, Arizona. Many of its older patients now reside in these communities during the winter months. Recognizing the competition in these regions, responding to customer convenience, the Mayo Clinic opened satellites in these cities. The Mayo Clinic also operates primary care clinics in the manufacturing facilities of the John Deere Corporation. The Ochsner Clinic, a 350-person physician group in New Orleans, several years ago also opened a satellite in Baton Rouge, Louisiana to increase its distribution intensity.

VERTICAL MARKETING SYSTEMS

Among traditional organizations and now in the health care industry, the longstanding concept of a channel consisting of separate organizational entities, such as a manufacturer, wholesaler, and retailer, is undergoing change, with a noticeable growth of vertical marketing systems. **Vertical marketing systems** can be defined as channels in which the intermediaries are integrated so their functions are performed at the most efficient place within the channel.[5] Ideally, in a well-run vertically administered system, conflicts and differing goals should be eliminated so that the system performs well.

Several factors have been cited as driving vertical integration in health care:

1. production cost savings
2. transaction cost savings and improved coordination of services (i.e., continuity of care)
3. overcoming market imperfections
4. management and internal factors
5. environmental changes that affect market conditions, production technologies, and transactional relationships.[6]

In this framework, transaction cost savings center on economies in the transfer and use of information across different care points. Market imperfections relate to regulatory constraints or market power on the side of the buyer or seller. Vertically integrated systems can help achieve countervailing power.

Vertical marketing systems can be formed by any entity within the channel. One approach to creating these entities is through **forward vertical integration**, in which operations are acquired or developed that are closer to the final buyer in the channel of distribution. For example, Health Dimensions, in San Jose, California, has vertically integrated forward. The hospital foundation operates health clinics in schools that provide primary care services to the community. An alternative strategy is to develop a vertical marketing system by backward integration, acquiring operations that are farther from the consumer. In this instance, the Ochsner Clinic vertically integrated backward by adding their Baton Rouge site several years ago. The multispecialty group practice of physicians purchased a small hospital in the community by which to deliver inpatient services. Table 9–1 shows a variety of vertically integrated health care organizational forms relative to the five factors previously mentioned.

In traditional industries, there are three common forms of vertical marketing systems: (1) corporate, (2) administered, and (3) contractual.

Corporate Vertical Marketing Systems

A **corporate vertical marketing system** combines both the production and distribution of a product or service under one corporate ownership. Companies can achieve this result by integrating either forward or backward depending on the position from the channel that they evolve. Levi-Strauss, for example, was originally a manufacturer of clothes. The company created a corporate vertical marketing system by integrating forward and opening its own retail clothing stores to sell its merchandise. A similar strategy is being used by the University of Michigan Hospitals of Ann Arbor. This tertiary center is buying up primary care medical practices within a 30–mile radius of Ann Arbor. Vertically integrating forward allows for greater control in a managed care environment.[7] This sample shows the strong benefit of a corporate vertical marketing system giving the manufacturer distribution control. Figure 9–3 shows several alternative vertical marketing systems.

Figure 9–4 shows examples of several vertical marketing systems being developed in health care. These systems are called **integrated delivery systems**, in which health care is coordinated and is delivered at the level of intensity needed. One of these systems, referred to as a closed health system model, is comprised of physicians, hospitals, and an insurer all vertically integrated in one system in which the functions are delivered at the optimum point and centrally managed.

In Miami, Florida, Affiliated Health Providers is comprised of eight hospitals with multiple physician group practices. This network plans to contract with several insurers to be able to assume risk.[8] This enables the network, in conjunction with the insurance companies, to act as a prepaid health care plan. The physicians in the hospital will be responsible for managing the care and will accept the premiums for the coverage of that care from subscribers. This arrangement is represented in Figure 9–4 as the closed health system.

Administered Vertical Marketing System

An **administered vertical marketing system** occurs when there is coordination between members of the distribution channel but there is not common

Table 9-1 Forms of Vertical Integration in Health Care

Form of Vertical Integration	Determinants				
	Production Cost Savings	Transaction Cost Savings	Overcoming Market Imperfections	Management and Internal Factors	Environmental Conditions
1. Closed staff-model HMO (common ownership, fully integrated value chain)	Primarily through utilization management of inpatient care	Continuity of care through integration of facilities and medical staff	Response to physician market power	Internal "culture" linking organizational and physician interests	Cost sensitivity of purchasers; necessary supply of physicians
2. IPA-model HMO (separate ownership; contracting between the "plan" and physicians, hospitals; contract-based integration of value chain)	Utilization management; less-rigorous utilization management incentives than in closed-staff HMO	Still essentially market in contracting between plan and physicians, hospitals	Potential for more competitive physician pricing through contract and capitation incentives	Contracting largely supplants internal hierarchy	
3. Insurer-sponsored PPO (separate ownership; contracting on preferred vs. closed-panel or exclusive basis; contract-based integration)	Minimal; achieved primarily through unit cost reductions stimulated by price discounting	Replaces repeated contracting with one-time costs of establishing preferred provider network	Simulates competitive market's price network	Minimal	Minimal factor
4. Integrated hospital-multispecialty physician group practice (shared governance of the hospital and clinic; partially integrated value chain)	Not a prominent factor	Continuity of care benefits; referral and practice network; increased congruence of hospital and physician goals	Minimal factor	Internal culture linking hospital and physician interests	Similar to Form 3
5. Hospital-based ambulatory primary care group practice (shared-equity investment by hospital and physician group; internal staffing of semi-autonomous unit; partially integrated value chain)	Minimal factor	Some continuity of care gains due to tightened referral network between the hospital and primary care physicians (PCPs)	Minimal factor	Example: an internal corporate joint venture	Excess hospital bed capacity; increasing supply of PCPs

continues

Table 9–1 continued

Determinants

Form of Vertical Integration	Production Cost Savings	Transaction Cost Savings	Overcoming Market Imperfections	Management and Internal Factors	Environmental Conditions
6. Local-market-based managed care product (formation of "quasifirm" by short-term general hospital, multispecialty physician group, skilled nursing facility, and insurance carrier; partially integrated value chain)	Primarily through overall "case management" of utilization	Managed care via care manager; partially supplants arms-length market contracting; enhanced pre- and postdischarge services (visit, planning for hospital, ambulatory care, and long-term care); link to insurer enhances continuity between delivery and financing of care	"Backward" integration by insured into delivery; exerts buyer bargaining power on providers to reduce costs of services	Can deliver the product through variety of tightly or loosely "coupled" market or ownership mechanisms	Cost sensitivity of purchasers; excess supply of physicians; limited reimbursement for long-term care; (health) insurance underwriting cycle
7. McKesson's "value-adding partnership" (VAP) (with manufacturing, distribution, retailing, third-party insurance, and consumers for prescription drugs) (separate ownership of value chain components, contract-based integration)	Dramatic reductions in cost of order processing; reduced costs of restocking orders through conscious redesign of shelves	Enhanced monitoring through computer database of clinical-biological effects of alternative drug combinations	Minimal factor	Create management culture that monitors competitive dynamics throughout value chain and fixes weaknesses as they occur; use of computer systems and information technology for order entry, packing, shipping, shelf design (e.g., for quality assurance) (drug combination)	Increasing competition from large drugstore chains; eroding market share of independent drugstores served by McKesson

Source: Reprinted from Conrad, D.A., and Dowling, W.L., Vertical Integration in Health Services: Theory and Managerial Implications, *Health Care Management Review*, Vol. 15, No. 4, pp. 18–19, Aspen Publishers, Inc., © 1990.

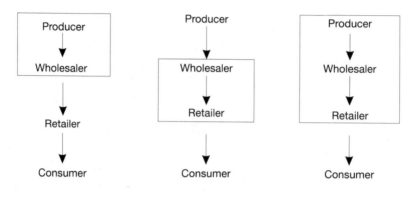

Figure 9–3 Alternative Vertical Marketing Systems

ownership. Typically, when one member of the distribution channel is more powerful, an administered vertical marketing system can occur. Scott Lawn Products is an administered vertical marketing system. Because of the manufacturer's power with its successful product line, it can demand its intermediary to give it better floor space, differential emphasis in selling, and adherence to pricing guidelines. In some administered vertical marketing programs, the manufacturer may take over the functions of pricing items, checking inventory levels, and servicing the account.

Administered vertical marketing systems are the growing form in health care. Increasingly, hospitals are employing their own physicians, and staffing their own outpatient facilities and diagnostic centers. As the health industry moves to contracting for care, hospitals have integrated forward, with the objective of owning the referral flow of patients. In a similar fashion, the Kaiser Foundation Health Plan, a multispecialty, prepaid group model HMO in Chula Vista, California, vertically integrated backward and has opened its own hospitals in several communities rather than trying to negotiate discounts from community hospitals. An interesting administered program was attempted by Mt. Sinai Hospital in Chicago in 1986. Primary medical centers owned and operated by Mt. Sinai were placed in Zayre department stores in the Chicago metropolitan area.[9]

Figure 9–4 shows a variation of an administered vertical marketing system appearing in health care—the physician/hospital organization (PHO) model, in which the physicians and hospitals merge and contract with third parties for administrative needs. An alternative variation of this model is also presented in Figure 9–4, in which the hospital and insurer merge and contract for the care to be delivered by providers (the HHS model). The most advanced state of the administered vertical marketing system in health care may be that represented in

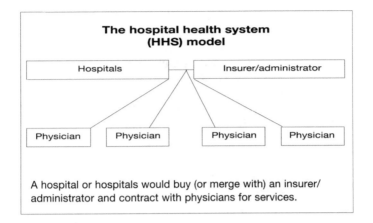

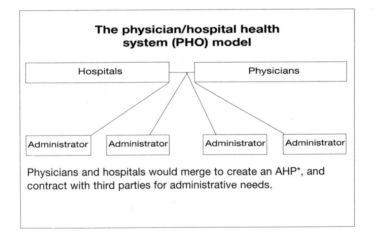

Note: AHP* stands for "accountable health partnership," a combination of hospitals and physicians that contract for care of a defined patient population.

Figure 9–4 Four Models of Integrated Delivery Systems in Health Care. *Source:* Reprinted from Findlay, S., How New Alliances Are Changing Health Care, *Business & Health,* October 1993, pp. 28–34, with permission of Medical Economics Publishing, Inc., © 1993.

Figure 9–4 continued

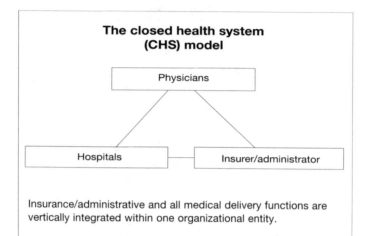

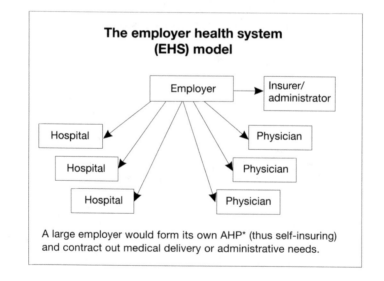

Figure 9–4 as the employer health system (EHS) model. In this instance, the administered program is formed by the employer, who then contracts out for care and administration of health needs. In Minneapolis–St. Paul, a coalition of 20 employers has formed, representing 80,000 workers. These employers are contracting with one consortium of providers to take care of their employees' health needs.

Contractual Vertical Marketing Systems

This form of vertical marketing systems consists of either a cooperative or a franchise. **Cooperatives** are agreements between members of the distribution channel who exist on the same level. For example, several retailers may band together in a retailer cooperative to act as a large purchasing group and to extract discounts or other concessions from suppliers. The I.G.A. (Independent Grocers Association) is a retailer cooperative of small grocery stores that bulk purchase from manufacturers.

In health care, a recent version of a cooperative marketing system is the National Cardiovascular Network, formed in 1993. Forty-one top heart programs were invited to join a cooperative venture to offer discounted, high-quality services at all-inclusive rates under contract to large employers and managed care organizations.[10]

Franchising, one of the fastest-growing forms of a vertical marketing system, is a contract that links elements of the manufacturing and distribution of a product or service.[11] Automobile dealerships are franchise arrangements, as are McDonald's restaurants and many Holiday Inn hotels. In these cases, independent businesses have signed agreements with the franchiser to deliver the product or service in a defined fashion. The franchisee pays a fee for the opportunity to deliver this service, and there is often a yearly payment as a function of the revenue generated by the outlet. Similarly, the franchiser often provides national advertising support, guidance for conducting the business, and ongoing training and product development. A relaxation response program developed under the auspices of Harvard University Medical School at Deaconess Hospital of Boston is being franchised to other medical centers around the country for $80,000.[12]

While franchising has been a fast-growing segment of the economy, it has not escaped criticism. A major issue has been the terms of contracts that exist for many franchisees. A growing number of lawsuits by franchisees cite nonsatisfactory performance by the franchiser, or an overselling of the possibilities of the business. A common complaint voiced by franchisees is that the franchiser promises a level of sales that is found to be unachievable. Or, the franchiser promises to provide advertising or marketing consulting support, but does not follow through with this promise.

CHANNEL LEADERSHIP

In many distribution channels there is often one member who is considered the channel commander. The **channel commander** can dictate or control the activities of the other members of the channel of distribution.

The manufacturer can be the channel commander when its product is very popular. Proctor and Gamble, for example, has several brand-name products that are well recognized and have significant market share. Ivory soap and Crest toothpaste are just two of Proctor and Gamble's many brands that retailers know are important to carry in their grocery stores. In this way P&G can control certain aspects of its product merchandising. A manufacturer can also be channel commander by providing intermediaries with significant rewards.

A wholesaler can be the channel commander if the product must be distributed to a large number of manufacturers or to a large number of retailers. In these instances, the consolidating function of the retailer becomes a key element in the distribution of the product. In the alcoholic beverage industry, Foremost McKesson is a wholesaler that exerts significant leadership in the channel of distribution.

The retailer is the channel commander when it has a strong image or extensive market coverage. K-Mart has a large number of outlets across the United States. As a large purchaser and ultimately distributor of products, manufacturers must consider K-Mart's needs when the retailer places an order.

This framework of a channel commander also applies in health care. M.D. Anderson is an internationally known cancer center in Houston, Texas, which is part of the University of Texas medical institution. As a result of its strong reputation, this organization can act as a channel commander in terms of cancer treatment. Likewise, in areas with several community hospitals, the intermediary (the physician) is often the channel commander. In the managed care environment, large HMOs increasingly play the part of wholesalers coordinating the needs of the many employers in the community with the services of available providers. Many of the larger HMOs such as US HealthCare of Blue Bell, Pennsylvania, and PruCare, an HMO that is part of the Prudential Insurance Company of America in Newark, New Jersey, can play the role of a channel commander and negotiate effective discounts with hospitals or doctors.

Using Power

There are several sources of power a distribution channel member can use to control other members of the channel.[13] Five specific sources have been identified: coercive power, economic power, rewards, referent power, and expertise.

Coercive

One negative source of power is coercive power. Threats can be effective in modifying behavior if they can be implemented. A manufacturer might threaten to pull its popular product from the shelves, or a retailer might withhold the kind of merchandising attention the manufacturer would like for its product. Typically, most members of the distribution channel prefer not to use this form of power since it has little positive impact on building long-term channel relationships. A hospital might threaten the physicians with the possibility of recruiting additional practitioners if the physicians do not comply with the hospital wishes. Yet the gains from this approach would, no doubt, be short-term if physicians developed an alternative organization or switched hospital allegiance.

Economic

A second form of power is economic power. If one member of the channel has significantly more economic resources than another, that firm has the power. General Motors can exert significant power over small manufacturers that supply it with auto parts. A large multispecialty health clinic could convince a small two-person medical group to sell its practice to the clinic or face stiff competition. Columbia/HCA–Healthtrust is now wielding great economic power with its suppliers. In February 1994, Columbia renegotiated several purchasing contracts and announced it would pay $160 million instead of the $220 million previously negotiated for these services.[14]

Reward

Power can always be gained by providing other intermediaries with a significant incentive to cooperate. In traditional industries, the margins or profit provided can be a useful mechanism for gaining cooperation. In March 1994, CIGNA Companies of Bloomfield Connecticut, an insurance and HMO company, rewarded Torrance Memorial Medical Center of Torrance, California by shifting 40,000 covered lives to this hospital from South Bay Hospital in Redondo Beach. Torrance agreed to offer a broader array of services than South Bay Hospital. The loss of business for South Bay Hospital was estimated to be 20 percent of its daily census.[15]

Referent

This form of power refers to the name or reputation of the organization. As was noted previously, an organization that has brand-name recognition in the marketplace can exhibit significant power over smaller competitors or intermediaries.

Expertise

Having a recognized expertise in a particular area is a fifth valuable source of distribution channel power. The *U.S. News & World Report* has developed a mathematical model to assess and rank the major tertiary hospitals in the country on a range of 12 clinical specialties. The rankings are based on a model that weighs reputation and mortality rate plus a combination of other factors such as the ratio of board-certified physicians to beds. A listing from the 1994 rankings of the top hospitals in cardiology are shown in Table 9–2. Having a recognized area of

Table 9-2 1994 *U.S. News & World Report* Rankings for Cardiology

Rank	Hospital	Overall score	Reputational score	Mortality rate	COTH member	Residents to beds	Technology score	R.N.s to beds	Board-certified M.D.s to beds	Inpatient operations to beds
1	Mayo Clinic, Rochester, Minn.	100.0	32.5%	0.64	Yes	0.37	8	0.73	1.49	21.5
2	Cleveland Clinic	95.6	32.7%	0.76	Yes	0.59	9	1.47	0.38	19.9
3	Massachusetts General Hospital, Boston	68.9	19.8%	0.77	Yes	0.47	9	1.14	0.66	17.5
4	Stanford University Medical Center, Stanford, Calif.	56.0	15.5%	0.95	Yes	0.79	8	0.86	1.81	13.9
5	Duke University Medical Center, Durham, N.C.	54.8	14.1%	0.86	Yes	0.43	9	1.60	0.66	15.3
6	Brigham and Women's Hospital, Boston	54.2	11.7%	0.75	Yes	0.64	8	0.79	1.24	20.0
7	Emory University Hospital, Atlanta	51.1	12.5%	0.84	Yes	0.31	7	1.28	0.68	17.2
8	Johns Hopkins Hospital, Baltimore	47.4	8.9%	0.78	Yes	0.45	9	1.43	0.66	15.5
9	University of California San Francisco Medical Center	45.5	6.8%	0.76	Yes	0.32	8	1.82	1.55	18.3
10	Texas Heart Institute (St. Luke's Episcopal Hospital), Houston	43.4	12.7%	1.16	Yes	0.19	8	1.36	0.62	19.3
11	New York University Medical Center, New York	41.5	2.2%	0.62	Yes	0.20	8	1.15	1.25	13.6
12	Barnes Hospital, St. Louis	39.9	5.3%	0.76	Yes	0.47	9	0.81	0.90	11.1
13	Indiana University Medical Center, Indianapolis	39.6	2.1%	0.69	Yes	0.37	9	1.86	0.90	17.3
14	Columbia-Presbyterian Medical Center, New York	39.2	5.4%	0.78	Yes	0.31	9	1.05	0.81	12.0
15	Cedars-Sinai Medical Center, Los Angeles	39.1	6.2%	0.81	Yes	0.26	8	0.83	1.19	13.4
16	Beth Israel Hospital, Boston	37.0	1.5%	0.75	Yes	0.54	8	1.93	2.08	14.5
17	New York Hospital-Cornell Medical Center, New York	36.5	2.7%	0.72	Yes	0.38	8	1.00	0.99	11.5
18	UCLA Medical Center, Los Angeles	35.3	2.2%	0.77	Yes	0.71	9	1.20	0.82	14.6
19	University of Illinois Hospital and Clinics, Chicago	35.2	0.0%	0.73	Yes	1.22	7	1.95	0.60	13.7
20	Thomas Jefferson University Hospital, Philadelphia	35.0	0.0%	0.70	Yes	0.68	8	1.44	1.12	16.3
21	Deaconess Hospital, Boston	34.7	0.0%	0.69	Yes	0.63	9	1.33	0.93	16.9

continues

Table 9-2 continued

Rank	Hospital	Overall score	Reputational score	Mortality rate	COTH member	Residents to beds	Technology score	R.N.s to beds	Board-certified M.D.s to beds	Inpatient operations to beds
22	Green Hospital of Scripps Clinic, La Jolla, Calif.	34.6	1.1%	0.69	No	0.00	8	1.99	0.51	23.1
23	University of Washington Medical Center, Seattle	34.0	0.0%	0.73	Yes	0.30	8	2.06	1.90	14.8
24	University of Wisconsin Hospital and Clinics, Madison	33.7	0.0%	0.71	Yes	0.65	9	1.24	0.74	18.9
25	Mount Sinai Medical Center, Cleveland	33.6	1.0%	0.72	Yes	0.40	7	0.86	1.09	15.2
26	University of Minnesota Hospital and Clinic, Minneapolis	33.5	1.2%	0.75	Yes	0.72	8	0.86	0.89	17.1
27	Presbyterian University Hospital, Pittsburgh	33.5	1.2%	0.82	Yes	0.72	7	2.10	1.27	17.2
28	Lahey Clinic, Burlington, Mass.	33.4	0.7%	0.70	No	0.28	8	1.22	0.80	22.4
29	Rush–Presbyterian–St. Luke's Medical Center, Chicago	32.8	0.8%	0.75	Yes	0.63	8	1.23	0.85	13.2
30	Mount Sinai Medical Center, New York	32.7	1.6%	0.79	Yes	0.50	7	1.50	1.11	12.3
31	University of Alabama Hospital at Birmingham	32.6	6.1%	1.03	Yes	0.46	8	0.92	0.60	13.7
32	Methodist Hospital, Houston	32.6	5.3%	0.98	Yes	0.18	8	1.33	0.65	17.6
33	Ohio State University Medical Center, Columbus	32.3	1.0%	0.75	Yes	0.58	8	1.11	0.68	12.1
34	Georgetown University Medical Center, Washington, D.C.	31.4	0.0%	0.75	Yes	0.34	8	1.59	1.28	15.4
35	New England Medical Center, Boston	31.3	0.0%	0.74	Yes	0.53	6	1.65	0.66	14.7
36	University of Michigan Medical Center, Ann Arbor	30.9	2.0%	0.85	Yes	0.41	9	1.29	0.66	16.8
37	Forster G. McGaw Hospital at Loyola Medical Center, Maywood, Ill.	30.8	2.0%	0.90	Yes	0.60	8	1.58	0.88	18.3
38	New England Baptist Hospital, Boston	30.5	0.0%	0.65	No	0.04	4	0.75	0.59	26.3
39	George Washington University Medical Center, Washington, D.C.	30.3	0.0%	0.82	Yes	0.78	8	1.16	1.71	14.9
40	Long Island Jewish Medical Center, New Hyde Park, N.Y.	30.3	0.0%	0.79	Yes	0.55	7	1.20	1.90	12.0

"Reputational score" is the percentage of doctors surveyed who named the hospital. "Mortality rate" is the ratio of actual to expected deaths (lower is better). "COTH member" indicates member of Council of Teaching Hospitals. "Residents to beds" is the ratio of interns and residents to beds. "Technology score" is a specialty-specific index from 0 to 9. "R.N.s to beds" is the ratio of registered nurses to beds. "Board-certified M.D.s to beds" is the ratio of doctors certified in a specialty to the number of beds. "Inpatient operations to beds" is the ratio of annual inpatient operations to beds.

Source: Adapted from America's Best Hospitals, *U.S. News & World Report,* July 18, 1994, pp. 54–88, with permission of U.S. News and World Report, © 1994.

expertise is a power basis for each institution. Many hospitals have attempted to develop centers of excellence in certain clinical areas. The objective is to have the power to draw patients around the intermediaries.

SELECTED CONCEPTS FROM RETAILING

There are many aspects of the distribution of health care services that involve basic aspects of retailing. In examining the distribution element of the marketing mix, then, concepts such as the retail positioning matrix, the retail mix, and the wheel of retailing can aid a health care organization in strategy development.[16]

The Retail Positioning Matrix

The **retail positioning matrix** shown in Figure 9–5 is a concept developed by the Chicago-based management consulting firm, MAC, Inc. (now called Gemini).[17] This matrix is a model for retail positioning based on the breadth of the retailer's product line and the value added. The breadth of the product line can be defined as the number of different products and services offered by the company. The value added refers to such things as location (7–Eleven, Health Stop neighborhood urgent care centers), the prestige or name recognition of the organization (Neiman Marcus or the Mayo Clinic), the product reliability (McDonald's), or personal service offered by a personal financial advisor or a medical group that might offer extended hours or even house calls.

In using this matrix, an organization can position itself in any of four quadrants. Whereas all organizations attempt to build a loyal base of customer support, the retail positioning matrix suggests that the medical organization can accomplish this goal through several alternative strategies.

1. The Neiman Marcus/Mayo Clinic position is one of four options. Organizations in this quadrant have a broad product line and a high degree of value-added. Organizations in this quadrant typically offer many services and are recognized as prestige organizations.
2. High value-added with a narrow product line can also be provided by organizations such as Boston's Children's Hospital and Tiffany's. The jewelry retailer is known for premium jewelry and a strong customer service orientation.
3. The position of the community hospital is similar to that of K-Mart. These organizations provide a reasonable range of products and services but not at the margins achieved by those with the prestige name and service delivery.

Broad

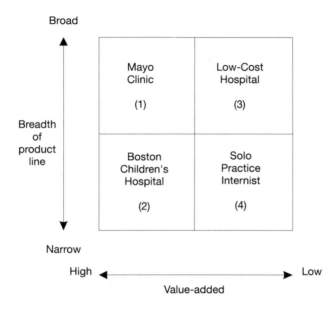

Narrow

High ◄─────────────────► Low

Value-added

Figure 9–5 Retail Positioning Matrix. *Source:* Reprinted from *Health Care Marketing Plans: From Strategy to Action,* 2nd ed., by S.G. Hillestad and E.N. Berkowitz, p. 114, Aspen Publishers, Inc., © 1991.

4. Low value-added with a narrow range is common to Kinney Shoes and the solo-practice internist. Both entities provide a narrow product line in a setting that is not often the most convenient (few sites).

In positioning an organization, no one quadrant is necessarily better than the others. The position must be chosen that offers an identity in the market relative to the competitors. Organizations can shift between quadrants in this matrix but the implications of moving up the value-added dimension is clear. Typically, there is a need to provide more services to the market. A lower value-added position implies fewer services and reduced prices to the market. Organizations should consider reviewing the following five steps to position themselves successfully in the market:

1. *Strategic Direction*—An organization must decide whether to be a full-service or part- (narrow) service provider.
2. *Current Positioning*—The organization must understand its current composition, using quantitative and qualitative information.
3. *Competitive Positioning*—Primary and secondary data should also be employed to understand competitors' positions.

4. *Alternative Evaluation*—An organization should compare its current position with competitors to identify gaps, weaknesses, and strengths.
5. *Plan Development and Implementation*—The position selected should reflect the organization's attributes and conventions. The chosen position must be reelected with a consistent marketing mix.[18]

Retail Mix

In developing a position for the organization, retailers can vary the components of the **retail mix**, which includes the goods and services the organization offers, the distribution of these services, and the communication strategies implemented.[19] Figure 9–6 shows the components of the retail mix with the health care alternatives.

Goods and Services

The goods and services component pertains to the breadth and depth of the product line, the prices, and the level of service delivery. An HMO, for example, may offer a traditional plan as well as a point-of-service option, which allows

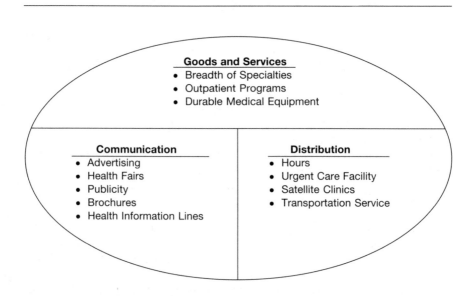

Figure 9–6 Health Care Organization's Retail Mix

subscribers to select physicians outside the HMO's panel at an additional fee. Within the goods and services mix is the service component. Organizations vary in the amount of services they provide to the customer. Some retailers, for example, provide home delivery, credit, extended hours, and personal shopper assistance. Likewise, some medical organizations will fill out insurance forms for seniors, have an on-site pharmacy service, and rent durable medical equipment in an attempt to be more customer service oriented.

Pricing, as noted in Chapter 8, is becoming a more critical factor in health care as organizations move away from cost-based pricing to value pricing. Health care organizations are increasingly dealing with the issue of markup, which refers to how much should be added to the cost of the service before it is offered to the final consumer. As in retailing, health care is experiencing the growing phenomenon of service discounting. Hospitals have had to offer discounts to HMOs in order to get contracts to provide certain services. This situation involves the retailing concept of "maintained markups," which represents the amount of the markup received from the original markup, less the final price at which the product or service is sold. In retailing, discounting a product is referred to as a "markdown."

In determining its goods and services mix, the organization must identify which elements to offer, and how this mix will affect the relative position, as noted in the retail positioning matrix.

Distribution

The number of locations, the hours open, and the transportation of products are all part of the distribution side of the retailing mix. The location decision for most physicians has historically focused on convenience for the practitioner. Most medical office buildings are located adjacent to inpatient facilities. In metropolitan areas, this location is usually downtown where there are few residential developments. As a result, facilities are finding ways to bring patients to the service. Columbia-Presbyterian Hospital in New York City has a satellite practice in midtown Manhattan with a shuttle that brings patients to the medical center in Washington Heights. Site location is a key element for any organization. The facility's location directly affects the profile of the customer who uses the organization.

Acknowledging the importance of location, health care organizations are turning to Geographic Information Systems (GIS). These systems overlay maps with demographics databases. Overlook Health System in Summit, New Jersey plans to use such programs to plot physician office sites with the addresses of employees. The organization hopes to position itself appropriately for direct contracting.[20]

Some retail organizations have based their competitive strategy on the distribution component of their retail mix. 7-Eleven convenience stores have multiple locations in any one community where they compete. This organization's goal is to have the customer drive no more than ten minutes to access one of its stores. So too, in health care, convenience is becoming an important component for customers. Multiple primary care satellites with convenient parking all play a major role in the mix of value provided to the patient.

In the retail setting, it is easy to observe another trend in terms of hours of availability. Many supermarkets are now open 24 hours a day in response to the changing household demographics with both spouses working throughout the day. Increasingly, many primary care physicians are scheduling regular office hours on weekends and evenings in response to the time-compressed consumer.

Communication

The communication component of the retailing mix includes advertising, personal selling, public relations, catalogs, and brochures. The 1980s saw a growing acceptance of health care advertising. Some hospitals also expanded their retail mix with the addition of physician relations personnel who call upon staff doctors as well as on potential referral services. Brochures have played a major role in hospital advertising. Some academic medical centers have expanded these brochures to resemble catalogs with detailed descriptions of services, access numbers, and biographical sketches of the personnel who deliver the service. All of these communication components provide additional value-added by delivering more information to the marketplace.

Related to the communication component is the issue of store layout and atmosphere. Retail research has demonstrated that the ambience of the retail setting can affect employees as well as customers.[21] Historically, many medical organizations viewed the atmospherics purely as an expense. Now many facilities are paying greater attention to the layout and design of the space in which the services are delivered.

The Wheel of Retailing

There are always new retailing forms that enter the market and seem to replace or capture some of the core business of an existing entity. The **wheel of retailing** describes the process of how new retail forms enter the market and how they evolve over time.[22] Figure 9–7 depicts this evolution.

According to this concept, the retail outlet enters the market at position 1 with low status, low price, and low margin. McDonald's first began with two brothers operating a hamburger stand in California. Operated as a drive-in restaurant, it had no seats for customers and a limited menu of hamburgers, French fries, and shakes. Over time, the restaurant added services and other outlets. McDonald's began to

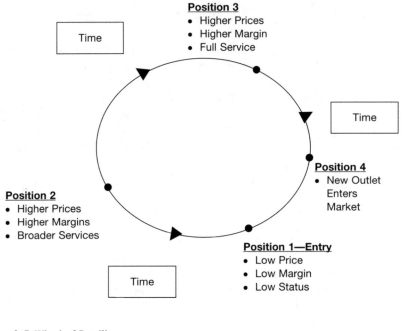

Figure 9–7 Wheel of Retailing

expand, by offering fish sandwiches on its menu and tables for customer seating
in multiple locations. At position 3, McDonald's no longer differs from the
restaurants and diners from which it originally stole market share. McDonald's
restaurants exist around the world. Services have been expanded to include
morning bingo games for seniors at some locations, and birthday parties for kids.
Menus have broadened to include pizza, salads, and even Mexican food. Some outlets offer home delivery. Margins and prices have also increased. At this point,
position 4, the wheel of retailing concept predicts that a new low-margin, low-
price, low-status organization will enter the market. In the hamburger business, a
relatively recent entrant is "Just Burgers." The wheel begins to turn anew.

The wheel concept also can be applied in health care. Consider how it has turned
for many former solo-practice primary care groups or hospitals. The solo-practice
physician adds a partner, opens a number of satellite offices, expands into offering other clinical specialties, and becomes a multispecialty group practice.
Margins increase, prices rise. Over time, another practice opens in the community
offering low-cost, convenient primary care in the shopping mall, and the wheel
turns again.

CONCLUSIONS

The channel of distribution is a central consideration in the formulation of health care marketing strategy. Understanding the flow of patient volume and the intermediaries who affect this flow is at the foundation of the marketing mix plan. Channels can be controlled and influenced by a variety of alternative strategies and depend on the respective power of any entity involved in the channel. As many health care organizations establish vertically integrated marketing systems, concepts common to traditional retail settings will play a more important role.

KEY TERMS

Channel of Distribution
Utilities
Functional Shifting
Channel Intensity
Vertical Marketing Systems
Forward Vertical Integration
Corporate Vertical Marketing System
Integrated Delivery Systems

Administered Vertical Marketing System
Cooperatives
Franchising
Channel Commander
Retail Positioning Matrix
Retail Mix
Wheel of Retailing

CHAPTER SUMMARY

1. The channel of distribution is the path a product takes as it moves from producer to end user, or the path a patient takes as he or she moves through the health care system to the appropriate level of care.

2. Within the channel of distribution, intermediaries (middlemen) provide value in the form of utility. While the intermediary can be eliminated, the function is only shifted elsewhere in the channel.

3. In establishing the channel of distribution, organizations must decide the level of intensity of service delivery—or how available their service will be to consumers.

4. In order to control the channel of distribution and obtain greater efficiencies, organizations can integrate either forward or backward.

5. The growing formation of integrated delivery systems in health care is a vertical integration strategy.

6. In any distribution channel, there is often a single entity or leader who can dictate or control policies with its intermediaries.

7. *There are several sources of power available to any distribution channel member. These sources can take the form of economic power, rewards, referent power, coercion, or expertise.*

8. *Organizations can be positioned perceptually in terms of the breadth of their product line and the perceived value-added.*

9. *Health care organizations, just as retailing businesses, have a retail mix that includes their pricing policies, distribution, services, and communication tactics.*

10. *In service industries, new market entrants tend to start as low margin, low status. As they mature and grow, this low-entry position is left open to new retail forms.*

CHAPTER PROBLEMS

1. In recent years, two nationally known health care providers established satellite facilities a great distance from their main clinic locations. The Mayo Clinic, of Rochester, Minnesota, opened facilities in Arizona and Florida. The Cleveland Clinic also opened a facility in Florida. Explain the changes in distribution intensity these actions represent.

2. Explain the vertical integration options and directions for the following providers: (a) a major academic medical center such as the University of Iowa, (b) a five-person general surgery group, and (c) a manufacturer of durable medical equipment.

3. In a recent contract negotiation session between a group of physicians and a managed care health plan, the parties disagreed about the level of reimbursement that the physicians would receive for treating subscribers. The physician group is the largest such organization in the community and represents 75 percent of all primary care providers in the area. What sources of power does this group wield in negotiating a managed care contract?

4. In examining Figure 9–5 containing the retail positioning matrix, explain how the community hospital in its present position (quadrant 3) could reposition itself to quadrant 2, and to quadrant 1.

5. Utilizing the wheel of retailing concept, explain the evolution in market growth of a neighborhood urgent care medical center that treats minor emergencies.

NOTES

1. E. Chapman and T. Wimberly, Looking Upstream, *Healthcare Forum Journal* 37, no. 3 (1994): 18–21.

2. S. Gelfond, Don't Leave Home Without Your Health Card, *Health Week* 5, no. 3 (1991): 29–30.

3. W.L. Trombetta, Channel Systems: An Idea Whose Time Has Come in Health Care Marketing, *Journal of Health Care Marketing* 9, no. 3 (1989):26–35.

4. B. Holcomb, Hospital HYPE, *New York* (August 3, 1987): 30–35.

5. L.W. Stern and A.I. El-Ansary, *Marketing Channels*, 4th ed. (Englewood Cliffs, N.J.: Prentice Hall, 1991).

6. D. A. Conrad and W.L. Dowling, Vertical Integration in Health Services: Theory and Managerial Implications, *Health Care Management Review* 15, no. 4 (Fall 1990):12.

7. University of Michigan Hospitals Adds Docs To Gird for Managed Care, *Modern Healthcare* 24, no. 46 (1994):18.

8. S. Findlay, How New Alliances Are Changing Health Care, *Business & Health* 11, no. 10 (1993):28–34.

9. R. Contreras, B. Greenspan, and R.C. Leventhal, Medical Care in the Discount Aisle, *Journal of Health Care Marketing* 9, no. 3 (1989):58–61.

10. G. Borzo and B. McCormick, Cardiovascular Network Receives Federal Approval, *American Medical News* (1993):4.

11. J.A. Tannebaum, Franchise Fever, *The Wall Street Journal*, 16 October 1992, R14–R15.

12. I. Albert, Unconventional Medicine . . . The Other Half of a Continuum, *Strategic Health Care Marketing* 11, no. 7 (1994):6–8.

13. J. Gaski, The Theory of Power and Conflict in Channels of Distribution, *Journal of Marketing* 48, no. 3 (Summer 1984):9–29.

14. L. Scott, Suppliers Feeling Effects of Columbia, *Modern Healthcare* 24, no. 11 (1994):22.

15. The Dynamics of Power in Healthcare, *Integrated Healthcare Report* (November 1993):1–7.

16. An early article suggesting the linkage of retailing concepts in health care was T. Paul and J. Wong, The Retailing of Health Care, *Journal of Health Care Marketing* 4, no. 4 (Fall 1984):23–35.

17. This discussion is derived from W.T. Gregor and E.M. Firars, *Mass Merchandising: Retail Revolution in Consumer Services* (Cambridge, Mass.: Management Analysis Center, 1982).

18. E.F. Goldman, The Power of Positioning, in *Responding to the Challenge: Health Care Marketing Comes of Age,* ed. P.D. Cooper (Chicago, Ill.: Alliance for Health Care Marketing and Strategy, 1986), 109–111.

19. W. Lazer and E.J. Kelley, The Retailing Mix: Planning and Management, *Journal of Retailing* 37, no. 1 (Spring 1961):34–41.

20. J. Morrissey, Geographical Software Aids Executives, *Modern Healthcare* 25, no. 2 (1995): 34.

21. M.J. Bitner, Servicescapes: The Impact of Physical Surroundings on Customers and Employees, *Journal of Marketing* 55, no. 1 (1992):57–71.

22. This theory was first proposed by M.P. McNair, Significant Trends and Development in the Postwar Period, in *Competitive Distribution in a Free High-Level Economy and Its Implications for the University,* ed. A.B. Smith (Pittsburgh, Pa.: University of Pittsburgh Press, 1958), 1–25; and M. McNair and E. May, The Next Revolution of the Retailing Wheel, *Harvard Business Review* 56, no. 5 (1978):81–91.

PROMOTION

After reading this chapter you should be able to:

- Understand the nature of the communication process

- Recognize the alternative components of the promotional mix and their respective values

- Appreciate the range of sales promotion strategies for both consumers and the trade

- Know the alternative promotional strategy approaches for controlling the channel of distribution

Promotional strategies that companies use to communicate their messages to the marketplace have four basic components: (1) advertising, (2) personal selling, (3) publicity, and (4) sales promotion. At the heart of all of these tools lies communication. With any promotional strategy, the ultimate goal is to communicate to a market. Before examining each of the four basic promotional tools of marketing, however, this chapter will first consider how communication occurs, and discuss the elements necessary for communication to take place.

THE COMMUNICATION MODEL

There are several factors that contribute to effective communication. Many of these essential components can be affected by a company's strategies and tactics. Successful communication with a target market depends upon the effectiveness of the major components of communication, as shown in Figure 10–1.[1] The components within this diagram include:

1. A *sender*, which can be a person or company who wants to communicate a message
2. A *receiver*, the target of the communication
3. The process of *encoding* or developing the message
4. The *message*, which is what is to be communicated
5. The *channel* by which the message is sent
6. The process of *decoding*, or interpreting the message encoded by the sender
7. The element of *noise*, which includes factors external to the message that affect how the message is interpreted
8. *Feedback*, which provides the sender with an assessment of the effectiveness of the communication between sender and receiver

Each of these elements determines whether effective communication occurs.

The Sender

The sender of the message is often referred to as the source. The sender can be a person, a company, or a spokesperson representing someone else. The *spokesperson* is the person in marketing communications who delivers the message. In an advertisement, the spokesperson can be a famous baseball player, for example; in personal selling the spokesperson is the company's sales representative.

An important element for the senders, or spokespersons, of any message is their *source credibility*, which is the target market's perception that the sender can be

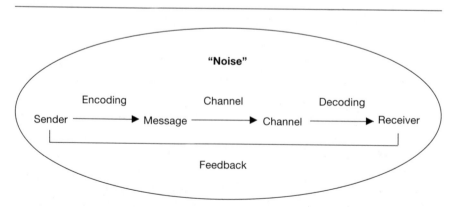

Figure 10–1 The Communication Process

believed. Elements that contribute to source credibility are dimensions such as trustworthiness, knowledge or expertise, experience, and to some degree the source's likability.[2] During the mid-1970s, an actor named Robert Young played the role of a physician, Dr. Marcus Welby, on a popular television drama. Young's acting role translated into a high degree of medical source credibility, which resulted in his being hired in 1978 to promote the positive benefits of Sanka, a brand of decaffeinated coffee. Similarly, popular movie actor John Wayne promoted Datril 500, a headache remedy, during 1979.

Encoding

Communication cannot occur without the process of **encoding**, which refers to translating the meaning to be communicated into words or symbols. For example, a family practice group might want to communicate that it is a caring organization that will meet the health care needs of the entire family. To encode this message, the group practice might use a picture of a physician caring for a child with the parents looking on. The message is encoded with a series of pictures and possibly a tag line that reads, "Your family's one-stop health source."

For communication to occur, the sender of the message must encode with symbols or words that are shared in a similar way by the receiver. In Chapter 11, on advertising, the issue of pretesting is discussed as a way to ensure that the shared meaning is occurring.

Increasingly in the United States, health care organizations are facing a multicultural marketplace. The interesting and challenging nature of this marketplace is the frequent absence of shared meaning between different cultural groups. This problem has been experienced in the international marketplace. For many years, Chevrolet tried to market its Nova automobile in Latin American countries, with dismal sales for its efforts. In Spanish, the word *nova* means "no go." Needless to say, promoting a car with this meaning makes gaining market acceptance an impossible challenge.

The Message

The **message** is the combination of symbols and words that the sender uses to transmit. There are several forms a message can take. Some varieties are:

Two-Sided vs. One-Sided Message

In a two-sided message, the sender presents both the pros and cons of the service being promoted. Prior research has shown that two-sided messages have a stronger impact on higher-educated consumers. A two-sided message also helps prepare the market for opposing messages, which they may hear about or read in competitors' presentations. The disadvantage of two-sided messages is that it may make the target market aware of negative product features that it might not have considered.[3]

Comparative Messages

Comparative messages involve direct claims relative to the competition. Prior research reveals that these types of messages work best when the product is noticeably different from the competition. Studies also show, however, that consumers generally find comparative advertising less credible and informative than advertising that just focuses on the product itself.[4] Organizations that engage in comparative advertising must have supportable evidence for any product claims to ward off litigation from the competitor whose product is being compared.

Emotional Appeals

The creation of any message involves determining its level of appeal. Messages can appeal to the product benefits or to emotions. Emotional appeals can take the form of fear, humor, or sentiment. In health care, there is some concern about using fear as an emotional appeal in advertising. Because concern about health is a basic issue for most consumers, a fear appeal could generate unnecessary anxiety or higher utilization rates—all due to an issue that, factually, might be true, but has a very small incidence rate.[5] For example, a medical group might run an advertisement, stating that the presence of a number of symptoms might indicate a heart attack. While there is a factual basis for any one symptom, a consumer would have to experience these symptoms with a degree of frequency combined with other factors before any diagnosis could be made. Such an advertisement could generate a large number of medical claims at a diagnostic clinic. In general, moderate fear appeals have been found to be more effective than either weak or strong appeals.[6]

Sentiment is also used in some health care–related advertisements. Manufacturers of Rogaine® show men looking into the mirror thinking about prior days when they had hair. Usually these reminiscences show them in the company of an attractive woman or as the focus of a party. The advertisement returns to the man looking at his head of thinning hair, and announces an available treatment. A similar concern with regard to personal appearance has led to many plastic surgeons placing an attractive person who has undergone cosmetic surgery in their advertisements. Such emotional appeals are viewed by some as testing the boundaries of what is acceptable for promotion within health care. The issue is whether such promotion is medically appropriate or necessary. Yet, since cosmetic surgery is a self-paid procedure, promotion of cosmetic surgery might be considered similar to any other product for which consumers pay directly out of their own pockets.

Occasionally, health care providers use humor to draw attention to negative aspects of a health care service. The advertisement typically will show how improved conditions are in the particular provider's setting. Humor is a useful emotional appeal, however, its major problem is that it is often very individual-specific. Funny to one person may be degrading to another. It is necessary in the use of humor to ensure that the encoding and decoding processes occur. Health care marketers need to exercise great care when using humor in advertising. Since most health care decisions are high involvement issues, as described in Chapter 4 on buyer behavior, consumers treat health care as a serious issue. Like religion, certain issues are less adaptable to humorous appeals. When using humor, it is also important that the theme doesn't so overwhelm the product that it goes unnoticed.[7]

The Channel

The **channel** is the means used to deliver a marketing message. It is the foundation of the promotional plan. In the promotional mix, companies can use mass media, personal salespersons, or publicity to communicate their message to the target audience. The latter portion of this chapter will review the advantages and disadvantages of each of these alternative channels in greater detail.

The major difference in channels is whether they involve interpersonal or mass communication. Interpersonal communication involves a salesperson or word-of-mouth communication among members of the target audience. A company can control the salesperson through training and supporting sales literature. Because interpersonal communication occurs between people, however, a company can never ensure total control over how its message is encoded or over the message's content. In health care, this lack of control has been a common source of complaint among physicians who work for some HMOs. These physicians often believe that the HMO's salespeople, in their enthusiasm to attract new subscribers, state claims that the providers cannot deliver. In this instance, the physicians believe that the communication is leaving misimpressions in the market. Yet, the sales personnel believe that in their communication they are highlighting the factors that are important in the selection of the health care plan by consumers. Such a source of conflict can indicate a lack of control of this interpersonal channel.

Historically, health care has relied upon word-of-mouth advertising by satisfied patients as its primary promotional channel. One friend telling another friend about a particular doctor or a positive experience at a sports medicine clinic has a high level of source credibility. Some organizations try to target specific people who play a vital role in the word-of-mouth process. These individuals are often recognized as **opinion leaders**, whose advice or experience is sought out by others. Typically, the opinion leader is someone regarded by peers or social group as having experience or expertise in a particular area. Pharmaceutical companies often try to identify which physicians in the medical group or hospital staff are the opinion leaders whom others turn to for advice. Pharmaceutical sales representatives target these physicians for the initial calls. These physicians might receive advance materials regarding the pharmacological aspects of a new medication.

Decoding

While a sender of a message must encode, the message's receiver must decode, or translate, the message. **Decoding** is the process by which the receiver interprets symbols and words. For communication to be effective, a message must be decoded the same way the sender has encoded. Decoding is based on the attitudes, values, and beliefs of the message's receivers.[8] Communication does occur when decoding differs from the encoding; however, the outcomes of this situation are not always positive. For example, the family practice group sent a message showing it as the source of care for the entire family. Yet, the target audience may have decoded the message (the picture and words) depicting the medical practice as a pediatric group. Communication occurred, but not effective communication.

Noise

Noise is anything that interferes with the effective communication of a message. Several sources can produce noise: the message, the channel, the environment, the sender, or the receiver. Noise from any source, however, creates problems.

The message can create noise that distracts the receiver from the intended focus. An advertisement that uses humor, for example, can be quite funny to the receiver. The focus of the message, however, might be lost while the receiver attends to the humor rather than to the service being promoted.

The channel can also create noise. A recent Harris & Associates poll indicated the physician, as channel, can create noise. In a survey of 2,525 women and 1,000 men conducted for The Commonwealth Fund, a national health philanthropy, 10 percent of the female respondents said they didn't discuss a problem with their physician because they found the physician to be squeamish about the issue.[9]

Noise can readily occur when using interpersonal channels. A salesperson who makes a poor presentation due to inadequate preparation or organization can create enough noise to prohibit effective communication.

Channel noise can also exist in mass communication. Advertising on television often faces the problem of clutter, with too many distracting messages. The noise of the medium inhibits effective communication. The environment is often a major source of noise. There are increasingly unfavorable reports about rising health care costs. This noise in the environment may negate an organization's attempt to communicate that it is a cost-efficient provider. Receivers can also create their own noise. Lack of attention or interest greatly inhibits the decoding process.

Feedback

The sender of any message is always concerned whether the message has been decoded exactly as it was encoded. In this regard, **feedback**, which is communication from the receiver to the sender, is essential. Feedback is communication in reverse. When the sender uses an interpersonal channel for a message, feedback is often immediate. A company's human resource director can communicate directly with the managed health care plan indicating that she doesn't understand a particular benefit. Feedback is more difficult when using mass communication. Many companies, however, will set up toll-free telephone lines to encourage customer response or feedback. WRNX radio station in western Massachusetts has established a listener call-in line. The audience is encouraged and solicited to call in with their thoughts or preferences regarding the station's song list. Chapter 11 on advertising will examine alternative forms of feedback mechanisms for mass communication channels.

THE PROMOTIONAL MIX

The promotional component of marketing involves four basic tools: advertising, personal selling, publicity, and sales promotion. **Advertising** can be defined as any directly paid form of nonpersonal presentation of goods, services, and ideas. **Personal selling** is any paid, personal presentation of goods, ideas, or services. **Publicity** can be defined as any indirectly paid presentation of goods or services. **Sales promotion** is any short-term inducement or offer for a particular product or service. Each of these promotional tools has unique aspects with inherent benefits and weaknesses. Before discussing these aspects, it is important to recognize that an organization might combine one or more of these particular tools to communicate with an intended market.

Advertising

Advertising is distinguished from the other promotional tools in the marketing mix in that it is both paid *and* nonpersonal. The directly paid component of advertising distinguishes it from publicity. Because an organization pays for space in a magazine or for television or radio time, the advertiser has the advantage of control. When paying for the space or time, the advertiser controls to whom the message is sent. This control is achieved wherever the advertiser places the advertisement. An advertisement run on the MTV channel will most likely attract a different audience than an advertisement placed on CNN World News. By directly paying for the space, an advertiser also can control *when* the message is sent. An advertiser can buy time during the 6:00 p.m. news broadcast, specifying that its advertisement for the hospital will be shown in that time slot. The advertiser also can control *what* is said. Because the advertiser pays for the space, the advertiser can (within the bounds of the law and good taste) create the exact message it wishes to convey. Finally, the advertiser can control *how often* the message is communicated. The frequency of advertising is determined purely by the advertiser's budget constraints. If a health plan wanted to purchase all the time on the Super Bowl broadcast, its greatest limitation would be the cost of the time relative to the advertiser's budget.

Another distinguishing feature of advertising is that it is nonpersonal. As discussed in the model of communication, this may be advertising's greatest limitation because it makes feedback difficult. Another important limitation to advertising is the noise created by the large number of advertisements that bombard the consumer each day. Finally, advertising is limited because most consumers recognize it as a self-promoting communication. In this regard, advertising messages often face credibility problems. Within health care promotional strategy, advertising has become a major focus. In 1993, the total marketing budget for all U.S. hospitals was estimated to be $1.81 billion, of which advertising represented $768 million.[10]

Advertising Effectiveness

Advertising can be more effective in some situations than in others. Advertising is most effective when buyer awareness about a service is minimal. This is when the differential impact of advertising tends to be the greatest. Advertising also works best when industry sales are rising. Advertising cannot stop a decline in industry sales. No amount of advertising, for example, can change the trend in pediatrics or in inpatient stays for the hospital industry. The factors that affect these aspects of health care—in one case demographics (pediatrics), and in the other technology and reimbursement (inpatient days)—are beyond the influence of advertising.

Advertising also works best when the service features are not normally observable, and advertising can demonstrate the outcome of using a particular service. Health New England, an HMO based in Springfield, Massachusetts, uses outdoor billboards showing a cross-country skier. Its slogan states, "Our definition of an outpatient." Another condition under which advertising works best is when the opportunities for differentiation are strong, and advertising can highlight a real point of difference between products. When there is no real differentiation, advertising can do little more than remind the consumer that the brand or service exists in the marketplace. Finally, advertising is effective when the service is new, or not commonly advertised. In the early days of hospital advertising, initial campaigns generated significant consumer attention since health care and hospitals were a novel product to advertise. In most communities today, hospital advertising is as common as McDonald's or Burger King promotions.

Personal Selling

The second major tool of the promotional mix is personal selling. The major difference between this tool and advertising is that it is a personal form of communication. The major strength of personal selling is that it allows for direct feedback from the receiver. A message can then be refined or explained in greater detail to correct any misunderstandings or difficulties that the receiver had in interpretation. Personal selling also has a greater advantage than advertising in that it provides more direct control over who receives the message. Advertising is a form of mass communication. People who see the message often were not part of the intended audience. With personal selling, a company can target directly the audience for its communication. Hospitals that use personal selling have reported several benefits, as shown in Table 10–1.

As with any promotional tool, however, personal selling also has its limitations. A major limitation is cost. Maintaining an effective sales staff requires expenses far beyond salaries. Costs for a sales staff also include individual benefits, travel costs, and technical and equipment support, to name a few. The number of sales calls a salesperson can make in one day is limited. In health care, sales calls to referral physician offices or companies can be very time-consuming. A salesperson may only be able to make four to six calls per day. Another limitation to personal selling is related directly to the strength of the interpersonal communication. Because sales involves a person, the message may vary as a function of the individual's training, disposition, or style. In these cases, a company can suffer from a lack of uniformity regarding its sales training and communications techniques.

Table 10–1 Benefits of Personal Selling for Selected Hospitals

Increased Facility Utilization	35.2%
Improved Medical Staff Relations	31.5%
Financial Benefits	26.5%
Increased Market Share	21.6%
Increased Market Presence	17.3%
Increased Organizational Marketing Sophistication	14.2%
Greater Customer Focus	12.3%

(Total sample: 279 hospitals)

Source: Adapted from Powers, T.L. and Bowers, M.R., Challenges and Opportunities for Personal Selling, *Journal of Health Care Marketing*, Vol. 12, No. 4, pp. 26–32, with permission of American Marketing Association, © 1992.

Advertising vs. Personal Sales Trade-Off

In developing promotional strategy, most companies often face a trade-off in the dollars to be allocated between advertising and personal selling. Table 10–2 shows some of the trade-offs to be made between advertising and personal selling, depending which tool a company chooses to emphasize in its promotional effort.

The more technologically sophisticated the service, the greater the need for personal selling. A salesperson might be needed to explain the intricacies of a particular diagnostic service or program. A medical center might use a personal sales representative to call on potential referral physicians regarding its hyperbaric medicine program. The uniqueness and newness of any services can warrant significant explanation regarding their use or applicability.

The second criterion shown in Table 10–2—number of potential customers—provides the rationale why most consumer product companies use advertising and industrial firms rely on personal selling. In health care, promoting a primary care group to all households within a particular zip code warrants a mass communication strategy such as direct mail. An occupational medicine program, however,

Table 10–2 Trade-Offs between Advertising and Personal Selling

Sales ◄	──────── Greater Emphasis ────────►	Advertising
High	Degree of Technical Sophistication	Low
Few	Number of Customers	Many
Complex	Size of Decision–Making Unit	Simple
High	Degree of Risk	Low

might be best promoted by targeting with a personal sales effort the companies who have employee assistance personnel.

The third criterion in Table 10–2 relates to the composition of the decision-making unit. The more people involved in making a corporate purchasing decision, the greater the need for personal selling. When numerous decision makers are involved, each one may have a distinct set of attributes upon which he or she bases a decision. Personal selling is necessary so that the message can be tailored to address each decision maker's unique concerns. When HMOs advertise their health plans to prospective enrollees, their ads can promote the benefits covered or the outcomes to be derived. Yet, a personal sales effort is required when the HMO persuades a company to offer the plan to the firm's employees. The chief financial officer, the union representative, the company president, and the human resources director may have different concerns that must be addressed before the company accepts the plan. A company that offers significant ancillary services with its product often finds the need to devote more effort to personal selling. In these instances, a salesperson can provide the service or explain its use.

The last criterion when deciding between advertising and personal selling involves degree of risk. The higher the risk, the more personal selling is necessary. This last criterion should make personal selling a key ingredient of most health care organizations' promotional strategy plans. A salesperson can provide the assurance or support that the service or product will meet the customer's expectations. Many academic medical centers have spent significant dollars developing glossy physician referral books. Typically, these booklets have photographs of the physicians on staff, their backgrounds, and areas of expertise. While helpful, these brochures have limited impact. Few decisions are riskier for a physician than making a referral. A personal sales call and follow-up with the potential physician to whom the referral will be made will have a greater likelihood of generating a referral.

Advertising vs. Sales in Decision Making

In addition to the criteria considered above in the trade-off between advertising and personal selling, these two promotional tools also can vary in impact, depending at which stage the buyer is in deciding to purchase. Figure 10–2 displays the levels of impact that advertising and personal selling have at different stages in the buying process.[11]

Unlike the buyer behavior model described in Chapter 4, the horizontal axis on this graph has delineated the decision to buy in three basic stages: prepurchase, purchase, and postpurchase. In the prepurchase stage, the consumer searches for information and evaluates alternatives. As seen in Figure 10–2, both advertising and personal selling are of equal significance at this stage. In the actual purchase stage, personal sales is the key—it is the salesperson who closes the sale. Only

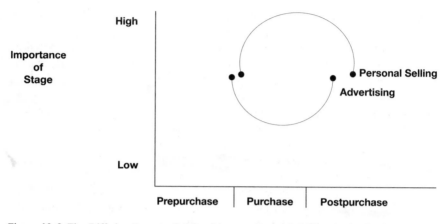

Figure 10–2 The Differing Impact of Advertising vs. Personal Selling in the Buying Process. *Source:* Adapted from Eric N. Berkowitz, Roger A. Kerin, Steven W. Hartley, and William Rudelius, *Marketing* (Burr Ridge, Illinois: Irwin, 1994) 4th ed., p. 504.

occasionally can advertising play this role, such as with direct-mail catalogs. Yet even in these instances, the prospective purchaser often seeks out additional information by dialing the toll-free number listed in the catalog.

Finally, there is the postpurchase stage. The consumer selects a particular health plan. Both advertising and personal selling play a role in the postpurchase stage. The importance of this stage is more significant when the buyer chooses between competing alternatives. The consumer often suffers from cognitive dissonance, which is postpurchase anxiety about whether the correct alternative was chosen. The consumer will seek out additional information to reconfirm that the selection was the best alternative. In this stage, the more personal the postpurchase communication, the more satisfied the buyer.

Publicity

This third promotional tool, publicity, is most common to health care organizations. As noted, this form of communication is an indirectly paid form of presentation of goods, ideas, or services. Most publicity is coordinated through the efforts of a public relations department. The public relations department encourages the media to print or broadcast stories about the organization or its accomplishments. The hospital, for example, that is discussed on the nightly news for having saved a person's life does not pay directly for that coverage. Such coverage is usually garnered through the efforts of the public relations director who contacts the media and provides them with the story. Many public relations departments will also develop news or story releases for dissemination to the media for potential publication or broadcast. The indirect payment involves the resources needed to staff a public relations organization.

In Wisconsin, Physicians Plus is a multispecialty medical group that relies heavily on publicity generated through strong media relations. The marketing director sets up media interviews with the group's specialists who comment on nationally reported health care stories. The group also assists reporters in localizing national stories or trends. In five years of following this publicity-driven promotional strategy, the physicians have participated in 49 radio interviews, 71 television interviews, and have assisted in 188 magazine and newspaper stories.[12]

The greatest advantage to publicity is its credibility. Most consumers who read a story in a newspaper or magazine or watch a television report do not understand that the organization often worked hard to obtain favorable coverage. These communications are seen, instead, as unbiased presentations about the firm. Yet, the indirect payment aspect of publicity is also its greatest weakness. The organization does not control how or when the message gets out. And, to most media, a story is only good once and then it is old news. Thus, a medical group that works hard to obtain publicity may find its story told on the Saturday evening television news when viewership is light and the target audience who watches the news differs from the desired audience. Because of this lack of control, publicity is only useful as a supplemental tool in the promotional plan. It is the rare promotional strategy that can be fully successful by relying totally on this tool for dissemination of its message.

Negative Information

Occasionally, the publicity that an organization receives is not the result of a planned attempt to have its name or accomplishments mentioned in the media. An area of growing importance for public relations and publicity is how to deal with negative information. In 1985, the Health Care Finance Administration (HCFA), a division of the U.S. Department of Health and Human Services, began to publish morbidity statistics for hospitals. Not every hospital fared well in these initial presentations. Many hospitals claimed their outcomes were less favorable than competitors because of difficulties with the data or because of the severity of the patient mix that they treated. These statistics often received great attention in many local media markets. Hospitals with unfavorable ratings had to mount publicity endeavors to counter these negative impressions.[13]

There is a growing need for almost every company to prepare a public relations response plan to deal with any unforeseen negative information. The cases in business are classic, from the early days of the Ford Pinto (exploding gas tanks), to Tylenol (product tampering), to the Pepsi-Cola scare (hypodermic needles in the cans). All these cases show the value of being able to respond effectively to negative information.[14]

Public Relations/Marketing Interaction

In many health care organizations, the delineation between marketing and public relations is often unclear. There is a significant overlap between these two functions since both deal with target markets. Figure 10–3 shows some overlapping areas of responsibility between marketing and public relations. Circle B within the diagram shows the areas where there is often overlap between both departments. When marketing first appeared as a functional area within the management structure of hospitals, there was significant conflict between marketing and public relations over departmental responsibilities. Both marketing and public relations contribute greatly to the organization's presence among key market segments. The essential ingredient is that there be coordination of the promotional plan by the marketing and public relations departments.

Sales Promotion

The fourth tool in the promotional mix—sales promotion—involves temporary inducements to buy. These efforts can be directed to the end user or to the intermediary who carries a product. Most readers of this text are familiar with the common sales promotions of coupons, sweepstakes, or premiums, each of which will be described briefly later in this chapter. Traditional businesses spend more money on sales promotion than they do on advertising. In health care, limited

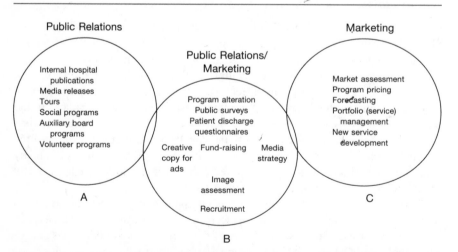

Figure 10–3 The Marketing/Public Relations Interface. *Source:* Reprinted from Berkowitz, E.N., Hillestad, S., and Effertz, P., Marketing/Public Relations: A New Arena for Hospital Conflict, *Health Care Planning and Marketing*, January 1982, pp. 1–10, Aspen Publishers, Inc., © 1982.

attempts at sales promotion have been implemented. Some organizations, like hospitals, have used sales promotion to induce consumers into engaging in a health screening activity. Pharmaceutical companies also have used sales promotions to induce trial of medications. Yet, to some degree, the limited use of sales promotion has been due to a concern that such activities might lead to unnecessary utilization of health care services. Although not used to date with any great frequency, it is useful to understand the two broad types of sales promotions that have been incorporated by traditional industries.

Promotions to Consumers

A large number of sales promotions are directed to the end user of the product. There are numerous sales promotion objectives, as shown in Exhibit 10–1. For each of these sales promotion objectives, a different promotional tactic might be applied. Following are examples of sales promotions commonly directed to individual consumers.

Coupons. Coupons is one of the most common forms of sales promotions, and is one of the few that have been used in health care. Some hospitals have offered coupons for a free blood pressure screening or for a pamphlet on a particular medical problem. Some coupons occasionally will have a discounted offer as part of their appeal. For example, $10 off the price of a mammogram might encourage some first-time triers whose insurance coverage requires a significant co-payment.

Cash Rebates. This sales promotion involves providing consumers with a monetary incentive if they purchase a particular brand. It is an indirect way of discounting a product's price without giving the appearance of a price reduction.

Exhibit 10–1 Sales Promotion Objectives

1. To encourage trial usage of the product by consumers
2. To encourage intermediaries to utilize the facility
3. To encourage customers to buy more than one unit of the product
4. To encourage intermediaries to devote more effort to selling the product or service
5. To acquaint customers with service changes
6. To identify new customers
7. To build customer loyalty
8. To encourage customers to switch facilities or providers
9. To gain entry into new markets

Contests. Contests are sales promotions that require the consumer to participate actively in the promotion. The consumer might have to solve a puzzle or provide a slogan in order to enter a chance to win. Many retail outlets use contests to encourage the consumer to keep returning to acquire more game pieces or clues to a puzzle.

Premiums. Premiums are products given to the consumer in return for a particular action. Many premiums are often tied to the product being purchased. Marlboro cigarettes, for example, markets as premiums a line of western clothes. These premiums are an attempt to reinforce the image of the rugged cowboy who smokes Marlboros. McDonald's restaurants provide children with small toys related to particular themes, such as pumpkin pails on Halloween.

Samples. Samples are products disseminated to the consumer free or at a greatly reduced cost. Companies frequently manufacture smaller-packaged versions of a product to be promoted in a special trial size. Samples are a valuable form of sales promotion because they allow the consumer to try an item with less risk. Since the product is often given free or at a greatly reduced price, the consumer's investment is minimal. Pharmaceutical sales representatives give physicians samples of new medications as a way to encourage trial use. New mothers are often presented with a free sample kit of baby-related products upon discharge from the hospital.

Service businesses are at somewhat of a disadvantage in terms of sampling. One cannot create a smaller version of the service. Yet it is possible to create a sample by allowing the consumer a free visit or a first-time visit at a greatly reduced price. Sampling, however, is costly. For sampling to be effective, the product or service being tried should be noticeably better than the competition's.

Promotions to the Trade

There is a second level of sales promotions, which is directed to intermediaries within the channel of distribution. For example, traditional businesses such as Proctor and Gamble may direct sales promotion efforts at retailers, with the goal of encouraging retailers to stock more of a particular product in inventory. Two of the most commonly used sales promotions in the distribution channel are allowances and cooperative advertising.

Allowances. A common trade promotion is the allowance, which is a discount based on some particular criterion. For example, a manufacturer might give a case allowance based on a minimum amount of product ordered. Another common allowance is a merchandise allowance, which provides a discount or reimbursement to the intermediary who makes extra merchandising efforts for a particular product or line.

Cooperative Advertising. A second major trade allowance involves sharing or underwriting some portion of the advertising expense with an intermediary. Coca-Cola, for example, might pay Kroger supermarket up to $5,000 per quarter per region for advertisements that highlight Coca-Cola products. This is a form of sales promotion that could be used in health care. A hospital, for example, could pay some of the advertising for a medical group that is a loyal member of the institution. General Electric Co. has, for example, helped providers who offer mammography services by advertising those programs. At times, G.E. covers the cost of advertising.[15]

A cooperative advertising program is an acceptable form of a trade allowance. Yet, every organization must be careful that these arrangements are not viewed as tying arrangements, which would violate the Clayton Act (1914). Tying arrangements create situations in which a seller requires the purchaser of one product to also buy another product in their line. These arrangements, which would lessen competition, were specifically forbidden by the Clayton Act.

FACTORS AFFECTING SALES PROMOTION USE

There are two main factors to consider when emphasizing one particular promotional tool relative to another when developing the promotional plan. These factors include the stage of the product life cycle and the channel control strategy.

The Product Life Cycle

At each stage of the product life cycle there are distinct promotional considerations.

Introduction

A major factor to consider in determining the promotional mix is the stage of the product life cycle. In the introduction stage, as noted in Chapter 7, a key consideration is gaining awareness. At this stage advertising plays a major role. As a mass communication strategy, advertising can efficiently generate early recognition of the service among consumers. In the introduction stage of the life cycle, companies must often develop *primary demand*. This is purchase interest in a product class. Any early publicity to build credibility is of particular value at this stage. Depending on the product, sales promotion can also play a valuable role in this stage. In this regard, service businesses are often limited. A product-based company often has the opportunity to disseminate samples of the new item, offering consumers a low-cost way to try the product.

Growth

In the growth stage of the life cycle, competition appears, in which case product businesses try to lock up the channel of distribution. Personal selling efforts are directed to the intermediaries to tie in the buyer. This scenario also works in health care. As more competitors vie for referrals in the cardiac surgery, a physician referral sales force must focus efforts on the primary care referrers to lock up their patient base. At the growth stage of the life cycle, advertising efforts shift from generating awareness to highlighting the differences between competitors. Advertising at this stage develops *selective demand,* which is interest in and preference for the specific brand of product or service.

Maturity

At the mature stage of the life cycle, there are few new buyers. The major goal of promotional strategy is to maintain the buyers the company presently serves. The advertising is done mainly for reinforcement or reminder purposes. In industries where sales promotion is common, these efforts are directed at keeping the present customer base returning. Games or discounts for multiple purchases become more common. Within the airline industry, as business travel began to level off in the recessionary period of the late 1980s, frequent-flyer mileage programs evolved as a new sales promotion tool to encourage repeat business.

Decline

The decline stage of the product life cycle is one where little promotional effort occurs.

Channel Control Strategies

Chapter 9 presented the concept of the channel of distribution. For any organization, the ultimate goal is to control the channel of distribution. There are two basic strategies involving promotional tools that are used to accomplish this: These are referred to as push and pull.

Push

A **push** strategy involves controlling the channel of distribution by working through the channel. Figure 10–4 shows the channels of distribution for a typical consumer goods manufacturer and for an acute-care hospital. For the consumer

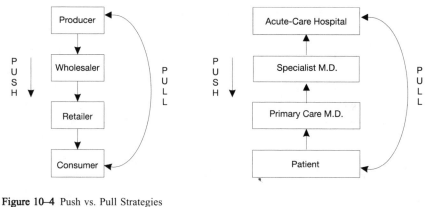

Figure 10–4 Push vs. Pull Strategies

goods company, the product moves to the consumer. For the hospital, the patient moves to the facility. In a push strategy, the manufacturer influences the intermediaries to carry the product. A manufacturer might offer the wholesaler a discount if it orders so many cases of a new brand of soft drink. The wholesaler, in turn, may employ a push strategy by offering the retailer a similar inducement to order. When consumers go to the retailer to buy their regular soft drink, the retailer might encourage the consumer to buy the new brand. Because of the discount provided by the wholesaler, the smart retailer knows it will make more money if the new brand is purchased.

A similar push strategy is familiar in health care. A hospital has a medical staff that also has practice privileges at competing facilities. The hospital administrator wants these doctors to admit patients to her particular facility. In order to encourage the physicians, the administrator might provide them with preferential parking, free lunches in the doctors' lounge, and office space in an attached medical office building. The goal is that physicians will refer patients to the hospital at which the physicians feel most comfortable.

Pull

An alternative to the push strategy is **pull**. In this strategy, the organization appeals directly to the consumer by bypassing or controlling the intermediary. Again, in Figure 10–4, the manufacturer may find, in trying to introduce a new product, that the wholesaler is not interested in carrying the item in spite of incentives offered. If wholesaler acceptance is not gained, retailer acceptance will be unlikely. As a result, the manufacturer may try to pull the product through the channel by advertising the item to end uses. Consumers, seeing advertisements for the new brand, or receiving coupons for a dollar off a two-liter bottle, will seek out the item from retailers. Retailers, seeing consumer demand, will call the wholesalers requesting delivery. Wholesalers, learning of retailer interest, will call the manufacturer to place orders.

Many health care organizations often implement a pull strategy. A tertiary care center might find that local physicians do not want to refer to the medical center. In spite of efforts to generate referrals, patient flow is low. So the medical center begins to promote its new program directly to consumers. Many consumers in Arizona, for example, know about the Arizona Heart Institute. These consumers might bypass their local physician or cardiologist to whom their doctor has referred them, in order to seek out care at the Arizona Heart Institute. In the mid-1980s, many hospitals began to establish centers of excellence—specialty clinical programs touted to consumers to generate self-referred business, or to influence the decision making of intermediaries to use the facilities on patient request. In this fashion, the patients (end users) were pulled around the intermediaries or traditional referral sources. In July 1993, the American Physical Therapy Association launched an advertising

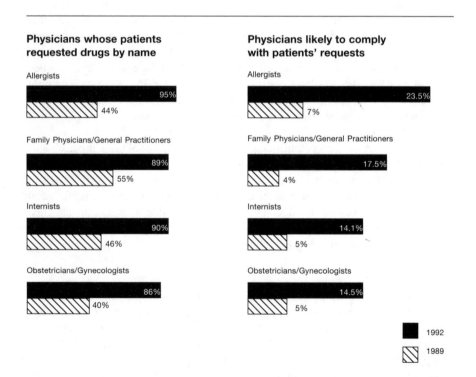

Figure 10–5 The Pulling Power of Patients. *Source:* Reprinted from Are Your Patients Telling You What To Prescribe?, *Medical Economics,* November 8, 1993, p. 18, with permission of Scott-Levin Associates, © 1993.

campaign in the *Ladies Home Journal* and *Good Housekeeping* magazines to educate female baby boomers to the benefits of physical therapy. The goal was to have these consumers either request a referral from their physicians to such therapists when they had a problem, or to have these individuals self-refer themselves for an evaluation and possible treatment by a certified physical therapist.[16]

The pull strategy is being used more often in health care, for example, for pharmaceutical products and even for surgical procedures. CooperVision advertised its "Natural Eyes" pigmentation implant procedure in women's magazines to encourage patient requests.[17] Many health care providers question whether the pull strategy does, in fact, work. Figure 10–5 shows that many physicians are reporting a dramatic increase in the number of patients requesting specific drugs by name. The data also show that physicians are more likely to comply with these requests. Slightly more than 23 percent of allergists report complying with such requests in 1992 compared to only 7 percent in 1989.[18]

CONCLUSIONS

Promotional strategy encompasses far more than advertising. Increasingly, health care providers are turning to personal selling and sales promotions as ways to compete more effectively. At the foundation of a good promotional strategy is the understanding of the components essential for effective communication. A sender and receiver must be able to encode and decode often in the midst of significant noise. Successfully communicating can ultimately lead to controlling the channel of distribution for market share.

KEY TERMS

Encoding	Advertising
Message	Personal Selling
Channel	Publicity
Opinion Leaders	Sales Promotion
Decoding	Push
Noise	Pull
Feedback	

CHAPTER SUMMARY

1. Several factors are necessary for effective communication. There must be a sender, receiver, encoding, decoding, a channel, and feedback. Communication often is affected negatively by noise.

2. *Messages can take several forms; they can be one-sided, two-sided, or emotional. Because of the unique nature of health care, emotional appeals to fear must be used with caution.*

3. *The promotional mix for an organization consists of advertising, personal selling, publicity, and sales promotion.*

4. *A major advantage of advertising over publicity is in terms of what is said, to whom it is said, how often it is said, and when it is said. Publicity has greater credibility than advertising.*

5. *Advertising and personal selling each have distinct values. The decision to use one promotional tool more than the other is based on the risk of the decision, size of the decision-making unit, the complexity of the service, the size of the market, and the geographic dispersion of the market.*

6. *Advertising and personal selling have differing levels of impact in each stage of the consumer's decision-making process. The more personal the post-purchase contact with the buyer, the more satisfied the buyer.*

7. *Sales promotion has been an underused tool of the promotional mix within health care. Sales promotion tactics can be directed to consumers or to the trade.*

8. *In a push strategy, the promotional efforts are directed to the intermediaries in the channel, while in the pull strategy, promotional efforts are directed to the end user.*

CHAPTER PROBLEMS

1. After a recent presentation of health plans at her company, Julia Brouck made her first visit to her new HMO with her son, Arthur, and daughter, Emmy Lou. After seeing the pediatrician, she was told that there was a $5 co-payment for the visits. "I don't understand," Julia said, "I thought all doctor visits were free." Explain the potential source of this misconception.

2. At a local hospital, a decision was made recently to downsize the nursing staff. The local television station sent a reporter and camera crew to interview the administrator regarding the impact of this action on patient care. After 20 minutes filming the interview, the reporter left. That evening a 15-second segment of the interview was shown, which left an unfavorable impression regarding the impact on quality. The administrator wondered what went wrong. Explain how more control could have been used to send out the message about the down-sizing.

3. Explain the relative emphasis that would be placed on advertising or personal selling in each of the following situations: (a) a manufacturer of an

infusion pump therapy kit for use in hospitals, (b) a hospital offering a nutrition workshop for seniors, and (c) an academic medical center offering a helicopter service for trauma cases within a 200-mile radius of the facility.

4. In recognition of the post-purchase role of promotion, what strategies would you suggest for: (a) a busy hospital emergency room, (b) an executive fitness program that provides health screening and fitness evaluation, and (c) an occupational medicine program that contracts its services to companies?

5. The University of Chicago Hospitals recently ran an advertisement in *The Chicago Tribune*, showing an intensive care nurse employed at the hospital saying, "Personally, I'd be concerned if my health insurance plan didn't offer the University of Chicago Hospitals." Explain the channel control strategy being used with this advertisement, and the logic of the approach.

NOTES

1. W. Schramm, How Communication Works, in *The Process and Effects of Mass Communication*, ed. W. Schramm (Urbana, Ill.: The University of Illinois Press, 1955), 3–26.

2. H.C. Kelman and C.I. Hovland, Reinstatement of the Communication in Delayed Measurement of Opinion Change, *Journal of Abnormal Psychology* 48, no. 3 (1953):327–335.

3. C.I. Hovland, A. Lumsdine, and F.D. Sheffield, *Experiments in Mass Communications* (New York, N.Y.: John Wiley & Sons, Inc., 1949), 182–200.

4. W.L. Wilkie and P.W. Farris, Comparison Advertising: Problems and Potential, *Journal of Marketing* 39, no. 4 (1975):7–15.

5. M.S. LaTour and S.A. Zahra, Fear Appeals as Advertising Strategy: Should They Be Used?, *Journal of Consumer Marketing* 6, no. 2 (Spring 1989):61–70.

6. M.L. Ray and W.L. Wilkie, Fear: The Potential of an Appeal Neglected by Marketing, *Journal of Marketing* 34, no. 1 (1970):54–62.

7. M.G. Weinberger and C.S. Gulas, The Impact of Humor in Advertising: A Review, *Journal of Advertising* 21, no. 4 (1992):35–39; and B. Sternthal and C.S. Craig, Humor in Advertising, *Journal of Marketing* 37, no. 4 (1973):12–18.

8. H. Hyman and P. Sheatsley, Some Reasons Why Information Campaigns Fail, *Public Opinion Quarterly* 11, no. 3 (1947):412–423; and J.T. Klapper, *The Effects of Mass Communication* (New York, N.Y.: Free Press, 1960), 166–205.

9. Are Doctors Sexist? Women Seem To Think So, *Medical Economics* 70, no. 16 (1993):18.

10. J. Burns, Hospitals Splurge on Selling Efforts, *Modern Healthcare* 24, no. 10 (1994):92.

11. E.N. Berkowitz, et al., *Marketing*, 3rd ed. (Homewood, Ill.: Richard D. Irwin, Inc., 1992), 473–474.

12. A.T. Beal, How Physicians' Plus Grew into the Video Age, *Marketer's Guidepost* 3, no. 4 (Spring 1993):1, 4–5.

13. An interesting discussion of these issues has been presented by B.P. Roberts and B. Allen, Data Driven Quality Differentiation: Using Pro Mortality Data To Market Your Hospital, in *Marketing Is Everybody's Business*, ed. P. Sanchez (Chicago, Ill.: Alliance for Health Care Strategy and Marketing, 1988), 165–170.

14. M.G. Weinberger and J. Romeo, The Impact of Negative Product News, *Business Horizons* 32, no. 1 (1989):44–50.

15. S. MacStravic, Reverse and Double Reverse Marketing for Health Care Organizations, *Health Care Management Review* 18, no. 3 (Summer 1993):53–58.

16. E. DeNitto, Medical Groups Find Ads Fit the Bill, *Advertising Age* 64, no. 28 (1993):12.

17. CooperVision Begins Marketing Eyeliner Procedure for Physicians, *Physician's Marketing* 2, no. 1 (1986):1.

18. Are Your Patients Telling You What to Prescribe?, *Medical Economics*, 70, no. 21 (1993):18.

11

ADVERTISING

After reading this chapter you should be able to:

- Recognize the differences between the two basic forms of advertising: product and institutional

- Describe the steps followed when developing an advertising campaign

- Know various ways to develop an advertising budget

- Understand the value of alternative media

No element of the marketing mix has been more visible in health care than advertising. "Advertising" may be defined as any directly paid form of nonpersonal presentation of goods, services, or ideas by an identified sponsor. The key aspects of this definition are: (1) that it is paid, which distinguishes advertising from publicity; and (2) that it is nonpersonal, which separates advertising from personal selling.

Concerns have long been raised regarding health care advertising. Yet, as seen in Table 11–1, consumers respond favorably toward this aspect of marketing. In two separate studies, Hite, Bellizzi, and Andrus examined the differences in attitudes toward advertising between consumers and psychiatrists, and between consumers and dentists. In Table 11–1, the lower the value, the more agreement there is with the statement. Thus, when considering each statement for psychiatrists and the issue of advertising, more consumers than psychiatrists consistently agreed with the statement that was favorable toward advertising. In the next two columns, a similar study was done with regard to these issues and dentists. Again,

Table 11–1 Acceptance of Advertising in Health Care

	Mean[1]			
	Consumers	Psychiatrists	Consumers	Dentists
It is proper for psychologists (dentists) to advertise?	2.05*	3.61	2.07	3.65
I would like to see more psychologists (dentists) advertise.	2.16	4.21	2.48	4.49
Advertising can be done tastefully by psychiatrists (dentists).	1.59	2.78	1.93	2.80
Advertising would help consumers make more intelligent choices between psychiatrists (dentists).	2.06	3.92	2.51	4.23
Advertising will tend to increase the overall quality of psychiatric (dental) services.	2.59	4.17	3.13	4.47
I presently have a high image of psychiatrists who advertise.	2.38	4.28	2.47	4.35
The public would be provided useful information through the advertising of psychiatric (dental) services.	1.85	3.41	2.25	3.60
Advertising would make consumers more aware of the qualifications of psychiatrists (dentists).	2.01	3.46	2.68	4.27

(Sample = 251 psychiatrists, 196 consumers)
1 = all means significantly different at .0001
(Sample = 388 dentists, 290 consumers)
* Lower value indicates more agreement with the statement.

Source: Data from *Journal of Health Care Marketing,* Vol. 8, No. 4, pp. 21–29, December 1988, and from *Journal of Health Care Marketing,* Vol. 8, No. 1, pp. 30–38, March 1988.

consumers were more favorably disposed to these statements compared to the dentists.[1] Also, another study of 400 consumers found that 70 percent indicated approval of hospital advertising.[2]

COMMON CLASSIFICATIONS OF ADVERTISING

There are many alternative forms of advertisements with the two common advertising classifications being *product* and *institutional*. Product advertisements focus on a particular product or service, while institutional advertisements build up or enhance an organization's image rather than a particular product. There are several variations within each form of advertising.

Product Advertising

Product advertising can assume one of several forms: informational, competitive, or reminder. Informational advertisements are used in the early stage of a new product or service introduction. These advertisements help to explain the service, how it can be accessed, or what its objectives are.

Competitive product advertisements are persuasive—they try to generate selective demand for the organization's service over that of competitors.[3] In traditional industries, this form of advertising has often been conducted in a comparative fashion, where specific comparisons are made between competing products. Few comparative advertisements have been seen in health care.

A final version of product advertising is purely reminder. For example, hospitals often have implemented nurse information lines on which consumers can call and talk to a nurse regarding a medical question. When necessary, these nurses will provide callers with the names of health care providers to call for further examination or consultation. For this type of "ask-a-nurse" program, hospitals like St. Vincent Health System, a 580-bed institution in Erie, Pennsylvania, have used billboards in the community to remind people of the availability of the service.

Institutional Advertising

Institutional advertising is frequently used in health care. These advertisements are used to build goodwill and to enhance the public's image of a particular organization. There are several variations of institutional advertising; some introduce or announce the opening of a new company or facility, some compare programs, and some advocate public policy positions.

The advertisement shown in Figure 11–1 is an example of a pioneering institutional advertisement. Similar to ads for products, it is used to announce a

Harvard Community Health Plan:

1) Developed an innovative pediatric asthma outreach program.

2) Established a non-profit foundation for medical education, research and community service.

3) Assessed the quality of life in breast cancer patients receiving chemotherapy.

4) Developed a cystic fibrosis carrier screening program.

5) Established the Department of Ambulatory Care and Prevention with Harvard Medical School.

6) First health plan in New England to fully cover a heart transplant.

7) Instrumental in discovering new ways to reduce the need for hospitalization.

8) Developed a program with a major teaching hospital to reduce unnecessary C-Sections.

9) Established the first department in an HMO responsible for measuring quality-of-care.

10) Developed ground-breaking programs on alcohol awareness and violence prevention.

11) Researched the relationship between myopia and glaucoma.

12) Ranked number one HMO in New England four years in a row by the HMO Buyers' Guide.

13) Developed innovative teen AIDS and pregnancy prevention programs.

14) Pioneered usage of computerized medical records.

15) Developed new teaching methods for better relationships between doctors and patients.

Lahey Clinic:

1) Pioneered the safe use of frozen blood in surgery.

2) Developed techniques for repairing damaged bile ducts.

3) Performed the first operation to replace the entire aorta in one stage.

4) Pioneered safe and effective techniques of radiation therapy for cancer.

5) Pioneered laser therapy to treat superficial bladder cancer.

6) Invented the first portable chemotherapy infusion pump for cancer patients.

7) Discovered techniques of kidney surgery to restore function to viable shut-down kidneys.

8) Pioneered electron beam therapy for the skin disorder mycosis fungiodes.

9) Developed techniques for creating new bladders from intestines.

10) Acquired leading expertise in electrical abnormalities of the heart.

11) Developed techniques of laser surgery to treat chronically infected sinuses.

12) Developed leading expertise for rectal reconstruction for ulcerative colitis patients.

13) Performed the first successful removal of the right lung on a cancer patient.

14) Developed the first endoscopic examination of the middle ear.

15) Established the first multi-specialty group practice in the Eastern United States.

JUST IMAGINE WHAT'S

Two leaders that have revolutionized medical care and its delivery. Visionaries. Pioneers. Discoverers.

POSSIBLE NOW THAT WE'VE

They are one of the nation's leading HMO's and a nationally renowned medical center. Harvard Community Health Plan

DISCOVERED EACH OTHER.

and Lahey Clinic. And now, for the first time, they are working together. In fact, many Lahey physicians will now practice

at Harvard Health's Burlington Center. Which means beginning on the first of the new year, members can choose either

location as their primary care facility and have access to the physicians and services at Lahey. Of course, there are over

sixty other locations to choose from. So call 1-800-848-HEALTH for the one nearest you.

And discover for yourself what health care should be.

Harvard Community Health Plan
WE'RE WHAT HEALTH CARE SHOULD BE™

Figure 11–1 Pioneering Institutional Advertisement. *Source:* Courtesy of The Lahey Clinic, Burlington, Massachusetts.

new organization or entity. The ad shown in the figure promotes a new health care alliance between the Lahey Clinic and Harvard Community Health Plan in Massachusetts. Institutional advertisements occasionally can be competitive. These advertisements compare two or more organizational forms, showing one to be more effective than the others. In health care, this variation often appears with advertisements touting prepaid health care plans vs. more traditional indemnity insurance programs.

As in product advertising, institutional advertising occasionally serves as a reminder to reinforce previous impressions in the target audience.

Another common form of institutional advertising is referred to as *advocacy*, in which an organization publicizes its position regarding a particular issue. For example, Figure 11–2 shows an advertisement paid for by the American Chiropractic Association, asking consumers to contact their congressional representatives about including chiropractic care in President Clinton's health care reform proposal.

DEVELOPING THE ADVERTISING CAMPAIGN

The development of an advertising campaign begins with the preparation of a **media plan,** which outlines the analysis and execution of the advertising campaign.

Define the Target Audience

Essential to a successful media plan is the first step—a definition of the **target audience**. The target audience specifies the group or groups to whom the organization is trying to communicate. This step is an organizational decision, determined by earlier market research and based on prior market segmentation decisions. The more detailed this section of the media plan, the easier subsequent decisions will be regarding placement of advertisements and advertising copy design. As in the earlier discussion of market segmentation, a target audience description will include demographics and, possibly, attitudinal profiles and lifestyle descriptions. Upon defining the target audience, the media plan must then specify the advertising campaign's objectives, budget, message, communication program, and manner for evaluation. These steps are shown in Figure 11–3 and are described in detail in the following pages.

Determine the Advertising Objectives

Advertising objectives are critical to any successful campaign. In setting objectives, it is best to consider how advertising works. Consumers do not view an

Find Out If Anyone Here Has A Backbone.

The health care reform bills are getting ready to come through Congress. And most don't include safe, cost-effective chiropractic care as a *guaranteed* benefit—something the big insurance companies couldn't take away.

For 20 million Americans who receive chiropractic care every year, that's more than bad policy. It's bad politics.

That's why we're asking everyone who believes chiropractic care ought to be a *guaranteed* benefit to give Congress a piece of their mind.

Send copies of the coupon on the right to your Senators and Representatives and let them know you want chiropractic care included in whatever health care reform bill they ultimately pass.

Who knows. For once, maybe we'll see some backbone in this town.

Watch My Back! I expect you to stand up for my rights and lower health care costs by voting to include chiropractic care as a *guaranteed* benefit in any health care reform bill approved by Congress.

Name _____
Address _____
City _____State _____ Zip ____

Mail to:
(Your Senator or Patrick Moynihan)
U.S. Senate
Washington, DC 20510

(Your Representative or Dan Rostenkowski)
U.S. House of Representatives
Washington, DC 20515

Or call 202-224-3121

AMERICAN CHIROPRACTIC ASSOCIATION • 1701 CLARENDON BLVD. • ARLINGTON, VIRGINIA 22209 •1-703-276-8800

Figure 11–2 Sample advocacy advertisement. *Source:* Courtesy of the American Chiropractic Association, Arlington, Virginia.

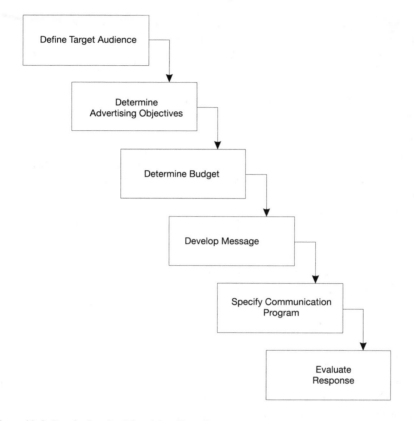

Figure 11–3 Developing the Advertising Campaign

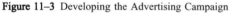

ad and then buy a product or use a service. Rather, advertising facilitates moving consumers along a sequence of steps that have been described as a **hierarchy of effects**—the stages a buyer moves through from first seeing an advertisement ultimately to buying the product or using the service.[4] These stages include: awareness, interest, evaluation, trial, and adoption.

Awareness

This level of the hierarchy is necessarily the first. The consumer must recognize the ad or be cognizant of the fact that it exists. Canonsburg General Hospital of Canonsburg, Pennsylvania, for example, selected consumer awareness as the advertising objective for its newly remodeled mammography center. The hospital conducted a five-week advertising campaign in several newspapers. Advertisements were also reprinted as flyers distributed to new residents.[5]

Awareness was also the advertising objective for Mission Hospital Regional Medical Center of Orange County, California. The hospital wanted to target residents new to the area. The hospital purchased a mailing list of new arrivals and directly mailed a marketing package to residents in 13 zip codes. It also sent newcomers two cards. After sending out 8,980 brochures in 1992, the hospital received a 2.7 percent response rate requesting more information.[6]

Interest

After developing initial awareness, a consumer must have some inclination to seek additional information about the product. The organization's goal at this level of the hierarchy is to provide some information that will motivate further deliberation or action.

Evaluation

Before consumers will buy a product or seek out a service from a particular provider, they must compare that product or service with other available options. Organizational advertising must include dimensions that are important to the target market.

Trial

The initial use of a service is called trial. Advertising can only move a person to this level of the hierarchy. In order to have repeat purchases, a service must meet the customer's expectations. No amount of advertising can correct a bad experience with a hospital or medical group.

Adoption

This is the highest level of the hierarchy and the ultimate goal of advertising— the stage at which the customer becomes a regular user. If trial was satisfactory, reminder advertising plays an important role in this level of the hierarchy of effects.

Determine the Budget

Several methods are generally used to determine the appropriate amount to spend on advertising. Since there is no absolute formula, these methods tend to include one of the four following categories: percentage of sales, competitive parity, "all you can afford," and objective and task.

Percentage of Sales

This method involves determining a fixed percentage of sales or revenue to use as the basis for advertising allocations.[7] For example, a hospital might decide that one half of one percent of last year's net revenue will be allocated to the current year's advertising. The advantage of this method is its simplicity. This method also provides some fiscal safeguard in tying advertising expenditures to organization resources. In spite of these advantages, however, this method has an inherent flaw that implies that sales or revenue causes advertising. Advertising should be seen as contributing to sales, not the other way around. Using this method, a company would reduce advertising expenditures when sales drop. In fact, this may be the period when additional monies must be spent to generate new sales. Hospitals that have large fixed-asset bases cannot afford to exist with large, idle capacity.[8]

Competitive Parity

This method is common in industries where there is a significant amount of trade data. The hospital sets the advertising budget based on industry norms or what it perceives the competitor is spending. Logic demands that an organization consider the competitor when determining any advertising budget.[9] Table 11–2 shows an example of such competitive comparison data collected in a recent study by Sutter Health of Sacramento, California, a health system consisting of hospitals, physicians, and a managed care plan. This study was conducted to determine norms regarding system advertising spending. Except for consideration of the competitor, the logic of this method is weak. It may well be that the competitor is trying to reach a different target market or has different goals. Moreover, this method assumes that the competitor knows what it is doing.

All You Can Afford

This approach is obvious by its name. Common to organizations that really don't believe in the value of advertising, it involves first allocating the budget to all important operations within the organization. If any money is left over, it might then be allocated to advertising.[10] While this method might address an organization's fiscal reality, it could lead to too much, as well as to too little, being spent on advertising. No consideration is given to the objectives of these methods.

Objective and Task

This fourth method is the most appropriate way to determine the advertising budget. The **objective and task** approach involves setting objectives along the hierarchy of effects and determining the tasks necessary to accomplish these objectives. The costs of these tasks ultimately determine the final budget needed.[11]

Table 11–2 Competitive Parity Advertising Expenses in Health Care

Advertising Expense Included

Entity	Communications budget as a percent of system net patient revenues	Communications budget as a percent of system expenditures	Communications expenditures per system employee
Henry Ford Health System, Detroit, Mich.	0.12%	0.13%	$138
Group Health Cooperative, Seattle, Wash.	0.14	0.15	142
Sutter Health, Sacramento, Calif.	0.23	0.23	156
Baylor Health Care System, Dallas, Texas	0.25	0.27	184
AVERAGE	0.52	0.55	355
Health Midwest, Kansas City, Mo.	0.53	0.55	390
EHS Health Care, Oak Brook, Ill.	0.89	0.95	477
Alliant Health System, Louisville, Ky.	1.48	1.54	1,000

Source: Adapted from Jaklevic, M.C., Benchmarking Study Targets Communications Departments of Systems, *Modern Healthcare,* October 3, 1994, pp. 88–90, with permission of Crain Communications, Inc., 740 N. Rush Street, Chicago, Illinois 60611, © 1994.

Exhibit 11–1 offers examples of advertising objectives for each level of the hierarchy.

In using this method, for example, a marketing director must decide how to accomplish the first objective of getting referral physicians in the upper peninsula to be aware of helicopter service. In this instance, the director must determine the following tasks and costs:

One physician referral brochure (6,000 copies at $2.00 each)	$12,000
One full-page advertisement in *Michigan Medical Society* monthly magazine	1,500
One open house at medical center for area physicians	6,000
Total cost	$19,500

The total cost is the proposed budget. At this point, however, the marketing director determines how much can be afforded, and adjusts the budget accord-

Exhibit 11–1 Advertising Objectives for the Hierarchy

Awareness: To have 25 percent of the physicians in the Upper Peninsula of Michigan aware of the University's emergency helicopter service within six months.

Interest: To have our program director for industrial medicine be invited to make three new presentations a month to companies interested in our packaged occupational/industrial medicine service.

Evaluation: To have 25 percent of the women between the ages of 21 and 40 rate the labor and delivery unit as the most modern and technologically advanced in the community.

Trial: In the next 30 days, to have 15 percent of the users to the new urgent care facility on the west side be first-time users.

Adoption: To have half the callers to the health information line define themselves as regular users of the program within one year of opening the service.

---

ingly. Any adjustment in the budget, then, must be reflected in what can be accomplished regarding the objectives. The tasks will be redefined, and the budget subsequently adjusted further.

In examining the objectives listed in Exhibit 11–1 it is important to note the ingredients for good, useful objectives. All of these objectives specify the target market. Each objective is time-based, whether it be 30 days or a quarter of a year. Finally, each objective is measurable. This last component is essential in order to prove the value of the campaign. In health care marketing, a common criticism of advertising has been whether or not it achieved its objective. This concern is a result of not beginning with a measurable objective.

Develop the Message

The third step in designing the advertising program is the development of the message. Marketing research is essential at this stage to determine the attributes that are important to the consumer. In developing these messages, varying appeals are often used, including rational, emotional, and moral/social appeals.

Rational. These messages are directed at distinct functional attributes of the product. The purpose is to explain the value in using the particular service.

Emotional. An increasingly common advertising appeal is emotion, with fear and humor being used most often.[12] The use of fear in health care advertisements has some troubling ethical dilemmas, as noted in an earlier chapter. In fact, the Alliance for Health Care Strategy and Marketing (formerly operated as the

Academy for Health Services Marketing) developed a set of ethical guidelines for advertisers (reviewed later in this chapter). The group specifically noted that advertising should not use emotional appeals to take advantage of individuals who are vulnerable due to health care needs.[13] Within limits, however, fear appeals can be effective. One study used fear appeals in advertisements for AIDS prevention to college-age students. Results of the study showed that an ad with a strong fear appeal generated tension, energy, and a more positive cognitive response than the milder version of the ad.[14]

Moral/Social Appeals. These messages focus upon causes or issues. Hospitals mount advertising campaigns to solicit funding for their medical foundation research. Likewise, the American Red Cross appeals to the community for participation in blood donation.

Pretesting

Any good advertising message should first be pretested. **Pretesting** involves assessing advertising copy options before their general use. Effective pretesting requires that it be conducted with the intended target audience.

In the earlier chapter on marketing research (Chapter 5), focus groups were discussed as one data-gathering methodology. Focus groups are used extensively in the early stages of advertising development and pretesting. Initially, focus groups can be used to identify the important dimension for the advertisements and alternative appeals that could be utilized. Other pretesting methods can be implemented, once a draft version of the advertisement is created. Pretests can be conducted to ensure that the target audience can interpret the advertisement, is interested in it, and prefers it over other versions. There are several ways to pretest an advertisement, including the use of portfolio tests, jury tests, and theater tests.

Portfolio Tests. This form of pretesting involves testing alternative copy. The test advertisement is placed in a grouping with other sample advertisements. Consumers are then asked to review all the samples. Upon completing the review, consumers are then asked to judge the advertisements on a series of dimensions such as interest, attention, likability, and informative value. When Fallon Health Plan in Worcester, Massachusetts initially embarked on its first HMO advertising campaign, it pretested four different advertisements among consumers who belonged to traditional indemnity plans. In conducting the portfolio test, the Fallon HMO also showed variations of the advertisements to subscribers of a competing HMO.[15]

Jury Tests. In this version of a pretest, the advertisement or variations are shown to a panel of consumers. Similar to a portfolio test, researchers solicit consumer reactions on several dimensions in the advertisements.

Theater Tests. The most expensive and elaborate form of pretesting is the theater test. For example, consumers are invited to a special viewing of a new television show or movie. Inserted into the show are sample advertisements. When the viewing is over, consumers are asked to rate the show and provide reactions to the advertisements. In the most sophisticated theater tests, consumers can react immediately to the commercials and record their intensity of like or dislike by using a hand-held device while they view the advertisement.

Regardless of the degree of sophistication applied to the pretest, it is an essential step in advertising. In health care, pretesting often involves showing the advertisements to the physicians on staff or in the medical group to gain their approval. This step is important to ensure that any advertisement intended for the consumer be factually correct regarding any intervention or treatment discussed. Yet, unless the advertisement is directed to other physicians outside the organization, this kind of pretest would not be entirely valid. The advertisement also must be pretested with the target audience of intended consumers.

Specify the Communication Program

Once an advertisement's message is developed and pretested, the next step in the advertising campaign is to select the appropriate medium and vehicle for delivering the message to the target market. Related to this decision is determining the timing of the messages to be communicated. **Medium** refers to the form of communication selected, whether it be newspapers, radio, television, direct mail, or magazines, to name a few. The **vehicle** is the advertising alternative chosen within each medium. For example, an advertiser might use magazines as the medium and *Modern Healthcare* magazine as the particular vehicle within that medium.

In selecting the appropriate medium, there are two objectives that often conflict within the constraints of any advertising budget. These are the goals of reach and frequency. **Reach** refers to the unduplicated audience that an advertising vehicle will deliver. The more people exposed to the message, the broader the reach. **Frequency** refers to the number of times the same person receives a message within a defined time period. The value of frequency was best shown by the advice to prospective advertisers from the 1800s shown in Chapter 4. Ideally, a company tries to maximize the reach and frequency of its advertising; however, based on definitions alone, it is easy to see that this would incur significant cost.

In addition to reach and frequency, advertisers must also consider the amount of waste, which refers to the people reached by a particular medium who do not belong to the intended target market. A magazine, for example, which counts family practitioners among its subscribers, as well as pediatricians, may have wasted coverage if the target is only pediatricians.

Most media advertising space is priced based upon the size and the purchasing power of the audience. The larger the audience of a radio station, the greater the charge to advertise on that particular station. Likewise, magazines that target an upscale audience, such as *Architectural Digest*, might charge more money for advertising than *Backpacker*.

Scheduling

After the organization determines the balance between reach and frequency, it must decide the timing for its messages. There are many variations by which an advertising campaign can deliver messages; the three most common are seasonal, steady, or flighting.

Seasonal. Some products and services have a seasonal pattern to their demand. For example, cold medicines have heavier demand in the winter months; a travel clinic might experience greater demand in the summer months. Advertising, therefore, is scheduled in heavier amounts at the onset of the peak demand period.

Steady. This schedule involves maintaining the same level of advertising exposure through the selected time period. Physician referral lines sponsored by hospitals often follow this scheduling pattern. On any given day, any number of people might need to avail themselves of this service. Maintaining a constant level of product or service awareness is necessary to reach each new consumer entering the adoption stage of the market.

Flighting. A common advertising schedule is called **flighting**, which involves a heavy amount of advertising for short time periods. Figure 11–4 shows three diagrams to represent flighting and two other alternative scheduling patterns that are discussed below. The flighting approach has distinct periods when there are a large number of exposures. The logic of this approach is that advertising will have sufficient carryover effect to maintain awareness when there is little or no advertising. The risk of losing product awareness is represented by the gaps before the next burst in expenditures.

An alternative scheduling strategy is **concentration**, in which a company spends its advertising dollars and achieves exposure within a defined, relatively short time period. Or, an organization can follow a **pulsing** approach, in which advertising expenditures occur at a constant level with occasional, short, heavy expenditures.[16]

Selecting the Most Cost-Effective Approach

In choosing which medium to use, advertisers select the most cost-efficient vehicle possible. Every advertiser wants to minimize the amount of wasted coverage. In calculating the most cost-efficient advertising medium, advertisers

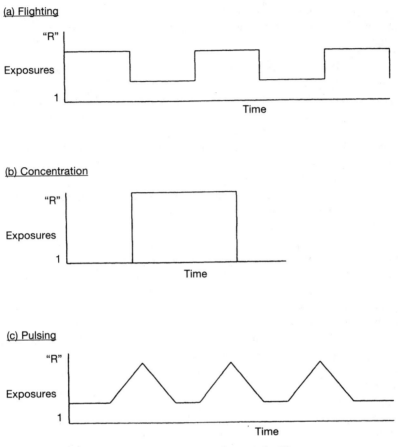

Note: "R" = Some finite level of exposures greater than one; 1 = First exposure

Figure 11–4 Variations in Media Scheduling Patterns

can select one of several formulas based upon the particular medium being considered. These formulas vary as a function of the medium selected.

Cost-Per-Thousand. A common frame of comparing the cost of advertising media is the **cost-per-thousand**, or CPM formula. This measures the cost of a medium to deliver an audience. The formula is:

$$CPM = \frac{\text{Cost of the Advertisement} \times 1,000}{\text{Circulation}}$$

Circulation is the number of people reached by the magazine or the newspaper. Using this formula, the advertiser can compare the cost of advertising in different magazines.

Cost-per-Point. In considering the cost of television advertising, advertisers use a different standard than the cost-per-thousand. The cost index in this medium is based on the audience which is delivered, or the rate. The rate is the program audience as a percent of the total television audience. In buying television advertising, however, advertisers schedule a package of advertisements across a number of different programs. The schedule is then determined in terms of its **gross rating points**, a measure of advertising reach calculated by multiplying the number of spots or ads times the rating.

Assume, for example, that Monday Night Football has a rating of 4.3 and the advertiser purchased 14 insertion spots during the season. The number of gross rating points would then be $14 \times 4.3 = 60.2$. The gross rating points are a measure of the reach times the frequency. The reach is reflected by the show's rating and the frequency by the number of insertions, or spots, purchased. This gross rating points system provides a common base that accounts for different sized markets. The same gross rating points in two markets of very different sizes cannot be considered equivalent.

In buying advertising, advertisers often use the cost per rating point to make comparisons. Yet, the following example shows the caution which must be taken with that approach. One point appears to cost more in New York City than in Salt Lake City, yet, a point in New York has far greater reach than a point in Salt Lake City.

Consider the data below, which show two very different settings:

	Households with Televisions	Average Cost per Spot	Average Prime Time Rating
New York City	7,800,000	$3,200	19
Salt Lake City	925,000	$2,600	17

Assume the advertiser buys five spots:

$$\text{Cost-per-Point (CPP)} = \frac{\text{Cost of Schedule}}{\text{Gross Rating Points}}$$

$$\text{In Salt Lake City: CPP} = \frac{\$13,000}{85} = \$152.95$$

$$\text{In New York City: CPP} = \frac{\$16,000}{95} = \$168.42$$

Ultimately, in any comparison of rating points or costs, the advertiser must consider that the audience being delivered by any medium is the target audience that the organization wants to attract.

Picking the Right Medium

Advertisers have a variety of media from which to choose to place their message. Each of these media has distinct characteristics that must be assessed in the final advertising plan.

Television. Of all media available, television has the advantage of communicating sight, sound, and motion. These components afford the potential advertiser significant flexibility in the creation of the advertising copy. Today, almost 98 percent of all homes in the United States have a television, providing the potential for enormous reach. Television's major disadvantage is its cost. Prime time spots can easily exceed $100,000. The production costs of television commercials also add significantly to the budget expense. Except for large national companies such as CIGNA, Prucare, or Blue Cross/Blue Shield, national advertising costs are not part of the average budget for most health care organizations.

In recent years, however, the advancement of local cable stations has made television advertising accessible and affordable for local advertisers such as hospitals or medical groups. The challenge of local market television advertising is in identifying the correct television station that will reach the desired target audience. As more households are wired for cable television, the number of station alternatives expands dramatically to 20, 40, or, in some markets, 80 channels, making vehicle selection all the more difficult for the local advertiser. Local television advertising is generally purchased by the part of the day rather than by a specific program. Because of this difference with national network advertising, local advertisers must again know the viewing habits of their target market by time of day.

Another disadvantage of television advertising is the degree of clutter or competing messages that exists. It is difficult for one advertisement to stand out when so many commercials are packaged within a station break.

Radio. There are 10 times as many radio stations as there are television stations in the United States. Since the mid 1970s, the radio's major growth has been on the FM rather than the AM band. A wide array of formats and programs make radio a highly segmented medium for potential advertisers. Also, on a cost basis, radio compares very favorably to television. The average cost-per-thousand for radio is $4.00. The cost of producing a radio commercial in local markets is often included in the rate charged to the advertiser.

The production of radio ads can usually be completed in a short time period, and St. Joseph's Hospital in Milwaukee has capitalized on this advantage. The hospital ran radio advertisements highlighting the birth of babies at its facility. The advertisements began with an announcer reporting the news of the day, followed by announcements of recent births at the hospital.[17] A final major advantage to this medium is that it reaches consumers out of their home. Peak listening times for radio are the morning and evening drive times.

Radio's major limitation is its lack of a visual means of communication. Also, because so many radio stations and varying formats are available, a potential advertiser has almost too many options. The advertiser must also accurately target the radio station that attracts its particular target audience.

Newspaper. Of all media available, newspapers receive the most advertising dollars. In health care, this medium has been the most popular, since the strength of newspapers is their coverage of local markets in which most health care organizations compete. Of all media, newspaper advertising is typically the best for generating immediate response. Coupons and special offers are common to newspapers. Newspapers are the medium of choice for physician referral lines or nurse information lines. Another advantage of newspapers are their cost. Newspaper rates are very reasonable compared to other mass media like television, making it the medium of choice for local advertisers. Although in recent years, with the advent of cable television, the rate advantage of newspapers has been somewhat negated.

The segmentation possibilities in local newspapers is relatively limited. In recent years, however, most large metropolitan newspapers have developed zone editions that target specific geographic areas within their circulation. *The New York Times,* for example, has a national edition sold in airport terminals throughout the United States. An additional advantage of newspapers is the short lead time required to place an advertisement. A hospital often will only need to wait a day or two before its advertisement can be run in the local newspaper.

Newspapers do have some disadvantages. Newspaper readership tends increasingly to be concentrated among older consumers. To overcome this problem, many local newspapers have followed the pattern of *USA TODAY*, using a glossy four-color approach and succinct writing to appeal to a younger, more visually oriented audience.

Magazines. Few media have grown as dramatically in recent years as magazines.[18] For the advertiser there is a vast array of specialized publications that allow an organization to target a specific market segment. Environmentally concerned consumers read *Garbage*, outdoor enthusiasts might peruse *Backpacker*, health-oriented consumers might subscribe to *Men's Health, Organic Gardening, Women's Health*, or a host of others. Within the magazine industry there is significant competition as varying publications compete for advertising dollars. And, like newspapers, many national publications have developed both zone and demographic editions targeted to particular subsets of their readership. All of these variations allow advertisers who know their target market to spend their advertising dollars efficiently.

Magazines have other advantages beyond the selectivity that they can deliver. Many publications have a long shelf life, meaning readers will keep them for weeks, months, or, in the case of the *National Geographic*, years. An advertisement in these publications may be read several times over the course of a publication's shelf life. An additional advantage of magazines is their excellent reproduction capabilities for advertisements. The quality of the printing and color separation in magazines far surpasses anything achieved to date by newspapers.

Like all other media, however, magazines have some disadvantages. The sheer number of magazines makes it more difficult to select the specific publication in which to advertise. Some publications also have a long lead time for the placement of an advertisement, often requiring delivery of ad copy four to six weeks prior to publication. Magazine advertisements thus must be used to support a longer running campaign rather than one needed to generate an immediate response.

Outdoor Advertising. Outdoor media consist of a couple of variations, namely billboards or transit. Because of space and time exposure limitations for these media, outdoor advertising is typically viewed as a supplemental medium to support exposures in other media. Outdoor advertising is useful for its reminder appeal or in the introduction stage of a service to generate brand name or service recognition. This medium has also been useful in generating calls to referral lines or health information lines.[19] According to the Outdoor Advertising Association of America, the health care industry is the fastest growing segment of its business.[20]

The major advantage of outdoor advertising is the repetition it can provide through broad exposure of the message. Yet, its limitations are significant in terms of the degree of selectivity and the message that can be communicated. As a medium, outdoor advertising has an image problem. There are community concerns that billboards, in particular, are a form of visual pollution. Some communities have placed constraints on the presence and size of billboards. Four states (Alaska, Hawaii, Maine, and Vermont) have banned all outdoor billboards. Fewer constraints have been placed on transit advertising. These ads are common in larger communities that have public transportation.

Direct Mail. Over the last 10 years there has been phenomenal growth in direct-mail advertising. Most U.S. households receive countless catalogs advertising clothes, sporting goods, novelty items, and even food. As the creation of customer databases becomes more sophisticated, advertisers use direct mail increasingly to target a particular market segment. This targeting ability is the major advantage of direct-mail advertising. Direct mail also serves as a direct response form for the customer. Toll-free phone lines or prepaid return forms encourage the consumer to reply to the organization. With increasing computer sophistication, many direct advertising pieces can make a highly personalized appeal to the recipient.

Critical to a successful direct-mail approach is having a good list of prospects. There are two approaches most companies can use. The first is to develop their own refined lists of customers or prospects. Increasingly, companies are paying attention to what is referred to as database marketing, the process of developing and updating information about prospective customers. In effective database marketing, companies develop detailed profiles of their target market and can refine the list or access names based on qualifying variables such as income, age, or prior purchasing of particular products. A second approach is to purchase a list from a commercial list broker who can provide a customer database based on several classifications.

In a recent hospital survey, the prevalence of direct marketing efforts was clear. Almost 90 percent of hospitals surveyed indicated that their direct marketing budgets had increased. In citing their reasons for using this medium, hospitals reported four common objectives:

1. To increase hospital awareness,
2. To generate leads for current programs,
3. To promote special events, and
4. To enhance a facility's image.[21]

Direct mail's limitations are its image and cost. Many consumers regard direct mail as junk mail. As consumers are increasingly deluged with a large amount of such material on a daily basis, getting one piece to stand out from the competition is difficult. Direct mail's cost must also be considered as its level of sophistication increases. Historically, the major cost of direct mail was postage. While this factor continues to be a concern as rates increase, production costs must also be factored into the cost equation. To attract attention, direct-mail marketers have significantly increased the use of color, paper quality, and repetition to gain attention, all of which add greatly to total cost.

Evaluate the Response

Testing of advertising effectiveness occurs at two stages. As discussed earlier, the first form of evaluation, known as pretesting, ensures that the target audience receives the message in the way it is intended. Pretesting also determines preference and attention-getting value.

After selecting the media and placing advertisements, most organizations also conduct posttesting to determine the effects of their campaign. Testing formats vary, depending on the media used for advertising.

Regardless of the medium, however, attitude tests are used for posttesting. Companies often assess whether the advertising campaign has resulted in a large change in attitudes toward the product or service being promoted.[22]

Broadcast

A common form of posttesting for television or radio is day-after recall. Typically, after a commercial is aired on television or radio, the advertiser conducts telephone surveys to determine whether people remember the advertisement. Recall can be either aided or unaided. In unaided recall, the telephone interviewer might ask, "Have you seen any advertisements on television for a women's health program?" The recall of the particular hospital's program could then be assessed. In aided recall, the interviewer would ask, "Have you seen any ads lately for St. Mary's Women's Health Center?"

Print

In the magazine industry, posttest scores are often collected through a syndicated data service referred to as Starch. The Starch company conducts personal reader interviews to determine the number of people who read a particular issue and whether they read the ad, the signature, or whether they read most of the advertisement. Starch provides companies with scores for the advertisements for the issues in which they were placed.

Direct Mail

The advantage of direct-mail advertising is that customer response can be directly measured through follow-up inquiries or purchase orders. This direct form of measurement has led to the medium's growing appeal.

WORKING WITH ADVERTISING AGENCIES

Many hospitals and health care organizations do not have the in-house resources needed to develop their own advertising materials. Those that do not can hire the services of an advertising agency. Advertising agencies vary in size and in the scope of the functions that they perform. A health care organization must identify the types of services needed to select the appropriate agency.

Alternative Advertising Agencies

Full Service Agency

The most comprehensive advertising agency, the **full service agency**, provides all the elements necessary to assume the total advertising function. These organizations typically offer sales promotion, public relations, direct marketing, consulting on design and identification, and even television programming.

The full service agency typically has several departments organized around creative services, account services, marketing, and administrative services. The creative department is responsible for producing all the advertising design and copy. Account services deals with the client—the health care organization. This professional has to understand the health care business and how to translate the client's goals and objectives to the creative department. The purchasing of media space and time is the responsibility of the marketing services department. Full service agencies often have marketing research functions residing within this area. The administration and finance department handles billing and agency management.

Boutique Agency

Opposite of the full service agencies are the boutique, or specialized, firms. A **boutique agency** may offer a limited range of services, such as creative services or media buying services; or will act as a contractor to put together the range of services needed by the organization.

Agency Compensation

Advertising agencies are compensated in one of two ways: fees and commissions. Agencies paid by commission are, in effect, being paid by the media. In commission compensation, the agency places $200,000 of advertising in selected publications and in television. The agency keeps 15 percent of this billed amount as standard compensation. The media then provides $200,000 worth of advertising space. Although the client is paying the agency, the media is, in effect, subsidizing the commission by providing the full amount of media space or time.

A major buyers' concern about the commission system is that it provides agencies with an incentive to recommend more advertising than is necessary. Agencies have also felt that the commission-based compensation system may not be providing them with a fair return for the work they provide to a client. As a result, in recent years commissions have declined and some agencies have moved to a fee-based structure.[23] The fee is agreed upon by the agency and the client and is based upon the amount, type, and scope of work being provided.

ETHICS IN ADVERTISING

Few aspects of marketing were of greater concern to health care professionals than the onset of advertising. Because of the sensitive nature of health care and the often precarious position of the health care buyer, there is heightened sensitivity to the use of this tool. The Alliance for Health Care Strategy and Marketing, in Chicago, Illinois, is the largest national association of professionals involved in health care marketing. This organization has developed a set of voluntary guidelines regarding the concerns and issues that should be considered in health care advertising, shown in Exhibit 11–2.

Exhibit 11–2 Health Care Advertising Guidelines

- Advertising should state and imply only documentable, normally expected outcomes.
- Advertising related to clinical outcomes should use the actual words and images of actual patients who have experienced the procedure or treatment being promoted.
- Advertising should place the good of the patient above other interests—especially a provider's economic interest, prestige, or image building.
- Advertising of health care services, including physician referral services, should acknowledge criteria used in identifying the list of service providers.

Source: Reprinted from *Ethical Guidelines for Healthcare Advertising*, with permission of the Alliance for Health Care Strategy and Marketing, © 1993.

Nonprofit Concerns

One final aspect of health care advertising warranting attention is the matter of an organization's nonprofit designation. Federal, state, and local government agencies have examined whether advertising by these organizations is excessive. Twenty of Pennsylvania's 224 nonprofit hospitals were required to provide services in place of property taxes to various taxing agencies after being judged as acting more like for-profit organizations in light of their advertising expenditures.[24]

CONCLUSIONS

Advertising is an important ingredient of any health care organization's promotional strategy. Developing an effective media plan begins with a specification of its objectives. From this foundation, a budget and appropriate tactics for media selection and scheduling can be determined. Any effective advertising requires that there be a mechanism both to pretest and posttest the campaign. Because of the serious nature of health care and the vulnerabilities of consumers engaged in the selection of health care services, significant attention is due to the ethical dimensions of the advertising strategy ultimately implemented.

KEY TERMS

Media Plan	Frequency
Target Audience	Flighting
Hierarchy of Effects	Concentration
Objective and Task	Pulsing
Pretesting	Cost-Per-Thousand
Medium	Gross Rating Points
Vehicle	Full Service Agency
Reach	Boutique Agency

CHAPTER SUMMARY

1. Advertising can take one of several forms: It can be product-based or institution-based.

2. The basis for an advertising campaign is the media plan, which is built on the definition of the target audience.

3. Advertising objectives are based on the hierarchy of effects model. A well-written objective is measurable, time-bound, and targeted to a well-specified audience.

4. Advertising budgets are often derived on a percentage of sales, competitive parity, or "all-that-can-be-afforded" basis. The most effective basis for determining the budget is an objective and task method.

5. The creation of effective advertising copy requires pretesting of the message with a sample similar to the target audience.

6. In selecting the media for use in an advertising campaign, an organization often must make trade-offs between reach and frequency.

7. There are several patterns by which advertising exposures can be scheduled: steady, seasonal, or flighting.

8. Advertising media must be selected to minimize wasted coverage. Media choices can be compared on a cost-per-thousand or cost-per-point basis.

9. Cable television has greatly reduced the cost of television advertising, while technological advances have affected both print and direct mail. Environmental constraints limit outdoor advertising.

10. Advertising agencies differ in the structure, fee, and range of services provided. In recent years, there has been a trend away from commission payment to a fee payment system.

CHAPTER PROBLEMS

1. Outline the advertising copy an HMO would use in advertisements that are: (a) competitive, product-based, (b) pioneering institutional, and (c) reminder institutional.

2. Write an awareness objective for a newly formed adolescent chemical dependency program whose target market consists of judges and social workers who refer to the facility. How would this objective change for the trial level of the hierarchy of effects?

3. As the newly hired hospital marketing director, you have your first meeting with the administrator. "Okay," he says, "We need to advertise our physical rehabilitation program. I'll give you a couple of days to tell me how much you'd like to spend. Is $5,000 enough? I think we can afford a little more if you need it. And, based on what I've seen in the newspapers, St. Mary's seems to be spending a little less than that. Give me your thoughts in two days." Two days are up.

4. Recently, the physician marketing task force at State University Medical Center developed a physician referral directory and advertisement. The target was primary care physicians in the region who could refer patients to State University for tertiary care. A cardiologist who was an undergraduate English major chaired the committee and drafted the materials. Three months after distribution of the advertisement and directory, responses were disappointing. Explain how this process could have been improved to increase likely response.

5. The director of a cardiac rehabilitation program was recently approached by a sales representative from the community newspaper selling advertising space. The sales representative underscored the fact that the paper had the largest circulation of any of the three papers serving the area, and it had the lowest cost-per-thousand. Before deciding to use this medium, what other factors should the program director consider? 3 1 9

6. Robbinsdale Hospital is the only one of two hospitals among the six in the city to have an intensive care (Level III) nursery. This facility is tailored to treat infants suffering from severe medical complications upon delivery. The program director is deciding whether to use an emotional or rational appeal in advertising copy. What are the considerations in this decision?

NOTES

1. R.E. Hite, J.A. Bellizzi, and D.M. Andrus, Differences between Consumers and Psychiatrists in Attitude toward Advertising of Psychiatric Services, *Journal of Health Care Marketing* 8, no. 4 (1988):21–28; ___, Consumer Versus Dentist Attitudes Toward Dental Services, *Journal of Health Care Marketing* 8, no. 1 (1988):30–38.

2. C.M. Fisher and C.J. Anderson, Hospital Advertising: Does It Influence Consumers? *Journal of Health Care Marketing* 10, no. 4 (1990):40–46.

3. W.L. Wilkie and P.W. Farris, Comparison Advertising: Problems and Potentials, *Journal of Marketing* 39, no. 4 (1975):7–15.

4. R.J. Lavidge and G.A. Steiner, A Model of Predictive Measurements of Advertising Effectiveness, *Journal of Marketing* 25, no. 2 (1961):59–62. See also, C.L. Bovee and W.F. Arens, *Contemporary Advertising*, 3rd ed. (Homewood, Ill.: Richard D. Irwin, Inc., 1989), 228–233.

5. Attention to Detail Pays Off, *Profiles in Healthcare Marketing*, no. 60 (1994):50–51, 54.

6. Finding New Families on the Block, *Profiles in Healthcare Marketing*, no. 52 (1993):8–10.

7. C.H. Patti and V. Blanko, Budgeting Practices of Big Advertisers, *Journal of Advertising Research* 21, no. 6 (1981):23–30.

8. E.J. McCarthy, How Much Should Hospitals Spend on Advertising?, *Health Care Management Review* 12, no. 1 (1987):47–54.

9. J.A. Schroer, Ad Spending: Growing Market Share, *Harvard Business Review* 68, no. 1 (1990): 44–48.

10. D. Seligman, How Much for Advertising?, *Fortune* 54, no. 12 (1956):123–126.

11. J.E. Lynch and G.J. Hooley, Increasing Sophistication in Advertising Budget Setting, *Journal of Advertising Research* 30, no. 1 (1990):67–75.

12. K. Deveny, Marketers Exploit People's Fears of Everything, *The Wall Street Journal*, 15 November 1993, B1,B6.

13. Ethical Guidelines for Healthcare Advertising (Position paper, Academy for Health Services Marketing, Chicago, Ill., February 23, 1993), 6.

14. M.S. LaTour and R.E. Pitts, Using Fear Appeals for AIDS Prevention in the College Age Population, *Journal of Healthcare Marketing* 9, no. 3 (1989):5–14.

15. B. Edelman-Lewis and G.W. Thomas, The Development and Evaluation of a Multimedia Advertising Campaign, in *Marketing Is Everybody's Business*, ed. P. Sanchez (Chicago, Ill.: Alliance for Health Care Strategy and Marketing, 1988), 89–97.

16. P. Kotler, *Marketing Management*, 8th ed. (Englewood Cliffs, N.J.: Prentice-Hall, 1994), 646.

17. K. Haley, The Birth of Fast Ads in Milwaukee, *Healthcare Marketing Report* 12, no. 9 (1994):10–11.

18. S. Pomper, The Big Shake Out Begins, *TIME* 136, no. 1 (1990): 50.

19. L. Gintz Jasper and E. Lueders Terwilliger, Advertising's Impact on Calls to a Women's Hotline, *Journal of Healthcare Marketing* 9, no. 3 (1989):62–66.

20. Madison Avenue and Managed Care, *Managed Healthcare* 14, no. 9 (1994): 37.

21. J.W. Peltier, A.K. Kleimenhagen, and G.M. Naidu, Taking the Direct Route, *Journal of Health Care Marketing* 14, no. 3 (Fall 1994):22–27.

22. D.A. Aaker and D.M. Stayman, Measuring Audience Perceptions of Commercials and Relating Them to Ad Impact, *Journal of Advertising Research* 30, no. 4 (1990):7–17.

23. Kotler, *Marketing Management*, 628.

24. J. Burns, Hospitals Made To Justify Marketing's Worth, *Modern Healthcare* 23, no. 44 (1993):52.

_12_

SALES

LEARNING OBJECTIVES

After reading this chapter you should be able to:

- Understand the range of alternative sales positions

- Know the sequence of the personal sales process

- Differentiate between alternative sales processes

- Recognize the elements in the management of a sales force

An integral part of the promotional mix is personal selling. Historically, personal selling involved direct, face-to-face communication between the buyer and the seller. In our age of advancing technology, personal selling now occurs via telephone, video conferencing, and computer networks.

In the health care industry personal sales often had a somewhat negative connotation. The image of the salesperson was either that of the loud huckster on television or the medical detail representative rarely recognized for providing real value to the product. While few would dispute that the first image is less than desirable, the medical detail representative is an integral part of effective marketing strategy at a pharmaceutical company. This type of sales position represents just one of many variations of the sales functions that exist.

Personal sales representatives perform more than just the selling role. Personal sales jobs are multifaceted. An effective sales representative will be engaged not only in selling, but will also conduct important relationship-building activities with customers. Salespeople also serve as a source of ongoing market research information as they call upon their accounts. It is often the salesperson who first learns from physicians that a new PPO plan is being developed or that a competing hospital is establishing a physician-hospital organization. Health care organizations are wise to embrace this broader view of the sales function when developing a marketing program to maximize this component of the promotional mix.

TYPES OF SALES JOBS

There are many variations to the sales job, several of which have particular relevance in health care settings.[1]

New Business Selling

When most individuals think of sales they consider only this type of situation. This sales job requires a salesperson to go out and make calls to seek new business. The salesperson's primary responsibility is to identify, contact, and sell new accounts. New account selling is the most difficult aspect of sales, yet is becoming increasingly important in health care as the industry shifts to a managed care environment. University MEDNET, one of Ohio's largest multispecialty groups in Cleveland, has a sales force to handle contracting with employers and with third-party payers.[2]

Trade Selling

A second variation of the sales job is trade selling, which focuses sales efforts on the intermediaries in the channel of distribution. Trade selling's goal is to gain intermediaries' support for the company's products. This sales function is common to many consumer food product companies whose sales forces make regular calls on their wholesalers and retailers. In health care, this aspect of sales has often been found in tertiary hospitals and academic medical centers. Sales representatives call on referral physicians to attract more business and to reinforce the existing referral base.

Missionary Selling

A major aspect of many sales jobs is the missionary task, in which the primary goal is to maintain business from existing customers. Hospitals with established physician relation departments have been performing this missionary task. Gundersen/Lutheran Medical Center in LaCrosse, Wisconsin has a three-person staff that call upon referral physicians on a regular basis in order to maintain a positive relationship for referrals.[3]

Technical Selling

Another type of sales job is the technical representative. This sales person generates volume by providing technical expertise and support to potential customers. A sales representative for an occupational medicine program often conducts this type of sales activity. This representative might analyze a company's workers' compensation claims and develop a package of occupational medicine services to help reduce these claims.

These descriptions all underscore the point that sales involve more than just selling to a prospect. Maintaining relationships, servicing customers, reinforcing experiences, monitoring service performance, and selling are all part of most sales jobs. The medical detail representative provides clients with information and often asks questions as an early part of the market research process. Most medical detail representatives do little actual selling. Rather, the bulk of their efforts focuses on the missionary aspects of their jobs. The historical attitude that personal selling is wrong for health care reflects a naivety about the scope of sales functions that exist.

THE PERSONAL SALES PROCESS

Personal selling involves several steps beyond just getting the customer to agree to the sale. Figure 12–1 shows the six steps in the sales process. Each step in this figure shows the sales process as it pertains to an HMO sales representative selling this plan to a company.

Prospecting

Prospecting is the step in which the salesperson targets likely buyers, or **leads**, for sales calls. This is a difficult part of the sales process because it usually involves making **cold calls** by telephone or in person.[4] Cold calls are contacts with prospective buyers who did not initiate the process. For example, HMO sales-people make calls on large companies located in the HMO's business area. Doctors' Hospital in Columbus, Ohio uses a nonclinician to generate the vast majority of the leads for its occupational health program.[5] As expected, cold calls can yield many rejections before turning up an interested party.

In this stage, the salesperson identifies **qualified prospects**, individuals who have a need for the product or service or are likely to buy. In generating leads of

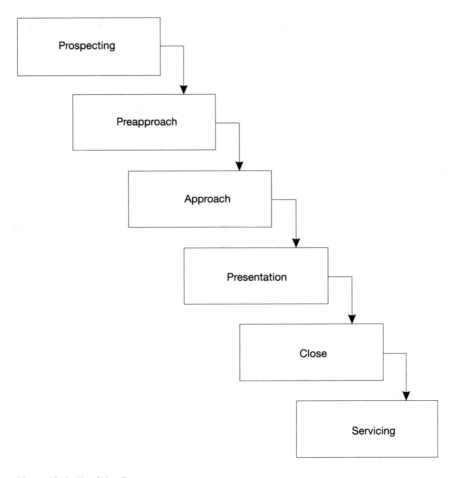

Figure 12–1 The Sales Process

qualified buyers, companies use several sources, one of the most effective of which is personal references. For example, one physician might recommend that a salesperson call another doctor who also might be interested in new diagnostic equipment. A reference from a knowledgeable source regarding another prospect reduces the salesperson's need to qualify the prospect. Advertising is often another source used to generate leads. For example, a hospital might advertise its industrial medicine program, and include in the ad copy a toll-free phone number for consumers to call for further information. A salesperson would receive the names of all callers and target these individuals as prospects.

At the prospecting stage, the salesperson tries to answer three key questions in qualifying the prospect:

1. Does the prospect have a need for my product or service?
2. Can I make the people responsible for buying so aware of that need that I can make the sale?
3. Will the sale be profitable to my company?[6]

Preapproach

The second step in the sales process is the preapproach. This is an information-gathering step in which the salesperson learns more about the customer and the customer's requirements. The more decision makers involved in buying the product, the longer and more complicated will be the preapproach stage. A corporation picking a health care plan for its employees might use a committee comprised of the chief financial officer, the human resources director, and an employee representative to make this decision. Each committee member might have very different concerns regarding the selection of the health care plan. The salesperson's goal in the preapproach stage is to identify the issues for the buyer or buyers and to learn about the prospect's needs. Effective salespeople try to acquire as much information at this stage from secondary sources. The more knowledgeable the salesperson is about the prospect, the greater credibility he or she will have when trying to make the sale.

Approach

The **approach** stage of the sales process involves the initial meeting with the buyer. At this point, the HMO's sales representative tries to generate interest in the plan's offering and address the buyer's concerns and questions. This stage involves establishing trust and credibility with the buyer.

Presentation

The *presentation* stage is when the salesperson makes the pitch for the product or service. This step is where the actual selling effort occurs. The presentation is more difficult in service businesses than in product businesses. Usually, the best way to make a presentation is to demonstrate the product; however, this is difficult to do for a health care program.

In the presentation stage, the salesperson must become adept at handling buyer objections. Objections often take one of several forms. Timing objections are when the buyer delays the decision to purchase. The salesperson needs to identify the reasons for the delay and highlight the benefits the company could realize by immediate use of the HMO plan. A second common objection involves price. At this point, the salesperson must underscore the program's values and benefits relative to the price. Competitive objections are a third common form, when the buyer expresses satisfaction or loyalty to the health care provider presently under contract. It is essential for the salesperson to be familiar with competitive plans to focus the sales presentation on the differential advantages of the particular service being presented.

Another type of objection is called the logical objection, which is when buyers perceive a difference between their needs and the solution offered by the salesperson. These objections are usually focused on price, service characteristics, the salesperson's organization, or the firm's past experience. In most cases, such objections are negative. The salesperson must reestablish a positive set of objectives by getting the prospect to clarify the objection. A last set of objections are psychological, which have no real logical basis. These objections often are based on the prospect's desire not to change existing habits or on the prospect's dislike of the sales process. The salesperson needs to minimize the degree of change. Citing testimonials from other new customers often can help reinforce the satisfaction others have felt since buying the service.

Within the presentation stage, a salesperson must learn how to counter any and all such objections. Several basic methods have been proposed for handling buyer objections.[7] These are:

1. Agree and counter: The salesperson agrees with the customer's concerns and then offers support for his or her own position.
2. List advantages and disadvantages: The sales representative specifically counters each negative with a positive perspective.
3. Positive conversion: The customer's objection is turned into the reason why the customer should buy the product. For example, the customer says, "We can't afford to change health care plans now." The salesperson responds, "Because of the real savings you are going to achieve, you cannot afford to stay with your existing plan."

The essential component of each method is that a well-trained salesperson must be able to diagnose the source of the objection. The sales representative must be adept at using one or more methods to counter the objection and move the prospect to the next stage of the sales process.

Close

The **close** is the stage of the sales process that involves asking the buyer for a commitment to purchase. All other steps of the sales process are irrelevant if the salesperson does not proceed to the close. Occasionally, a salesperson will use a *trial close* in which the salesperson asks the buyer for an opinion regarding the proposal. In this way, the salesperson can assess the buyer's readiness to decide without moving too quickly.

An alternative approach to closing is known as the *assumptive close,* which involves asking the buyer to chose payment terms, delivery location, or the like, before there has been an actual agreement to purchase.

Servicing

The last step in the sales process—servicing—is often ignored by salespeople. This involves providing the buyer with post-sales follow-up and support. Table 12–1 shows the differing views of what a sale means to a buyer and a seller. From the buyer's perspective closing the sale is not the end of the process, but the beginning of a relationship. In order to maintain repeat business, post-sales service and follow-up is essential.

SALES APPROACHES

There are several different approaches that are actually used in selling. Four common methods are the stimulus-response approach, the selling formula, the need satisfaction method, and consultative selling.

Table 12–1 Two Perspectives of a Sales Interaction

The Seller's View	The Buyer's View
Culmination of a long sales negotiation	Initiation of a new relationship
Closure opens the way to cultivating new potential clients	Concern about the support a new vendor will provide
Shift account from sales team to production team	How much attention and help will be received after the purchase decision
	Desire to continue to interact with the sales team

Source: Reprinted from *Aftermarketing* by T.G. Vaura, p.15, with permission of Business One Irwin, © 1992.

Stimulus-Response Sales Approach

The **stimulus-response sales approach** to sales presentations is based on psychological research conducted by Pavlov. As most introductory psychology students can recall, these experiments demonstrated that dogs who were given a stimulus (food) would yield a response (salivation). If the food was offered at the same time a bell was rung, the dog would begin to associate the bell with the food. And, if the bell alone was provided, the response of salivation would still occur even in the absence of food.[8] In effect, then, the bell became a substitute stimulus.

These experiments form the foundation of a sales approach in which the salesperson usually follows a canned presentation. A *canned presentation* is a set script through which the salesperson leads the prospect.[9] Following the stimulus-response method, then, the salesperson inserts questions within the presentation to encourage a particular response from the client.

For example, an HMO representative may follow a script such as the following:

Salesperson: Health care coverage is important to you and your family, isn't it?

Prospect: Yes.

Salesperson: You wouldn't want your family not to have comprehensive coverage, would you?

Prospect: No.

Salesperson: Don't you think you should sign up for ABC HMO?

Prospect: Yes, you're right.

In reading this abbreviated version of a canned presentation, it is easy to discern that the salesperson dominates most of the discussion. The advantage of this approach is that it ensures that the salesperson will convey the intended corporate message. Sales training is relatively simple following a canned sales presentation. With practice, a canned sales presentation can be delivered relatively smoothly. The problems of this approach, however, are evident even in the abbreviated presentation. It does not require or encourage significant prospect involvement. It is not oriented to the prospect's concerns or specific issues. It also assumes that each prospect will react in the same way to a particular set of stimuli or questions. As a result, this type of presentation is best suited for low-priced products where the decision issues are relatively simple and similar. Selling products door-to-door, such as magazine subscriptions, is an example of a commonly used version of the stimulus-response approach.

The Selling Formula

The selling formula approach assumes that before customers agree to buy a product, they go through a series of steps. Figure 12–2 shows the formula for these steps, often referred to as "AIDA," which stands for attention, interest, desire, and action. The last step—action—is when the prospect agrees to buy. A trained sales professional recognizes the preconditions represented by these other steps and develops the potential customer's attention, interest, and desire in the service.

The AIDA approach's advantage is that the customer plays a more active part in the sales process. To gain customer interest and desire, the salesperson must engage the customer in conversation to assess how the product might match the customer's needs. Unlike the canned presentation, the salesperson has greater flexibility to direct more effort to the buyer's stage in the sales process. The challenge of this approach is that it does require a highly skilled sales-person. Buyers do not necessarily move through each stage in distinct or timely fashion.

Need Satisfaction Method

This third sales method may well be the most marketing oriented. This approach focuses on identifying the customer's needs.[10] There are three stages of this sales method: need development, need awareness, and need fulfillment. In the first stage, the salesperson tries to identify the problems the customer is trying to solve.

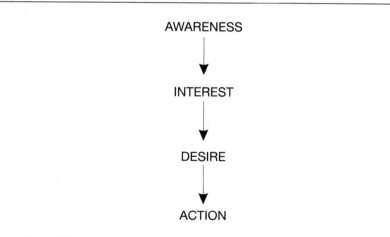

Figure 12–2 AIDA

A hospital sales representative might ask a corporate health benefits officer questions such as:

1. What are the most common reasons why workers' compensation claims are filed at your company?
2. Is there one division of the company where employees suffer more on-the-job injuries than they do in others?
3. Are there particular aspects of your company's business that workers have had physical difficulties accomplishing?

At the second stage of need awareness, the salesperson must ensure that the customer recognizes the same needs as the salesperson. For example, after assessing a company's needs, the salesperson might say something, such as:

> It appears that most employee injuries are back-related, but these injuries don't occur on the loading dock. It seems from the data I've gathered and from the supervisors with whom I've met, that workers on the production line are suffering the greatest number of back injuries. These problems may not be due to lifting but rather to the ergonomics of their work stations.

At this stage, the salesperson will begin to highlight solutions available for resolving the customer's problems.

The last stage of this sales approach is need fulfillment. The salesperson now demonstrates how his company can meet the customer's needs. The presentation is customized to the customer's needs rather than to what the selling organization wants to highlight. If ergonomic solutions are needed, talking about the industrial medicine toxicology components will not be helpful and may confuse the presentation.

Of the three sales approaches discussed so far, the needs satisfaction approach is the most customer-oriented and flexible. It requires a well-trained, sophisticated sales professional. The customer is an active participant in the sales process, but the salesperson must know how to engage the customer in the process and acquire the information necessary to ensure a match between the service being sold and the customer's needs.

Consultative Selling

This fourth sales approach focuses on problem identification. In this type of a sales strategy, the salesperson serves more as a consultant with a defined area of expertise.[11] A computer systems representative, for example, develops a proposal describing how a company can network its offices and explaining the potential values of such a network. Within the proposal, the sales representative provides a detailed specification list of the hardware requirements, as well as the necessary support services. Consultative selling will likely be used with greater frequency in health care as more organizations establish integrated delivery systems. For these organizations, a sales representative or consultant can analyze a business's specific health needs and tailor a package of services to meet the unique requirements of each customer.

MANAGING THE SALES FUNCTION

A health care institution just establishing a sales force must address many dimensions and concerns inherent in sales management including sales force organization, sales force size, recruitment and selection, training, compensation, and sales force evaluation and control.

Sales Force Organization

There are several ways a sales force can be structured. These variations include geographic, product, or customer organization.

Geographic Organization

This structure is the simplest way to organize a sales force. National companies can divide their sales forces by region, state, or even areas within states. The major advantage of this method is that it reduces the travel time and cost of sales personnel. And, within each sales territory only one company sales representative calls on customers.

The major disadvantage of this sales force organization is that salespeople must have a broad knowledge about all of the company's products and services. No sales specialization can be offered in this type of a structure. Sales representatives must also develop an ability to deal with a wide range of customers within their sales territory. Previously, this method had little applicability in health care. Most health care providers competed in relatively constrained geographical markets. Now, however, as more regional health care provider networks are being formed, geographic sales force structures might become more common.

Product Organization

Figure 12–3 shows a product organization structure for an integrated delivery system. In this design, there is a separate sales force for the Visiting Nurse

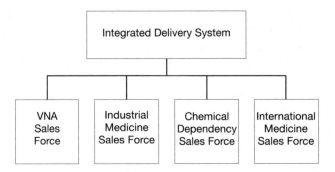

Figure 12–3 Product Organization Sales Structure

Association (VNA) and separate sales forces for several clinical programs. Compared to the previous method, the primary benefit is that of product specialization. Since many of the clinical services require detailed technical or clinical knowledge, this structure allows the salesperson to develop the needed expertise in a particular field.

The disadvantages of this design can be readily appreciated. One customer could receive multiple calls by sales representatives from the same organization. Not only can this lead to potential ill will among customers, but it also results in duplication of sales efforts, which could increase sales costs.

Customer Organization

The third method of sales force structure is customer organization. As shown in Figure 12–4, this health care system has organized its sales force around its major customers: referral physicians, third-party payers, employers, and long-term care

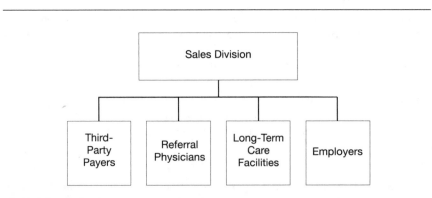

Figure 12–4 Customer Sales Force Organization

facilities. The major advantage of this structure is that the sales force can develop an expertise regarding customer requirements and concerns. Also, only one sales representative from the organization is assigned to call on a particular customer.

The major disadvantage to this sales force organization is that it requires the sales force to have a broad understanding of the product and service mix of the health system. A company can compensate for this by having a sales team make a presentation to a customer when specific technical knowledge is required. This sales structure seems to be the most appropriate way for health care organizations to serve their diverse customer bases.

Sales Force Size

The most common method for determining the appropriate size of the sales force is called the **workload method**.[12] To use this method, management needs to estimate the work effort required to service the market. It does this by calculating the number of accounts to be called upon, the frequency with which each account is to be called, and the length of each sales call. To implement the workload method typically requires six steps.

The first step in the process requires that the organization classify its customers into sales volume categories. For example, a tertiary hospital might target the referral physician market and classify referrers as follows:

> Class A physicians—heavy referrers: 550 doctors
> Class B physicians—medium referrers: 700 doctors
> Class C physicians—light/nonreferrers: 850 doctors

The second step requires a company to establish a call frequency for each class of account and the amount of time for each sales call. A hospital might decide that the heavy referral doctor offices should be called upon six times per year. Class B physicians' offices should receive four calls per year. Doctors who are categorized as Class C will receive two calls per year. For the Class A accounts, the sales calls might involve significant missionary work with the office and nursing staff, so these calls require 30 minutes. Classes B and C typically will require 15 minutes per call. With these call frequencies and call requirements established, each account class will require the following effort per year:

> Class A—6 calls/year x 30 minutes per call = 3 hours
> Class B—4 calls/year x 15 minutes per call = 1 hour
> Class C—2 calls/year x 15 minutes per call = 1/2 hour

The third step involves determining the work required to cover the entire market.

Class A—550 accounts x 3 hours/account = 1,650 hours
Class B—700 accounts x 1 hour/account   =   700 hours
Class C—850 accounts x 1/2 hour/account =   425 hours
                                             2,775 hours

The fourth step is to determine the time available for each sales person. A company must estimate the number of hours per week and the number of weeks per year that the salesperson works. Assume that the typical salesperson, working a 40-hour week, has 36 hours of effective selling time, which accounts for lunches and breaks. The salesperson might work a 48-week year:

$$36 \text{ hours} \times 48 \text{ weeks} = 1,728 \text{ hours}$$

The fifth step is to determine the amount of time the salesperson spends in selling. As noted earlier, not all of a sales representative's time involves productive selling or account contact time. Some portion of the day is spent traveling or is involved in nonselling activities such as report completion, telephoning, and following up on problems.

Selling/account contact   60% = 1,036 hr/yr
Traveling   20% =   346 hr/yr
Nonsales activities   20% =   346 hr/yr
                                   1,728 hr/yr

The sixth and final step involves calculating the number of salespeople needed. This is determined by dividing the number of hours needed to cover the accounts by the number of hours that is available for selling or account contact.

$$\frac{2,775 \text{ hours}}{1,036 \text{ hr/yr}} = 2.7 \text{ salespersons}$$

This number indicates that approximately three salespeople would be needed to cover the accounts for this medical center.

The workload method is one of the most common ways to determine sales force size. Its advantage is the relative ease at which estimates of size can be made. The disadvantage is that it does not account for differences in response by accounts if given varying levels of sales effort. Nor does it recognize that certain accounts within classes may still require higher levels of contact in order to maintain the existing relationships. The method also assumes that the cost of treating each account is identical, and that all salespeople use their time with the same level of efficiency. There are other methods for sales force size determination that go beyond the scope of this text. Suffice it to say that these methods all require a sophisticated level of knowledge about customer response and the costs of accounts.

Recruitment and Selection

The effectiveness of any sales force ultimately is related to the quality of the individual recruited for a sales position. It is essential that the right person be matched with the position's job requirements.

The first step in identifying the type of individual to be recruited is an analysis of the sales job. This analysis must review the activities and tasks to be performed and their relative importance. From this perspective, a company can determine what traits are helpful in choosing the type of candidate to be recruited. Often it is valuable to analyze the characteristics of the existing sales force and those persons who either left their positions or were terminated for unsatisfactory performance. Studies have been unable to demonstrate that specific personality traits are useful predictors of successful salespeople,[13] although there is some evidence that the following indicators have been found frequently among salespeople who fail. These are:

1. instability of residence
2. failure in business within the last two years
3. unexplained gaps in the person's employment record
4. excessive personal indebtedness.[14]

Recruitment

After a firm analyzes the types of sales skills needed for its sales positions, the next step involves recruiting qualified personnel. There are a variety of sources for finding qualified candidates, including educational institutions, other companies in the industry, professional associations, other departments within the company, and staff recommendations. Most universities, for example, have extensive placement services, and professional associations such as the Alliance for Health Care Strategy and Marketing have newsletters that frequently list job placement opportunities at various health care organizations. Depending on the level of the position being staffed, professional recruiting firms and employment agencies can be hired to match qualified applicants with the position.

Selection

Once a reasonable number of applicants is generated, an organization must have a strategy in place to select the best job candidate. Typically, selection involves several steps, as shown in Figure 12–5. These include preliminary screening, personal history form, in-depth personal interview, testing, and background investigation.

The preliminary screening interview serves as a way to eliminate the most unqualified applicants. These interviews normally are conducted by a member of

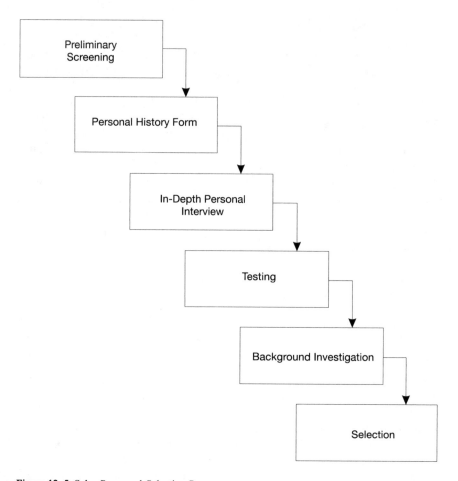

Figure 12–5 Sales Personnel Selection Process

the human resources staff. The second step in the process is the personal history form. This form typically is more detailed than the initial application. Information collected on this form should relate only to the performance of the position being sought. Questions regarding race, sex, religion, age, and national origin are considered illegal discriminatory acts under federal equal opportunity guidelines.

A third step is the in-depth personal interview. This interview usually is conducted by the individual who will supervise the salesperson. In addition to obtaining insight into the candidate's background, the interview allows for judgments to be made about the candidate's communication style, personality, and mental abilities. Firms tend to use one of three interview methods. One method is the **structured interview**, which follows a set list of questions. The advantage of this approach is that it allows all candidates to be compared on the same dimensions. Its weakness is that the manager often cannot deviate from the list without compromising the interview process. As a result, many organizations have switched to **unstructured interviews**. In this interview format, the applicant is encouraged to talk freely on a range of subjects. The interviewer acts almost like a focus group moderator (as discussed in Chapter 5), asking a few probing questions. Similar to focus groups, unstructured interviews require a well-trained interviewer. The third variation of the interview process is a **stress interview**. The interviewer places the applicant under stress using role playing exercises such as handling multiple customer objections or a rude customer. The goal is to assess how the candidate will behave under actual on-the-job conditions.

Candidates who succeed in the screening and interview stages often may be required to take tests. Tests can include any of three forms: intelligence, aptitude, or personality tests. Because of concerns regarding discrimination, the Federal Equal Employment Opportunity Commission requires that tests used for selection be validated by focusing strictly on the job requirements and on tasks related to successful performance of the position.

Intelligence tests measure an individual's mental abilities to reason or to learn. Aptitude tests are designed to test a person's ability to learn to perform certain tasks or job requirements. One well-known aptitude test is the Strong Vocational Interest test, which asks candidates which type of setting they are most comfortable working in. The third type of test—personality—measures traits such as assertiveness, sociability, independence, and empathy. While all these tests provide some insight, companies must correlate test results with the successful performance by sales personnel. To avoid major issues regarding testing discrimination, it is suggested that tests only be one part of the selection process.

A final step in the selection process is the background investigation. This typically involves reference checks, credit information, and in some instances, lie detector tests. In the pharmaceutical industry, for example, background checks are an important part of the selection process. Since medical detail representatives have access to samples of prescription drugs, the applicant's integrity is an issue of paramount concern.

Training

Sales training is an ongoing activity for companies that want to maintain an effective sales force. Training begins when the candidate is first hired and often continues with ongoing on-the-job training.

Training the New Recruit

Most companies have a formal training program for new recruits. Large companies, such as consumer food product companies or life insurance firms, maintain a centralized sales training staff with a prescribed program for ongoing selection and recruitment of sales personnel. In smaller companies or in organizations that have smaller sales requirements, training activities are less formal and often are conducted within the marketing department.

The scope of the sales training typically involves issues such as the sales process. Salespeople receive information about the company and the industry, as well as about the organization's policies and procedures. Sales training for new recruits must focus on time and territory management and on customer requirements and product knowledge. Many organizations will also have a new salesperson shadow a more experienced representative in the field prior to the completion of the sales training. After this mentoring experience, sales training can focus on what was observed in real on-the-job settings.

Ongoing Training

Ongoing training of experienced personnel varies little from that of the new recruit. Companies typically provide annual updating of new services or changes within existing programs. This training helps to improve morale and refine existing sales techniques.

Compensation

A major issue in the management of any sales force is determining the compensation system. In developing an effective compensation plan, there are specific requirements important to the salesperson and valuable to the company.

Salespeople need to be assured that the compensation plan is equitable for the entire sales force. A well-designed plan should provide salespeople with a stable income, yet offer the motivation or incentive to perform. Finally, a sound compensation plan should be understandable, meaning the sales staff should understand the dimensions on which they are to be rewarded and what the organization values.

The design of the compensation plan should allow the company to attract and retain good salespeople. A well-designed plan should also provide to the company the ability to encourage or focus the sales force's efforts on specific tasks. A good plan allows for recognition of the differences between good and bad performers and provides the necessary balance between costs and results. While a good plan ultimately should be easy to administer, it must be constructed in such a way to ensure long-term customer relationships. Three basic types of compensation plans are used: the straight salary, the commission plan, and the combination plan.

Straight Salary

The **straight salary** compensation plan provides salespeople with a fixed salary. This plan's advantage is that it allows the salesperson to focus upon the nonsales aspects of the job. For the organization, another benefit is that the sales costs are easily determined and budgeted. The plan is also appropriate when it is hard to determine the effect of the salesperson's efforts on resulting volume. For example, a sales position that is primarily missionary in its focus might receive straight salary compensation.

One of the plan's disadvantages is its direct effects on motivation. Financial reward is not tied to any particular aspect of sales performance. As a result, the rationale for salary increases may not be easy to communicate. Also, the fixed-cost nature of the straight salary plan, while cited as an advantage, is also its limitation. When sales are rising and volume is high, compensation costs become a smaller percentage of total revenue. With declining sales volume, however, the fixed salary costs become a significant overhead expense.

Commission Plan

An alternative to a straight salary program is one that pays on **commission**, in which the salesperson is paid based on sales performance in terms of volume, net revenue, or margin. The advantage of this plan is that the salesperson is clearly focused upon the sales task. It also has the advantage of equity in that good performers are rewarded more highly than those who are less proficient. Unlike straight salary plans, commission compensation plans vary directly with the organization's revenue, allowing the firm a built-in cost advantage.

Commission plans have some major limitations, however, one being that the salesperson focuses too heavily on the sales tasks alone. Nonsales activities and missionary functions may not receive warranted attention in the short term as the salesperson tries to maximize income. Salespeople also have concerns about the security of a commission plan. These type of programs can lead to a high degree of variability in income from one pay period to the next.

Combination Plans

A **combination plan** for a sales force consists of a base salary plus commissions and bonuses. The base salary gives the salesperson some financial security as well as the motivation to perform the nonsales aspects of the job. The salesperson also receives a bonus, or commission, based on achieving particular sales quotas or other, prior, specified levels of performance. A **bonus** is a payment made for achieving a particular level of performance.

In developing a combination compensation plan, companies must consider the size of the incentive portion of compensation relative to that which is fixed. The incentive portion must be large enough to motivate the sales staff. The more important actual selling skills are to the salesperson's role, the higher should be the incentive proportion of the compensation plan. A second issue in any combination plan is whether it should set limits on incentive earnings. Limitations are often imposed so that the high performer's income is not so great as to affect the morale of those with lower performance ratings. Another concern is that a new service might be so positively received when first introduced in the market that the sales staff will be rewarded, even though their efforts contributed little to actual sales. Whenever a company implements a compensation plan with an incentive component, it is always useful to pretest the plan with past performance data. The company should assess what the relative compensation levels of the sales force would have been if the incentive plan was in place. This pretest can determine whether the plan reflects the performance levels of the sales personnel.

Supplemental Incentives

A growing element in sales compensation is the use of supplemental programs, such as sales contests or nonfinancial incentives, as shown in Figure 12–6. In using sales contests, the purpose is typically to reward personnel for short-term, highly focused activities. For sales contests to succeed, sales people must believe they have an opportunity to compete for the prize. The objectives must be within the reach of each person. A contest that ties rewards to percentage improvement over last year's sales effort is one way to allow each person to compete. Programs should be simple and easy to communicate. Rewards should be attractive incentives, including cash, travel, or merchandise. With the use of nonfinancial incentives, the goal is to reward the salesperson through recognition such as a personal letter, an award, or other publicity. The value of a nonfinancial incentive is to reinforce the salesperson's higher-order needs, such as self-esteem, as presented by Maslow (see Chapter 4).

Sales Force Evaluation and Control

The final step in the sales management process is the ongoing evaluation and control of the sales force. Evaluation of the sales force is based on both input and output measures. *Input measures* assess the effort expended by salespersons to perform their job. These measures might include number of calls per day, product knowledge, hours worked per day, or number of phone calls made. *Output measures* assess the results of the salesperson's efforts. These measures often include sales, gross revenue, number of referrals generated, number of new users, and expenses.[15]

Organizations must decide whether to use single or multiple measures of performance. The advantage of a single measure is its administrative ease. In addition to being economical, single measure evaluation systems also are easy to

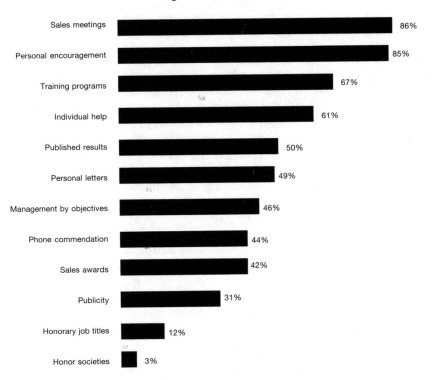

Figure 12–6 Nonfinancial Compensation Methods. *Source:* Reprinted from *Health Care Sales* by K. Mack and P.A. Newbold, p. 61, with permission of Jossey-Bass Inc., Publishers, © 1991.

communicate. Their chief limitation is that they often focus exclusively on sales. As discussed earlier in this chapter, selling is just one component of the salesperson's responsibilities.

There are many valuable sources of information that a company can use in the evaluation process. Company records are the primary source of evaluation data. Customers should also become part of the evaluation process, since it is the customer who might best be able to assess the salesperson's relationship-building methods and attitude. The limitation of this source is the validity of the information. Most consumer product companies have the sales manager accompany the salesperson on sales calls to assess on-the-job performance.

Regardless of the number of measures or sources used for evaluation, an organization needs to have an ongoing evaluation plan. The plan should be based on the requirements of the specific sales positions and selling and nonselling tasks should be weighted according to their relative importance.

CONCLUSIONS

Use of personal selling in health care has been limited to a few areas in the past 10 to 15 years. While a common strategy for pharmaceutical companies and managed care organizations, personal selling has been a smaller component of the promotional mix among other segments of the industry. Now, as the health care environment moves to a more fully capitated setting, personal sales will assume greater importance.

To utilize a sales force effectively requires understanding the dimensions of all the sales functions. This way, effective recruiting programs can be implemented, sales force size determined, and compensation and evaluation systems put in place.

KEY TERMS

Leads
Cold Calls
Qualified Prospects
Approach
Close
Stimulus-Response Sales Approach
Workload Method

Structured Interview
Unstructured Interview
Stress Interview
Commission
Straight Salary
Combination Plan
Bonus

CHAPTER SUMMARY

1. Personal selling is an ingredient of the promotional mix. Sales positions involve a range of sales functions—from selling to customer relationship building.

2. There are six steps in the personal sales process: prospecting, preapproach, approach, presentation, close, and servicing.

3. In the stimulus-response approach to sales, a canned presentation is often used as a script to generate a customer response, while in the selling formula approach, the prospect is moved through a sequence from attention, interest, desire, to action.

4. The need satisfaction sales method is the most marketing-oriented because it focuses on the customer's problems. With the consultative selling method, the salesperson acts as a problem solver.

5. Sales forces can be organized geographically, by product, or by customer type.

6. A common method for determining the size of the sales force is the workload method, which estimates the work effort required to serve the market.

7. Prior to recruitment and selection of the salesperson, the company should conduct a job analysis. The selection process then follows several steps, including an interview that can be a structured, unstructured, or stress interview.

8. Sales force compensation can be either straight salary, commission, or a combination plan.

9. Sales staff evaluation should be based on input measures (a salesperson's efforts) and output measures (sales results).

CHAPTER PROBLEMS

1. What type of sales position would you recommend for: (a) a four-person gastroenterology practice that wants to maintain strong ties to its primary care referral physicians, (b) an HMO trying to penetrate a new market and have its plan offered as an option to employees within any local company, and (c) a health care data management firm that provides a program to hospitals for billing and quality assurance?

2. Develop a short sales presentation about a chemical dependency program that you would make to an employee assistance professional of a large company. Show how the presentation would change using: (a) the stimulus-response approach, (b) the selling formula, and (c) the need satisfaction method.

3. What method of sales force organization would be most appropriate for: (a) a national company that sells a computerized billing system for small physician practices, and (b) a manufacturer of adhesive bandages and sutures?

4. A major tertiary care medical center has decided to establish a sales force to call on physicians practicing in the medical center's three-state region. The marketing director has classified the doctors into the following categories:

> Class A: loyal referrers—329 physicians
> Class B: moderate referrers—480 physicians
> Class C: potential referrers—620 physicians

She also estimates the following call pattern:

> Class A: 4 calls per year @ 30 minutes a call
> Class B: 3 calls per year @ 15 minutes per call
> Class C: 2 calls per year @ 15 minutes per call

The average salesperson works 48 weeks a year, 40 hours a week and spends 80 percent of his time selling. Calculate the number of sales representatives needed to service this market.

5. A manufacturer of prosthetic devices has decided to review his company's sales compensation system. Historically, salespeople were paid on straight salary. While the company has grown in recent years, the president is concerned that the sales force could generate more sales volume. A major part of the sales job is missionary, yet with the increasing number of physician groups expanding into rehabilitation medicine, a new target market is possible. The manufacturer is also concerned that not all the products in the line have the same margin. What form of compensation would you recommend?

NOTES

1. D.A. Newton, *Sales Force Performance and Turnover* (Cambridge, Mass.: Marketing Science Institute, 1973), 5.

2. W.S. Dempsey and S.H. Mandel, It's No Longer Words and Music: Marketing in a Capitated Environment, *Group Practice Journal* 43, no. 3 (1994):46–51.

3. Meet Needs of Segments of Physicians, *Physician Relations Advisor* 2, no. 11 (1993):143–146.

4. J.D. Lichenthal, S. Sikri, and K. Folk, Teleprospecting: An Approach for Qualifying Accounts, *Industrial Marketing Management* 18, no. 1 (1989):11–17; and M.A. Jolson, Qualifying Sales Leads: The Tight and Loose Approaches, *Industrial Marketing Management* 17, no. 3 (1988): 189–196.

5. E.O. Wogensen, Osteopathic Hospital Reaps Multiple Benefits through Occupational Health Program, *Strategic Health Care Marketing* 11, no. 7 (1994):4–6.

6. B. Shapiro, *Sales Force Management* (New York, N.Y.: McGraw-Hill Publishing Co., 1977), 160.

7. R.D. Balsey and E.P. Birsner, *Selling: Marketing Personified* (Hindsdale, Ill.: Dryden Press, 1987), 261–263.

8. I.P. Pavlov, *Conditioned Reflexes* (New York, N.Y.: Oxford University Press, 1927).

9. M.A. Jolson, Canned Adaptiveness: A New Direction for Modern Salesmanship, *Business Horizons* 32, no. 1 (1989):7–12.

10. M. Belch and R.W. Haas, Using Buyer Needs To Improve Industrial Sales, *Business* 29, no. 5 (1979):8–14.

11. R. Spiro and B. Weitz, Adaptive Selling: Conceptualization, Measurement, and Nomological Validity, *Journal of Marketing Research* 27, no. 1 (1990):61–69.

12. W.J. Talley, How To Design Sales Territories, *Journal of Marketing* 25, no. 3 (1961):7–13.

13. G.A. Churchill, Jr., et al., The Determinants of Salesperson Performance: A Meta-Analysis, *Journal of Marketing Research* 22, no. 2 (1985):103–118.

14. G.A. Churchill, Jr., N.M. Ford, and O.C. Walker, Jr., *Sales Force Management* (Homewood, Ill.: Richard D. Irwin, Inc., 1981), 305.

15. D.W. Jackson, Jr., J.E. Keith, and J. Schlacter, Evaluation of Selling Performance: A Study of Current Practice, *Journal of Personal Selling and Sales Management* 31, no. 2 (1983):43–51.

13

CONTROLLING AND MONITORING THE MARKETING STRATEGY

LEARNING OBJECTIVES

After reading this chapter you should be able to:

- Explain the value of monitoring market share compared to using absolute measure of performance

- Recognize the value of sales, profitability, contribution, and variance analysis

- Understand the array of specific marketing mix control procedures to monitor mix-specific activities

- Describe the scope of an organization's marketing audit and elements of that audit

CONTROLLING AND MONITORING MARKETING PERFORMANCE

Essential to an effective marketing organization is the ongoing measurement and monitoring of outcomes. In health care, this aspect of marketing is particularly important. As noted in Chapter 1, the health care industry for a long time viewed marketing as an unnecessary expense and limited to advertising. Even as there has been growing appreciation of marketing's role, concern still exists about whether the dollars spent on marketing are well invested. As health care organizations face more difficult resource allocation decisions, marketing managers will need to document their results. To accomplish this goal, marketing departments will need to have a system in place to monitor and measure results of marketing efforts continually.

To monitor marketing activities properly requires a multiple-step process, as shown in Figure 13–1. The initial requirement is to establish performance

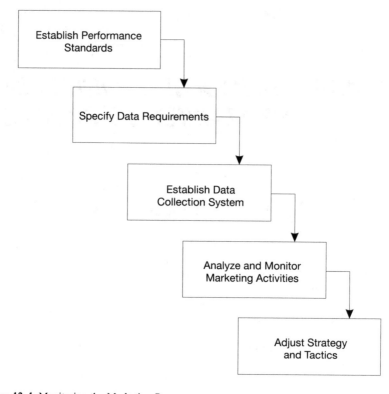

Figure 13–1 Monitoring the Marketing Process

standards on an *a priori* basis. These standards, once specified, allow for the appropriate data requirements to be developed, and the internal system require-ments to be established to collect data in a timely and accurate fashion. Data on the marketing activity can then be analyzed and corrective action taken or marketing strategy adjusted as needed.

Market Share Analysis

For some health care organizations, a major problem in developing an effective marketing strategy is complacency. Many health care providers believe they are doing well in the market simply by monitoring measures such as patient schedul-ing patterns for the physicians in the group. Many group medical practices often use measures of performance such as gross revenue, expense control, or net revenue that result in end-of-year payouts to the physicians. These measures are, in fact, all important indicators of performance. But, in a competitive market, these measures alone suffer from a major limitation—they are all absolute rather than relative indicators of performance. A group practice may believe it is performing well without fully understanding the dynamics of the marketplace or whether the revenue and patient increase it experiences is a result of its strategy or of a marketplace expansion.

Any organization in a competitive market must monitor its respective share of the market. Market share has the advantage of signaling when an organization needs to make changes. Market share is a measure of relative performance rather than an absolute indicator of performance. To understand the value of monitoring market share consider the graph shown in Figure 13–2. In this graph, "Hypothetical" HMO began its operation in 1975. This HMO was the first such plan to offer

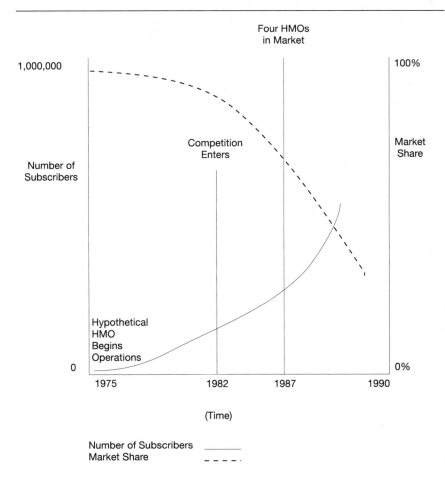

Figure 13–2 The Value of Market Share

a prepaid version of health care in this small, southeastern metropolitan community. After several years of slow growth (the introductory stage of the life cycle for managed care in this market), the number of subscribers began to increase as more consumers recognized this option as a viable way to pay for health care coverage. In 1982, this HMO saw its first organized competition from a large national HMO. As can be seen, the number of subscribers increased dramatically as both health care plans began to advertise. The second HMO served to legitimize this form of health care in the marketplace.

The graph shows that Hypothetical HMO was not concerned about the competition, since the number of subscribers was increasing. Little evidence existed for revising the organization's strategy. By 1987, four HMOs were operating in the market, yet Hypothetical HMO still saw its number of subscribers rise. Its monitoring of an absolute performance measure indicated little cause for concern. An examination of market share, however, indicated the time for a possible strategic change. In 1975, the original HMO had a market share of 100 percent. As seen in the graph, its market share did not change significantly by the time a competitor entered the market in 1982. By 1990, however, this original HMO is no longer a market leader. Monitoring absolute measures (sales, number of subscribers) never suggested the need for this HMO to revisit its marketing strategy. Yet, if market share had been monitored, Hypothetical HMO could have detected that, while its number of subscribers was growing, it may have had less to do with its strategy, and more to do with the fact that the entire market was expanding. If the company had been monitoring market share, it would have detected a fairly rapid erosion of its market position and recognized the need to reconsider its marketing mix. It could have opened a satellite office on the other side of the metropolitan area and changed its distribution mix. Or, the group could have offered an expanded benefit package including eye care (a product mix alteration), or changed the price of its premium.

Market share monitoring is an issue today in the health care marketplace. For many years, Kaiser Permanente Medical Group of Chula Vista, California experienced significant continuing growth in the number of its subscribers. No doubt this was due to the quality of the medical plan and the fact that Kaiser was an early entrant into managed care in California. Yet, in the past few years, Kaiser has met considerable competition from other organized managed care plans in the state. Monitoring market share earlier might have indicated the need for a substantial revision in its service mix. In 1994, Kaiser experienced its first major decline in the number of enrollees in the state of California. That same year, Kaiser began to offer a point-of-service (POS) plan as a way to boost share growth and compete against other POS plans that already existed in the market. With its POS plan, Kaiser was a late entrant into the market.

When measuring performance using market share, it is important to recognize that there are three types of market share measures to use:

1. **Overall market share:** This measure represents the company's sales as a percent of total industry sales. For a national HMO like CIGNA, market share would be calculated as the percentage of CIGNA HMO enrollees to the total number of HMO enrollees in the United States.
2. **Served market share:** This indicator is a measure of the organization's sales as a percentage of the total sales of the served market. The served market represents all the buyers who are able and willing to buy or use the service. For most medical organizations, the market share basis is really on the served market. For example, a hospital will calculate its served market share of coronary bypass procedures, which is its total number of bypass procedures performed as a percentage of the total number of bypass procedures done in its service area. An organization's served market share is always larger than its total market share.
3. **Relative market share:** This indicator of market share is a calculation of the percentage of the organization's sales compared to that of the largest competitor, or often the combined sales of the three largest competitors. When calculating market share to that of the largest competitor, a relative market share greater than 100 percent would indicate a market leader.[1]

There is no one correct market share indicator to use. It is important, however, for a company to determine a market share indicator and then track data using that same indicator. It is also essential to determine initially which market share indicator to use so that the appropriate data can be obtained. In health care, market data can often be obtained from state or local health regulatory agencies or federal statistics. There are also private, commercial organizations that provide data to health care organizations for market share measurement.

Sales Analysis

A common method for monitoring marketing performance is **sales analysis**, which compares the actual sales generated with the goals that were established. In conducting a sales analysis, it is useful to examine sales at a level below that of gross sales, such as by analyzing results on one or more criteria, such as: (1) product line analysis, (2) customer size, (3) geographic region, or (4) discount level.

Profitability Analysis

In Chapter 6, on market segmentation, the principle of heavy half segmentation was reviewed. As was noted, a large percentage of a product's sales is purchased by a small percentage of the customers. A useful method for monitoring marketing performance that incorporates this factor is **profitability analysis**, which examines the profitability of sales by customers, regions, products, or salespeople. For example, this type of analysis might reveal that there are some distinct differences among salespeople, as shown in Table 13–1. As seen in this analysis, salesperson A has the highest level of total sales. A more detailed examination of salesperson A's performance shows that, compared to salesperson C, A's level of sales resulted from selling possibly easier, less profitable products. This type of profitability analysis can help to refocus sales training efforts to encourage salespeople to sell more profitable items in the line. Profitability analysis can also indicate whether a company needs to redesign or change its sales compensation system to directly reward selling the more profitable products in the line.

In conducting an appropriate profitability analysis, a company needs to decide how to calculate costs. There are two options. One approach, referred to as **direct costing**, assigns only those costs to a product or service line that are directly associated with it. In **full costing**, both direct and indirect costs are assigned to the service unit and considered in the calculation of profitability.

Allocation of Costs

To conduct a full-costing analysis, a health care organization must assign both direct and indirect costs. Direct costs, as noted, pertain to costs directly associated with the program under analysis. Direct costs include any labor, technology, or supplies pertaining to the clinical program. There may also be direct marketing costs, if in fact specific advertisements were run for the program. Or, if a program manager made sales calls on possible accounts such as in an occupational medicine program, that person's salary would be a direct cost. **Indirect costs** are fixed costs that cannot be related to just one product line or service program. Indirect costs also include administrative management salaries unrelated to any specific program.

When using a full-costing method, a health care organization must decide to allocate costs to a particular program. While it is not incorrect to allocate costs, there are some concerns about what to use as the basis for the allocation. Is the allocation based on space utilized in the ambulatory building for a particular

---

Table 13–1 Looking at Product Profitability

Salesperson	A	B	C
Sales	$2,156,890	$1,768,925	$2,146,859
Direct selling expenses	$46,007	$57,809	$41,487
Gross margin of products sold	$1,113,873	$876,931	$1,246,701
Average gross margin percent	51.64%	49.57%	58.07%

program? Or, is the basis for allocation the percentage of total hospital revenue generated by the program?[2] Ideally, the basis of allocation should be fair and consistent. Since there often are no exact determinations for the appropriate allocations, however, management should not spend excessive amounts of time resolving issues of cost allocations. Marketing's major concern about cost allocations is that they often distort the real value or profitability of a particular product. The result is that a low-volume product can often be identified as more profitable than a high-volume product, purely as a function of the cost allocation.[3]

Because of the difficulties in assigning indirect costs, many companies prefer direct costing, which considers the contribution margin of a particular service. While overhead, or fixed costs, must be covered at some time, the contribution margin approach provides a clearer view of what would be gained or lost by dropping a particular clinical program.

Contribution Analysis

Another method for organizations to assess the market performance of a service or multiple services is contribution analysis. **Contribution analysis** considers the contribution of profit to fixed cost or overhead. Table 13–2 shows an analysis of four clinical services offered by a medical center and the percentage variable contribution margin per service. The **percentage variable contribution margin**

Table 13–2 Examining Contribution to Profit

	Product Profitability			
	Occupational Medicine	Substance Abuse	Rehabilitation Services	Executive Fitness
Number of Customers	375	222	97	75
Average Price per Employee	$127.00	$85.00	$320.00	$425.00
Variable Cost per Employee	$37.20	$22.50	$112.00	$97.00
Variable Contribution Margin per Employee Covered (Average Price- Variable Cost Per Employee)	$89.80	$62.50	$208.00	$328.00
Percentage Variable Contribution Margin (PVCM)	70.23%	73.53%	65.00%	77.17%

(PVCM) shows the percentage of each additional sales dollar available to the organization to cover its fixed costs. The calculation of this ratio is:

$$PCVM = \frac{\text{Average Unit Price–Unit Variable Cost}}{\text{Unit Price}}$$

The variable contribution margin is the price per unit sales less the variable cost per unit.

Insights from Contribution Analysis

The differences between using a contribution or full-cost approach are significant. Contribution analysis allows a marketing manager to calculate the incremental value of directing additional resources to a particular service line or customer account. Since contribution analysis only considers direct program costs, a company could estimate how much more sales or revenue would be obtained if additional, marketing efforts were committed. Table 13–3 shows the analysis of three departments using a full-cost method. As seen with the allocation of indirect costs (administrative expenses and overhead), clinical service # 1 is losing $5,000, while clinical service # 3 saw net profit of $78,000. Consider the difference, however, when the contribution method is applied, as shown in Table 13–4. Without the allocation of indirect costs, clinical service # 1 provides incremental value by contributing $50,000 to fixed costs, or overhead.

Recently The Beckham Company, a health care consulting firm in Whitefish Bay, Wisconsin, reviewed several community hospitals, and found an inverse relationship between total inpatient revenue and contribution to operating margin. Traditionally, high revenue-producing services such as cardiology, internal medicine, and pulmonary medicine were creating the greatest losses. Some of the lowest inpatient revenue services—family practice, rheumatology, and obstetrics—had the most positive contribution margins.[4]

Table 13–3 The Full-Cost Method

	Totals	Clinical Service #1	Clinical Service #2	Clinical Service #3
Sales	$1,000,000	$500,000	$300,000	$200,000
Direct Costs	$800,000	$450,000	$250,000	$100,000
Contribution Margin	$200,000	$50,000	$50,000	$100,000
Indirect Costs Allocated	$110,000	$55,000	$33,000	$22,000
Net Profit	$90,000	($5,000)	$17,000	$78,000

Table 13–4 The Contribution Method

	Totals	Clinical Service #1	Clinical Service #2	Clinical Service #3
Sales	$1,000,000	$500,000	$300,000	$200,000
Direct Costs	$800,000	$450,000	$250,000	$100,000
Contribution Margin	$200,000	$50,000	$50,000	$100,000
Indirect Costs Allocated	$110,000			
Net Profit	$90,000			

Variance Analysis

An important method for evaluating marketing efforts is through the use of **variance analysis**, which compares actual results to preestablished performance targets. Table 13–5 shows the results of a yearlong effort to enroll subscribers in a managed care plan. As seen in this table, the number of covered lives actually enrolled was 10,000 more than originally targeted. Yet, because there was intense competition from other managed care plans, the premium dollar received per subscriber was less than originally projected. Many competitors aggressively discounted to encourage new enrollment. As a result, the gross marketing contribution fell below the targeted level.

Examining these data, it's evident that the decreases in gross marketing contribution resulted from two factors: the increase in the number of subscribers and the decrease in the premium dollar received. Which factor contributed more to the decrease in gross marketing contribution? It is possible to get an answer by examining the data in Exhibit 13–1. In this exhibit, one can see that the company

Table 13–5 Variance Analysis

	Variance Analysis		
	Planned	Actual	Difference
Covered Lives	100,000	110,000	10,000
Premium per Subscriber	$1,400	$1,200	($200)
Direct Costs per Subscriber	$400	$400	
Subscriber Gross Marketing Contribution	$1,000	$800	($200)
Sales	$140,000,000	132,000,000	($8,000,000)
Direct Costs	$40,000,000	$44,000,000	($4,000,000)
Gross Margin Contribution	$100,000,000	$88,000,000	($12,000,000)

Exhibit 13–1 Sources of Variance

Differences Due to Changes in Gross Marketing Contribution:

Actual Gross Marketing Contribution =
  Actual Subscriber Level × Actual Subscriber Gross Marketing Contribution
  =110,000 × $800 = $88,000,000

Planned Gross Marketing Contribution =
  Actual Subscriber Level × Planned Subscriber Gross Marketing Contribution
  = 110,000 × $1,000 = $110,000,000

Variance Due to Failure To Get Subscriber Gross Marketing Contribution
  = $110,000,000 – $88,000,000 = $22,000,000

Differences Due to Changes in Volume:

Annual Gross Marketing Contribution =
  Planned Subscriber Level × Planned Subscriber Gross Marketing Contribution
  = 100,000 × $1,000 = $100,000,000

Planned Gross Marketing Contribution =
  Actual Subscriber Level × Planned Subscriber Gross Marketing Contribution
  = 110,000 × $1,000 = $110,000,000

Increase in Gross Marketing Contribution Due to Subscriber Enrollment Success
  = $110,000,000 – $100,000,000 = $10,000,000

enrolled more subscribers than anticipated. Such a difference between expected and real unit sales is called a **volume variance**. Yet because there was heavy discounting in the market, the contribution to gross marketing costs decreased. This difference between expected and real contribution margin is referred to as a **contribution variance** (or a price variance). By examining the variances calculated in Exhibit 13–1, one can assess which factor has a greater impact on the lower gross marketing contribution shown in Table 13–5. The analysis reveals that it was the lack of maintaining prices that resulted in the decreased gross margin contribution observed by the managed care plan.

Hospitals and other medical organizations have a wide array of products and services that they market. They can also assess market performance, therefore, by using a **product mix variance**, which refers to the difference between actual and targeted performance levels due to the composition of products or services offered. Consider the example shown in Exhibit 13–2. In this case, a hospital had established a company to sell durable medical equipment to nursing homes and long-term care facilities. The actual sales generated were $750,000. The exhibit also shows what the planned discounts and cost of goods sold were, based on the projected composition of products that were to be purchased. Exhibit 13–3 shows

Exhibit 13–2 Performance Targets for Durable Medical Equipment

Sales	$750,000	100.00%	Actual Sales Percent
Discounts	$37,500	5.00%	Planned Discount Percent
Net Sales	$712,500		
Cost of Goods Sold	$360,000	48.00%	Planned Cost of Goods Sold
Gross Marketing Contribution	$352,500	47.00%	Planned Gross Marketing Contribution Percent
Direct Marketing Costs	$51,300	6.84%	Direct Marketing Cost Percent
Net Marketing Contribution	$301,200		

the sales and actual cost of goods that were sold. As can be seen, a higher cost of goods sold resulted because a different composition of products was ultimately purchased by the customers. The results, then, can be assessed to determine the impact of the product mix on the gross marketing contribution, as seen in the bottom half of Exhibit 13–3.

Exhibit 13–3 Product Mix Variance

	Actual		
Sales	$750,000	100.00%	Actual Sales Percent
Discounts	$37,500	5.00%	Planned Discount Percent
Net Sales	$712,500	95.00%	Net Sales Percent
Cost of Goods Sold	$384,000	51.20%	Actual Cost of Goods Sold
Gross Marketing Contribution	$328,500	43.80%	Actual Product Mix Gross Marketing Contribution Percent
Direct Marketing Costs	$51,300	6.84%	Direct Marketing Cost Percent
Net Marketing Contribution	$277,200	36.96%	Actual Net Marketing Contribution Percent

Actual Sales	$750,000
Planned Discount @ 5.00%	37,500
Expected Sales	$712,500
Planned Cost of Goods Sold if Original Product Mix Sold @ 48.00%	360,000
Gross Marketing Contribution with Original Product Mix	$352,500
Gross Marketing Contribution with Actual Product Mix	$328,500
Decrease in Gross Marketing Contribution Due to Product Mix	($24,000)

This type of analysis could also be conducted to assess whether there is a **price variance**, which is the difference between the actual price received and the targeted level because of discounting. Consider the original data shown in Exhibit 13–2 (price variance # 1). In this case, the hospital planned to offer a planned discount level of 5 percent, or $37,500. In actuality, a new supplier of durable medical equipment entered the market, and, to retain customers and stay competitive, the hospital's actual discounts and allowances totaled $50,000. Results of this discounting are shown in Exhibit 13–4.

SALES FORCE CONTROL

Control and measurement of the sales force can take several forms. Sales force control is relatively more straightforward than other aspects of marketing, since the compensation system often is tied directly to the performance expected. This is particularly true when the organization uses a commission system or a salary with bonus incentives. Even with these compensation systems, however, sales performance can be monitored by considering the allocation of effort, the result of the effort, and the investment required to generate the output.

In monitoring sales staff performance, companies can use several objective measures based on input to the job, which includes aspects such as the number of customer calls, the number of calls on new accounts vs. existing accounts, the

---

Exhibit 13–4 Price Variance

		Actual	Planned
	Price Variance		
Sales		$750,000	$750,000
Discounts		$50,000	$37,500
Net Sales		$700,000	$712,500
Actual Cost of Goods Sold		$384,000	$384,000
Gross Marketing Contribution		$316,000	$328,500
Direct Marketing Costs		$51,300	$51,300
Net Marketing Contribution		$264,700	$277,200

Price Variance:

Actual Sales = $700,000
Planned Sales = $712,500
Price Variance = ($12,500)

number of presentations made, and where necessary, the individual's service record. This last component is important for sales positions that are primarily missionary in nature. Monitoring sales behavior often requires a formal solicitation of evaluation from the respective customer.

In evaluating salesperson performance, a common control mechanism is the **sales/expense ratio**. To a large degree this ratio indicates the efficiency of the salesperson in generating output. The sales/expense ratio considers the amount of input required in the form of sales expenses relative to the output achieved (sales). Sales expenses might include but not be limited to travel costs, entertainment expenses, trial samples of a product that are given away, or promotional costs.

Several subjective measures can be used to measure salesperson performance. These include items such as job knowledge, territory management, and personal characteristics. Job knowledge pertains to how well the person knows the service lines represented, the health care organization's policies and procedures, and possibly the details and complexities of contract requirements. Management of the territory includes aspects such as report accuracy and scope, customer complaint handling, and planning of calls and accounts. Personal characteristics relate to the individual's motivation, initiative, appearance, or personality. This last dimension, while often included on evaluation reports of salespeople, is difficult to assess. While several studies have examined the effect of personal characteristics on salesperson performance, results were disappointing.[5]

A reasonably comprehensive approach to evaluating salespeople is shown in the framework in Table 13–6. In this table, salespeople are evaluated in terms of sales potential, margin contribution, and expense. This analysis provides an overview that extends beyond just the gross sales achieved by the individual. By examining the sales relative to quota, one can examine sales potential. For health care organizations that do not have established quotas for their salespeople, it is possible to develop an index of territory sales potential. To estimate sales potential for a territory one needs to aggregate based on sales potential by accounts. This information requires a list of potential accounts in the territory and an estimate of potential sales for the product mix at each account. The sales staff can provide this information by obtaining estimates of the amount or volume of a particular item or service used by an account.[6]

ADVERTISING CONTROL

Compared to many aspects of the marketing mix, monitoring and review of advertising is easy. As noted in Chapter 11, however, it is essential to specify advertising objectives prior to the beginning of any promotional campaign. Specifying these objectives then provides a benchmark against which to measure performance.

Table 13–6 A Multidimensional Approach to Salesperson Evaluation

Salesperson	Number of Accounts	Sales Potential	Number of Sales Calls	Average Gross Margin	Sales	Sales Expense	Cost per Call	Percent of Potential
A	87	$1,568,000	198	37.80%	$839,000	$41,092	$207.54	53.50%
B	69	$2,098,000	202	41.20%	$1,230,083	$36,798	$182.17	58.63%
C	79	$989,000	272	40.02%	$424,084	$27,908	$102.60	42.88%

For most health care organizations, promotion and advertising are an ongoing process. They can establish a system that allows the comparison and review of a series of advertising campaigns with the use of media/service effectiveness ratios, as shown in Table 13–7. The table shows data for a hospital's advertising campaign for two new suburban primary care sites that were established in two different neighborhoods. A different ad campaign ran for three months in each service area. Initially, the campaign's objectives were to gain awareness for the site. Measure A is the total number of families in the target population. For both sites, this included all consumers over the age of 21 who lived within five miles of each new urgent care site. The hospital ran advertisements in local community shopping circulars and placed two advertisements on billboards on the major streets in each neighborhood. After four weeks, a telephone survey revealed an awareness level of 88 percent in neighborhood A, and 76 percent in neighborhood B. After eight weeks, a second random telephone survey revealed that 11 percent of consumers in neighborhood A had tried the new facility, 15 percent in neighborhood B had tried the other. At the end of the campaign, 4 percent of the consumers in neighborhood A said they were regular users, and 2.5 percent were regular users in neighborhood B.

Measures E through G are ratios that can be used to compare this campaign with other hospital campaigns. Ratio E is termed the media effectiveness ratio. This measure is the awareness over the total target population. This ratio suggests how well the organization did in identifying which media to use to reach the target population. As seen in neighborhood A, the media selection was more effective than in neighborhood B. Yet the creative effectiveness ratio indicates that the copy strategy employed in the advertisements in neighborhood B were more effective in moving people from the awareness level to the point of trial than in neighborhood A. The final ratio pertains more to the service itself than to the advertising. Advertising and promotion can move people through the hierarchy of effects (discussed in Chapter 11), but advertising and promotion cannot create regular

Table 13–7 Monitoring Advertising Campaigns

Media/Service Effectiveness Ratios

Measure		Neighborhood A	Neighborhood B
A	Total Families in Target Population	100%	100%
B	Aware of Service	88%	76%
C	Tried Service	11%	15%
D	Use Service Regularly	4%	2.5%
E	Media Effectiveness Ratio (B/A)	88%	76%
F	Creative Effectiveness Ratio (C/B)	12.5%	19.7%
G	Service Effectiveness Ratio (D/C)	36.4%	16.7%

customers. This objective can only be accomplished if the service meets customer expectations. The service effectiveness ratio indicates that the primary care site in neighborhood A is developing more loyal customers than that in neighborhood B. Now the objective of the marketing effort in the two neighborhoods will differ. In neighborhood A, a revision of the copy strategy is warranted based on the lower creative effectiveness ratio compared to neighborhood B (and, if this process is ongoing, based on other historical campaigns). In neighborhood B, the service itself must be analyzed relative to the customer satisfaction measures that are being obtained from the users at that clinic site.

The West Virginia University Health Science Center in Morgantown, West Virginia used a monitoring approach to track physician referrals. The hospital held tailgate parties in the fall in conjunction with university football games. Potential referral physicians were invited to attend along with alumni, donors, and faculty. In the six months after the last party, 11 physicians referred to the Health Science Center for the first time. These physicians sent $595,000 worth of insured patient business to the Center.[7]

CUSTOMER SATISFACTION CONTROL

A large number of health care organizations today conduct ongoing customer satisfaction surveys. This should be an essential ingredient of any successful marketing strategy, considering that the cost of a dissatisfied patient can be significant. The Technical Assistance Research Programs, Inc. of Arlington, Virginia, a research and consulting firm specializing in customer satisfaction, has estimated that the cost of dissatisfaction for a hospital with 5,000 annual discharges can be over $750,000.[8] Yet one recent study reported that only 20 percent of health care organizations conducting patient satisfaction surveys used them to provide feedback to clinical and administrative departments.[9]

Chapter 4 on buyer behavior presented a framework that showed how management should focus attention in the post-purchase evaluation stage of consumer decision making. As organizations monitor customer satisfaction, they can analyze these data by loyal or heavy half usage segments and determine how to change strategies.

The tendency in health care organizations, when dealing with medical staffs, is to respond to the physician who is the loudest complainer. Looking at physician satisfaction reports broken down by admission level (or, in managed care organizations, by utilization) might result in a different response to the customer dissatisfaction. Consider Table 13–8, which shows this provider satisfaction by utilization. One can see that scheduling is a major problem for the heavy utilizer. It might be incorrect for a managed care plan to respond directly

Table 13–8 Controlling Customer Satisfaction

Physician Utilization Level	Average Physician Satisfaction Levels		
	Scheduling Ease	Laboratory Service	Ease of Use
Light User	3.4	4.5	1.9
Medium User	2.5	3.6	2.8
Heavy User	5.2	2.8	1.7

Scale: '1'—very satisfied, to '7'—very dissatisfied

to this dissatisfaction. The more appropriate strategy might be to review the utilization pattern of this group of physicians and determine whether there is a way for these providers to be more efficient. This approach might reduce physician dissatisfaction with scheduling as well as save the managed care plan capitated revenue.

THE MARKETING AUDIT

Organizations should review periodically all aspects of their marketing operations. This process, called a **marketing audit**, is a systematic, critical review and appraisal of the total marketing operation. The audit reviews basic policies and assumptions, as well as procedures, personnel, and organization employed to implement marketing activities.[10] Because of the dynamic nature of the health care environment, health care organizations must periodically audit their total marketing activity and organization to ensure that it is responsive to market needs and preferences. A marketing audit has five major purposes:

1. It appraises the total marketing operation.
2. It centers on the evaluation of objectives and policies and the assumptions that underlie them.
3. It aims for prognosis as well as diagnosis.
4. It searches for opportunities and means for exploiting them, as well as for weaknesses and means for elimination.
5. It practices preventive as well as curative marketing practices.[11]

The marketing audit process has been described as a series of circles expanding outward from the consumer, as shown in Figure 13–3.[12] Beginning with the consumer market, a company examines how it is structured, how it can be divided, and how it is changing. To this information, a company can also add a review of

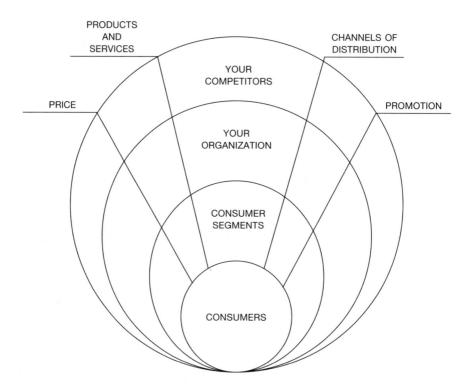

Figure 13–3 The Marketing Audit Process. *Source:* Reprinted from Berkowitz, E.N. and Flexner, W., The Marketing Audit: A Tool for Health Service Organizations, *Health Care Management Review,* Vol. 3, No. 4, p. 54, Aspen Publishers, Inc., © 1978.

its actions, policies, and plans. Internal constraints, organizational structure, and marketing programs can be reviewed. Within this context, the organization must conduct a detailed analysis of strengths and weaknesses. Finally, the audit must consider competitors and their respective programs, strengths, weaknesses, and trends.

As seen in this figure, the marketing mix variables—the controllable elements—cut across each aspect of this review. At each stage of the audit, the four marketing mix elements must be specifically considered: How are distribution channels changing for the market? Are new entities emerging that are gaining market share? How can functional shifting change the flow of patient volume?

The scope of issues reviewed in conducting the audit are far reaching. Exhibit 13–5 portrays a list of guiding questions that can be considered in a comprehensive audit of a health care organization.

Exhibit 13–5 Guiding Questions for the Marketing Audit

THE MARKET AND MARKET SEGMENTS

- How large is the territory covered by your market? How have you determined this?
- How is your market grouped?
  - Is it scattered?
  - How many important segments are there?
  - How are these segments determined (demographics, service usage, attitudinally)?
- Is the market entirely urban, or is a fair proportion of it rural?
- What percentage of your market uses third-party payment?
  - What are the attitudes and operations of third parties?
  - Are they all equally profitable?
- What are the effects of the following factors on your market?
  - Age
  - Income
  - Occupation
  - Increasing population ⎫

  ⎬ Demographic Shifting
  - Decreasing birthrate ⎭
- What proportion of potential customers are familiar with your organization, services, programs?
  - What is your image in the marketplace?
  - What are the important components of your image?

THE ORGANIZATION

- Short history of your organization:
  - When and how was it organized?
  - What has been the nature of its growth?
  - How fast and far have its markets expanded?
  - Where do your patients come from geographically?
  - What is the basic policy of the organization? Is it on "health care"? "Profit"?
  - What has been the financial history of the organization?
    - How has it been capitalized?
    - Have there been any account receivable problems?
    - What is inventory investment?
  - What has been the organization's success with the various services promoted?
- How does your organization compare with the industry?
  - Is the total volume (gross revenue, utilization) increasing? Decreasing?
  - Have there been any fluctuations in revenue? If so, what were they due to?
- What are the objectives and goals of the organization? How can they be expressed beyond the provision of "good health care"?
- What are the organization's present strengths and weaknesses in:
  - Medical facilities?
  - Management capabilities?
  - Medical staff?

continues

Exhibit 13–5 continued

- Technical facilities?
- Reputation?
- Financial capabilities?
- Image?
- What is the labor environment for your organization:
  - For medical staff (nurses, physicians, etc.)?
  - For support personnel?
- How dependent is your organization upon conditions of other industries (third-party payers)?
- Are weaknesses being compensated for and strengths being used? How?
- How are the following areas of your marketing function organized?
  - Structure
  - Manpower
  - Reporting relationships
  - Decision-making power
- What kinds of external controls affect your organization?
  - Local
  - State
  - Federal
  - Self-regulatory
- What are the trends in recent regulatory rulings?

COMPETITORS

- How many competitors are in your industry?
  - How do you define your competitors?
  - Has this number increased or decreased in the last four years?
- Is competition on a price or nonprice basis?
- What are the choices afforded patients:
  - In services?
  - In payment?
- What is your position in the market—size and strength—relative to competitors?

PRODUCTS AND SERVICES

- Complete a list of your organization's products and services, both present and proposed.
- What are the general outstanding characteristics of each product or service?
- What superiority or distinctiveness of products or services do you have, as compared with competing organizations?
- What is the total cost per service (in-use)? Is service over/under utilized?
- What services are most heavily used? Why?
  - What is the profile of patients/physicians who use the services?
  - Are there distinct groups of users?
- What are your organization's policies regarding:
  - Number and types of services to offer?
  - Assessing needs for service addition/deletion?

continues

Exhibit 13–5 continued

- History of products and services (complete for major products and services):
  - How many did the organization originally have?
  - How many have been added or dropped?
  - What important changes have taken place in services during the last 10 years?
  - Has demand for the services increased or decreased?
  - What are the most common complaints against the service?
  - What services could be added to your organization that would make it more attractive to patients, medical staff, nonmedical personnel?
  - What are the strongest points of your services to patients, medical staff, nonmedical personnel?
  - Are there any other features that individualize your service or give it an advantage over competitors?

PRICE

- What is the pricing strategy of the organization?
  - Cost-plus
  - Return on investment
  - Stabilization
- How are prices for services determined?
  - How often are prices reviewed?
  - What factors contribute to price increase/decrease?
- What have been the price trends for the past five years?
- How are your pricing policies viewed by:
  - Patients?
  - Physicians?
  - Third-party payers?
  - Competitors?
  - Regulators?

PROMOTION

- What is the purpose of the organization's present promotional activities (including advertising)?
  - Protective
  - Educational
  - Search out new markets
  - Develop all markets
  - Establish a new service
- Has this purpose undergone any change in recent years?
- To whom has advertising appeal been largely directed?
  - Donors
  - Patients
    - Former or current
    - Prospective
  - Physicians
    - On staff
    - Potential

continues

Exhibit 13–5 continued

- What media have been used?
- Are the media still effective in reaching the intended audience?
- What copy appeals have been notable in terms of response?
- What methods have been used for measuring advertising effectiveness?
- What is the role of public relations?
  - Is it a separate function/department?
  - What is the scope of responsibilities?

CHANNELS OF DISTRIBUTION

- What are the trends in distribution in the industry?
  - What services are being performed on an outpatient basis?
  - What services are being provided on an at-home basis?
  - Are satellite facilities being used?
- What factors are considered in location decisions? When did you last evaluate present location?
- What distributors do you deal with (e.g., medical supply houses, etc.)?
- How large an inventory must you carry?

Source: Reprinted from Berkowitz, E.N. and Flexner, W., The Marketing Audit: A Tool for Health Service Organizations, *Health Care Management Review*, Vol. 3, No. 4, pp. 55–56, Aspen Publishers, Inc., © 1978.

CONCLUSIONS

Health care organizations are facing an ever more competitive marketplace. Marketing strategies must be revised and changed continually to respond to the marketplace demands. In order to develop an ongoing marketing strategy that is effective, close monitoring and review of all marketing mix elements are necessary. Several control procedures and reports can be used to identify when strategies or tactics must be refined. Periodically, the organization must conduct a systemwide review of all marketplace and organizational marketing efforts to ensure that strategy is directed appropriately to respond to the changing dynamics of the health care environment.

KEY TERMS

Overall Market Share	Profitability Analysis
Served Market Share	Direct Costing
Relative Market Share	Full Costing
Sales Analysis	Indirect Costs

Contribution Analysis	Contribution Variance
Percentage Variable Contribution Margin (PVCM)	Product Mix Variance
	Price Variance
Variance Analysis	Sales/Expense Ratio
Volume Variance	Marketing Audit

CHAPTER SUMMARY

1. Market share provides a relative rather than absolute measure of performance. Market share can be either overall market share, served market share, or relative market share.

2. Sales analysis monitors sales performance relative to targets. It can be conducted on multiple bases for comparison.

3. Profitability analysis examines profitability by customers, regions, or products. The underlying premise is to monitor for a heavy half phenomenon.

4. A key issue in profitability analysis is the assignment of cost. It can be either a direct-cost or full-cost approach.

5. Contribution analysis considers performance of a service based on its contribution to profit or overhead.

6. Variance analysis compares actual results to targets. In conducting variance analysis it is possible to identify the source of the variance.

7. Variance can be due to volume, contribution, product mix, or price.

8. Multiple measures of input and output are used in the monitoring of salespeople. A common efficiency indicator is the sales/expense ratio.

9. To monitor ongoing advertising efforts, an organization can establish media effectiveness, creative effectiveness, and service effectiveness ratios.

10. Customer satisfaction control is at the foundation of any effective marketing program. Dissatisfied customers have been found to represent a real dollar cost to the organization.

11. Periodically, every health care entity should conduct a marketing audit, which is a systematic review of all policies, procedures, and structures used to implement marketing activities.

CHAPTER PROBLEMS

1. At a recent strategic planning retreat of a 40-person multispecialty group, the administrator made a presentation that focused on the coming year's plans to establish the organization's first two primary care satellites, which would be located in the two growing suburbs of the community. These new additions would require the hiring of four family practitioners and other support staff. When the administrator finished her presentation, one of the most senior physicians stood up and said, "This is a foolish expenditure. We're so busy now in this group, we can't even see another patient. Our revenue was up 14 percent according to the previous financial presentation we heard. There is no reason to change what we're doing." How might you respond to this physician?

2. The administrator of a small, acute-care hospital is faced with his first managed care contract. He meets with representatives from the prepaid plan to discuss the amount to be paid to the hospital. The administrator is concerned because the managed care business does not look profitable—the hospital will be reimbursed below its current reimbursement levels. In what ways might the administrator evaluate this new managed care business in terms of its economic value to his institution?

3. A large national HMO recently entered a major southwestern metropolitan market. The managed care plan anticipated that, with an intensive advertising campaign and sales effort, it would have 75,000 subscribers after two years. They planned on charging a premium of $1,800 per subscriber. Marketing and personnel costs directly related to this effort were anticipated to be $250 per subscriber. Prior to the HMO's entry into the market, two of the large tertiary facilities in the region began to offer their own managed care plans in a PHO arrangement with their medical staffs. The result was aggressive discounting of the managed care premiums. The national HMO chain dropped its premium to $1,400 per subscriber. Direct costs remained the same, yet because of the competition, the national HMO was only able to enroll 45,000 subscribers.

   1. What was the variance because of the failure to get the gross marketing contribution?

   2. What was the variance due to the lack of enrollment success?

4. The director of a large regional reference laboratory was reviewing the service's performance over the past year. The laboratory had gross revenues of $3,500,000. Some of the business was to managed care plans and to large-volume users that resulted in a discount of $350,000, which was $25,000 more than

anticipated due to intense competition. The cost of providing the lab testing was $1,400,500, which was $250,000 higher than expected. Direct costs for salaries was $870,000. What was the product mix variance experienced by the laboratory service? What was the price variance?

5. A medical group recently conducted an advertising campaign for its new pediatric orthopedics department. After four weeks, a telephone survey found that 42 percent of the families with children under the age of 18 years were aware of the service. Six months later, it found that 12 percent had actually used the service, and 3 percent said they were regular users of the facility for their children's orthopedic needs. Compare this organization's advertising performance to that of the hospital discussed in Table 13–7 in this chapter. How does this organization compare in terms of its media, creative, and service effectiveness ratios? Where might the medical group need to make adjustments?

NOTES

1. P. Kotler, *Marketing Management*, 8th ed. (Englewood Cliffs, N.J.: Prentice Hall, 1994), 742–766.

2. A procedure for allocating indirect costs has been proposed by Y. Goldschmidt and A. Gafai, A Managerial Approach To Allocating Indirect Fixed Costs, *Health Care Management Review* 15, no. 2 (Spring 1990):43–52.

3. R. Cooper and R. Kaplan, How Cost Accounting Systematically Distorts Product Costs, in *Accounting and Management: Field Study Perspectives*, eds. W.J. Burns, Jr. and R.S. Kaplan (Cambridge, Mass.: Harvard University Press, 1987), 204–228.

4. D. Beckham, Go Beyond Simple Revenues To Identify Best Specialties for Development, *Marketing To Doctors* (1990):1–2.

5. See for example, L.M. Lamont and W.J. Lundstrom, Identifying Successful Industrial Salesmen by Personality and Personal Characteristics, *Journal of Marketing Research* 14, no. 4 (1977): 517–529.

6. C.D. Fogg and J.W. Rokus, A Quantitative Method for Structuring a Profitable Sales Force, *Journal of Marketing* 37, no. 3 (1973):8–17.

7. V. Hunt, Tracking Physician Referrals through DocBase, *MPR Exchange* 19, no. 2 (1993): 2–3.

8. R.F. Ganey and M.P. Malone, Satisfied Patients Can Spell Financial Well-Being, *Healthcare Financial Management* 45, no. 2 (1991):34–42.

9. V.T. Dull, Evaluating a Patient Satisfaction Survey for Maximum Benefit, *The Joint Commission Journal on Quality Improvement* 2, no. 8 (1994):444–452.

10. A. Suchman, The Marketing Audit: Its Nature, Purposes, and Problems, in *Analyzing and Improving Marketing Performance*, eds. A. Oxenfeldt and R.D. Crisp (New York, N.Y.: American Management Association, 1950) no. 32, 16–17.

11. Ibid.

12. E.N. Berkowitz and W.A. Flexner, The Marketing Audit: A Tool for Health Service Organizations, *Health Care Management Review* 3, no. 4 (Fall 1978):51–57.

Appendix A

GLOSSARY

Administered Vertical Marketing System: A system in which there is coordination between members of the *channel of distribution* but not common ownership.

Advertising: Any directly paid form of nonpersonal presentation of goods, services, and ideas.

Alternative Evaluation: Comparison by the consumer of the various choices that may best meet the individual's need.

Antimerger Act (1950): Regulation that strengthened the *Clayton Act* by broadening the federal government's power to prevent intercorporate acquisitions that would substantially reduce competition.

Approach: The stage in the sales process involving the initial meeting with the buyer.

Aspirational Reference Group: The reference group to which one aspires to belong.

Assumptive Close: Asking the buyer to choose payment terms, delivery location, or the like, before there has been an actual agreement to purchase.

Attitudes: A consumer's enduring cognitive evaluations, feelings, or action tendencies toward some person, object, or idea.

Autonomous Decisions: Decisions of lesser importance that individuals make independently.

BCG Matrix: A model based on *market growth rate* and *relative market share* for focusing company strategies in firms with multiple product lines.

Baby Boomers: The segment of the population born between 1946 and 1964.

Backward Integration: A strategy of incorporating new products and services that makes the firm its own supplier.

Barriers to Entry: Technological, regulatory, financial, strategic, or other conditions that a company must overcome in order to pursue a business opportunity.

382

Barriers to Exit: The costs of leaving a particular business or product line.

Benefit Segmentation: The grouping of people based on the benefits sought from the product.

Blended Family: The joining together of two households through remarriage.

Bonus: A payment that is made for reaching a certain level of performance.

Boutique Agency: An advertising agency that acts as a contractor to put together services needed by an organization, or one that offers a limited range of services.

Brand: Any name, term, colors, or symbol that distinguish one seller's product from another.

Brand Equity: The added value which a name *brand* gives to a product through associations made by the consumer.

Brand Loyalty: A situation in which the consumer regularly chooses the same product or service to fill a recognized need.

Breadth: The number of different product lines in a *product mix.*

Break-Even Analysis: A mathematical determination of the level of sales required to cover *total cost* at a given price.

Bundled Pricing: A strategy that involves selling several items or services together for one total price.

Buying Center: The group of people involved in the decision to purchase a product or service.

Canned Presentation: A set script through which a salesperson leads a prospect.

Cannibalization: The situation when a company's own product steals share from other products within the company's line.

Census: A collection of data from an entire target population.

Channel: The means used to deliver a marketing message.

Channel Commander: The member of the *channel of distribution* who can dictate or control the activities of the other members.

Channel Intensity: The intensity with which a product is distributed that determines how available the product is to the ultimate consumer.

Channel of Distribution: The path a product takes as it goes from the manufacturer to the consumer.

Clayton Act (1914): Regulation forbidding certain actions likely to lessen competition, even if no actual damages occurred.

Close: The stage of the sales process that involves asking the buyer for a commitment to purchase.

Cluster Sampling: A sample in which the *sampling units* are selected in groups.

Cognitive Dissonance: A mental state of anxiety brought on because the consumer is unsure of the chosen alternative.

Cold Calls: Contacts with prospective buyers who did not initiate the process.

Combination Plan: A compensation plan for the sales force that consists of a base salary plus a *commission* or *bonus.*

Commission: Compensation to salespeople based on performance, in terms of volume, net revenue, or margin.

Competitor Orientation: Recognizing competitors' (and potential competitors') strengths, weaknesses, and strategies.

Complementary Products: Products or services for which the purchase of one will affect the purchase of another in that line.

Complex Decision Making: A decision-making situation requiring high involvement and extended search.

Concentration: An advertising schedule in which advertising dollars are spent and exposure achieved within a relatively short time period.

Concentration Strategy: (See *market concentration strategy.*)

Consolidation: A strategy of focusing a firm's business on a smaller set of markets, products, or services.

Consumer Decision-Making Process: A six-stage model of the decision-making process that includes problem recognition, *internal search, external search, alternative evaluation, purchase,* and *post-purchase evaluation.*

Consumer Goods: Products purchased by the ultimate consumer.

Consumer Price Index: A measure of monthly and yearly price changes for a broad range of consumer goods and services.

Contribution Analysis: An assessment of profitability of a product or service that considers the contribution of profit to fixed cost or overhead.

Contribution Variance: The difference between expected and real contribution margin.

Convenience Goods: Products that the consumer purchases frequently that require little deliberation or search prior to purchase.

Cooperatives: Agreements between members of the distribution channel who function on the same level.

Corporate Vertical Marketing System: A system that combines both the production and distribution of a product or service under one corporate ownership.

Corrective Advertising: Means of communications required by the Federal Trade Commission, by which a company must correct misimpressions formed in the marketplace.

Cost-per-Thousand (CPM): A common frame of comparing the cost of advertising media.

Culture: The values, customs, and conforming rules passed from one generation to the next.

Customer Contact Audit: A flow chart of the points of interaction between the customer and the service offering.

Customer Orientation: Having a sufficient understanding of the target buyers to be able to create superior value for them continuously.

Database Marketing: An automated system to identify people—both customers and prospects—by name, and to use quantifiable information about these individuals to define the best possible purchasers and prospects for a given offer at a given time.

Decoding: Translating the meaning of a message from words and symbols.

Demand-Minus Pricing: A pricing approach that involves determining what price the market is willing to pay and working backwards to compute costs.

Demand Schedule: A summary of the amounts of a product that are desired at each price level.

Demographics: Statistics to describe members of a population in terms of who they are, where they live, and the types of jobs they have.

Depth: The number of product items within each product line in a firm's product mix.

Derived Demand: The demand for one product or service that is derived from the demand for another product or service.

Differential Advantage: The incremental benefits of a product relative to competing products that are important to the buyer and perceived by the buyer.

Diffusion of Innovation: The rate at which a product is adopted by the market.

Direct Costing: An approach to costing in which only costs that are directly associated with the product or service are assigned to it.

Discretionary Income: The amount of money a consumer has left after paying for taxes and necessities.

Discrimination: The ability to determine differences between stimuli.

Disposable Income: The amount of money a consumer has left for food, clothing, and shelter after paying taxes.

Dissociative Reference Group: A reference group to which one does not wish to belong.

Diversification: A strategy of developing new products or services for new markets.

Divestment: The selling off of a business or product line.

Durable Good: A product that lasts over an extended period of time.

Encoding: Translating the meaning to be communicated into words or symbols.

Environment: The regulatory, social, technological, economic, and competitive factors to which the organization must be sensitive in developing strategy.

Evaluative Criteria: The criteria on which alternative products or services are judged, as determined by the consumer.

Exclusive Dealing: Condition under which a buyer is required to handle only the products of one manufacturer but not those of a competitor.

Experiment: A form of data collection where factors are manipulated to determine a causal relationship.

External (Information) Search: A consumer search for information from one or more sources after an internal search has failed.

Family Decision Making: Historical decision-making patterns within the traditional family life cycle.

Family Life Cycle: The stages the typical consumer passes through from childhood to the death of a spouse.

Federal Trade Commission Act of 1914: Legislation forbidding deceptive or misleading advertising and unfair business practices.

Feedback: Communication from the receiver to the sender.

Fixed Costs: Those costs that do not change based on the volume of product or service delivered.

Flexible Pricing Policy: A pricing approach in which a company charges different prices to different customers based on their ability to negotiate or on their respective buying power.

Flighting: Advertising heavily for short time periods.

Focus Groups: Interviews conducted with typically 8 to 10 people and a trained moderator following an interview guide for the purpose of examining and collecting data.

Forward Integration: A strategy of offering new products or services that are closer to the customer than existing products or services.

Forward Vertical Integration: The acquisition or development of operations that are closer to the final buyer in the *channel of distribution.*

Four Ps: Product, price, place, and promotion are the controllable variables that a firm uses to define its marketing strategy.

Franchising: A *vertical marketing system* in which a contract links elements of the manufacturing and distribution of a product or service.

Frequency: The number of times the same person receives a message within a defined time period.

Full Costing: An approach to costing in which both direct and indirect costs are assigned to the product or service unit and considered in the calculation of profitability.

Full Service Agency: An advertising agency that offers all the elements necessary to provide the total advertising function.

Functional Discounts: Discounts on price because the buyer agrees to perform or take over particular functions involved with the product or service.

Functional Shifting: The moving of different functions (credit, sorting, etc.) between the producer of a product or service and its intermediaries or the customer.

GE Matrix: A multidimensional model for focusing company strategies in firms with multiple product lines based on dimensions of market attractiveness and business strength.

Generalizations: Extensions of past reinforced behavior to other stimuli.

Going-Rate Pricing: A pricing strategy that involves setting prices relative to the prevailing market price with less consideration for internal costs or margin requirements.

Gross Income: The total amount of money earned by a person or family in one year.

Gross Rating Points: A measure of advertising reach that is calculated by multiplying the number of spots or ads times the rating.

Growth Market Strategy: A strategy of gaining more sales from an existing business line or attempting to penetrate new markets.

Harvesting: A consolidation strategy in which a firm gradually withdraws support for a product until there is little or no market demand.

Heavy Half Consumer: A phenomenon observed within marketing in which a small group of consumers accounts for a disproportionate amount of a product's sales.

Hierarchy of Effects: The stages a buyer moves through from first seeing an advertisement ultimately to buying the product or using the service.

High Learning Product: A product that requires a significant introductory period because the immediate benefits might not be seen by the consumer.

Indirect Costs: Fixed costs that cannot be related to only one product line or service program.

Industrial Products: Products purchased for use in the production of other products.

Inflation: The decline in buying power when price levels rise faster than income.

Input Measures: Measures to assess the effort expended by salespersons to perform their jobs.

Integrated Delivery Systems: Health care systems in which care is coordinated and delivered at the level of intensity needed.

Interfunctional Coordination: Coordinating and deploying company resources in a manner that focuses on creating value for the customer.

Internal (Information) Search: Attempt by an individual to determine the solution to a recognized problem.

Involvement: The level of the consumer's personal investment in the purchase decision.

Item Budget Theory: A theory suggesting that consumers set out with a predetermined price they are willing to pay for a particular item.

Joint Venture Business: A new corporate entity in which both partners have an equity position (often resulting from a strategic alliance).

Lanham Act: Legislation providing for the registration of a company's trademarks.

Leader Pricing: A strategy of attractively pricing an item in the product line and aggressively promoting it to encourage consumers to purchase it and other items in the line at the same time.

Leads: Likely buyers who are targeted for sales calls.

Learning: The changes in a person's behavior as a result of past experiences.

Lifestyle: The manner in which people live, as demonstrated by how they spend their time, what they think, and the interests they have.

Limited Decision Making: A decision-making situation involving extended search and low involvement.

Long-Term Focus: Adopting a perspective that includes a continuous search for ways to add value by making appropriate investments in the business.

Low Learning Product: A product for which the benefits are clearly seen by the consumer.

Majority Fallacy: The largest market segment is often not the most profitable due to its attractiveness to competitors.

Marginal Cost Pricing: A pricing approach based on the concept that the price per additional unit or service must equal or exceed the cost of the additional unit.

Markup Pricing: A pricing approach that involves calculating the per-unit cost of a product or service and determining the markup percentages needed to cover the cost of sales and profit.

Market Challenger: A firm that confronts the market leader.

Market Concentration Strategy: A marketing strategy in which only one segment of the market is targeted.

Market Development: A strategy of initiating sales of existing products and services in new markets.

Market Follower: A firm that competes in the market by following the market leader rather than by attacking it directly.

Market Growth Rate: The rate of sales growth in the market.

Market Leader: The firm that has the largest share and strives to dominate the competitors in the given market.

Market Modification: An attempt by a company to extend a product's life cycle by increasing use or creating new uses or users.

Market Niche: (See *niche strategy.*)

Marketing Orientation: The combination of *customer orientation, competitor orientation, interfunctional coordination, long-term focus,* and *profitability.*

Market-Oriented Organization: An organization in which every distinct major market has its own marketing organization.

Market Penetration: A strategy to increase sales of existing products and services in present markets.

Market Segmentation: The process of grouping into clusters consumers who have similar wants or needs to which an organization can respond by tailoring one or more elements of the marketing mix.

Marketing: The process of planning and executing the conception, pricing, promotion, and distribution of ideas, goods, and services to create exchanges that satisfy individual and organizational objectives.

Marketing Audit: A systematic, critical review and appraisal of a firm's total marketing operation.

Marketing Information System: A structured, interacting complex of persons, machines, and procedures designed to generate an orderly flow of pertinent information collected from inter- and extrafirm sources, for use as a basis for decision making.

Marketing Mix: The mix of controllable variables that the firm uses to pursue the desired level of sales. These variables are commonly classified as the *Four Ps*—product, price, place, and promotion.

Marketing Objectives: Quantitative measures of accomplishment by which the success of marketing strategies can be measured.

Marketing Research: A process in which there is a systematic gathering of data from customers to identify their needs.

Mass Marketing: A strategy of treating the entire market as one target market and appealing to the broadest group.

Media Plan: The analysis and execution of an advertising campaign.

Medium: Form used for communication (television, radio, direct mail, magazines, newspapers).

Membership Reference Group: The reference group to which one belongs.

Message: The combination of symbols and words that the sender uses to transmit.

Modified Life Cycle: A modernized view of the family life cycle.

Monopolistic Competition: A situation where many companies have substitutable products.

Monopoly: A situation where there is only one company that sells a particular product.

Motivation: The goals or needs that propel a consumer to action.

Multibrand Strategy: A branding strategy in which the company places a different name on each product.

Multichotomous Questions: Questions that present the respondent with a fixed alternative.

Multiproduct Branding Strategy: A branding strategy in which the company places one brand name on all the products in its line.

Multisegment Marketing: A strategy of targeting multiple segments in the market in which a distinct marketing strategy might be developed for each group.

Multivariate Statistical Analysis: A quantitative analytical approach that considers the impact of multiple variables on a dependent variable.

Need: A condition in which there is a deficiency of something, or one requiring relief.

Niche: A very small specialized market segment with a highly defined set of needs.

Niche Strategy: A strategy of targeting a narrow segment or segments in the market with specialized products or services.

Noise: Anything that interferes with the effective communication of a message.

Nondurable Good: An item that can be consumed in some defined period of time.

Nonprobability Sample: A sample that was collected without the use of chance selection procedures.

Objective and Task: A promotional budgeting method that involves setting objectives along the hierarchy of effects and determining the tasks necessary to accomplish these objectives. The costs of the tasks determine the final budget needed.

Observational Research: Marketing research conducted by observing consumers either through a camera or by another individual.

Odd Pricing: A pricing approach in which items are priced just below whole dollar amounts.

Oligopoly: A situation where a few companies control a majority of the industry sales.

One-Price Policy: A pricing approach in which the company charges the same price to all customers who buy the product under the same set of conditions.

One-Stage Cluster Sample: A sampling method in which all the population elements in the selected subsets are included in the sample.

Opinion Leaders: People whose advice or experiences are often sought by others.

Organizational Mission: The organization's fundamental purpose for existing, as defined by its values and the customers it wishes to serve.

Organizational Objectives: The long-term performance targets that the company hopes to achieve.

Output Measures: Measures that assess the results of a salesperson's efforts.

Overall Market Share: A measure of a company's sales as a percent of total industry sales.

Penetration Price: A pricing strategy involving a low initial price relative to competing goods or services.

Perceived Risk: The concerns or anxieties a consumer anticipates regarding a product or service purchase.

Percentage Variable Contribution Margin (PVCM): A measure that shows the percentage of each additional sales dollar that is available to the organization to cover its fixed costs.

Perception: The psychological process by which individuals organize, select, and interpret information.

Personal Selling: Any paid personal presentation of goods, ideas, or services.

Place: The manner in which goods or services are distributed by a firm for use by consumers.

Population: The description of all people or elements of interest to researchers and from which a sample will be selected.

Post-Purchase Evaluation: A consumer's post-purchase assessment of a product that affects the possibility of repurchase or endorsement.

Presentation: The stage in the sales process involving the pitch for the product or service.

Prestige Pricing: A pricing strategy in which a high price is established relative to the competition or the true cost of production, in order to give the image of exclusivity or value.

Pretesting: Assessing advertising copy options before their general use.

Price: (1) The level of monetary reimbursement a firm demands for its goods or services, or (2) the economic value which the buyer provides to the producer in exchange for a product or service, or (3) the amount a customer is willing to pay for a product or service.

Price Elasticity: The change in demand for a product relative to a change in its price.

Price Lining: A pricing strategy in which products in a line are priced within a distinct price range that is significantly different from the prices of substitutes in the next range.

Price Variance: The difference between the actual price received and the targeted level due to discounting.

Primary Data: Information that is collected for a specific research question.

Primary Demand: Purchase interest in a class of product or service.

Problem Recognition: The first step in the consumer decision-making process in which the individual perceives a difference between the desired state and the actual state, and is motivated to close this gap.

Product: The goods, services, or ideas offered by a firm.

Product Development: A strategy of providing new products to existing markets.

Product Differentiation: A strategy of altering one or more elements of the marketing mix to respond differently to the various wants or needs of different groups in a multisegment strategy.

Product Life Cycle: The stages a product goes through as it exists in the market from its first introduction to its final withdrawal.

Product Lines: Groups of related products or services offered by a firm.

Product Mix: The entire range of products a firm offers.

Product Mix Variance: The difference between actual and targeted performance levels due to the composition of products or services offered.

Product Modification: Altering the product in some fashion by changing its quality, features, performance, or appearance.

Product-Oriented Organization: An organization in which each distinct product or related set of products has its own marketing organization.

Product Positioning: How a product is perceived in the minds of consumers relative to defined attributes and competing products.

Production Goods: Goods that are used to become part of the final product.

Profitability: Earning revenues sufficient to cover long-term expenses and to satisfy key constituencies.

Profitability Analysis: An approach to monitoring marketing performance that examines the profitability of sales by customers, regions, products, or salespeople.

Promotion: Any way of informing the market that the firm has developed a response to meet its needs.

Pruning: A consolidation strategy in which a firm reduces the number of products or services that it offers to the market.

Publicity: Any indirectly paid presentation of goods or services.

Pull: A strategy that involves bypassing or controlling the *channel of distribution* by appealing directly to the consumer and bypassing intermediaries.

Pulsing: An advertising schedule in which advertising expenditures occur at a constant level with occasional short, heavy expenditures.

Purchase: The act of selecting one brand over the others.

Pure Competition: A situation where every company has the same product.

Push: A strategy that involves controlling the *channel of distribution* by working through the channel.

Qualified Prospects: Individuals who have a need for the product or service or are likely to buy.

Quasi-Experimental Design: Research in which the data gathering is set up similar to a laboratory experiment, although lacking in control over all variables.

Reach: The unduplicated audience that an advertising vehicle will deliver.

Reference Group: A group that influences an individual's thoughts or behaviors.

Regulation: The rules or restrictions placed on companies by federal or state governments.

Relative Market Share: The ratio of a product's share of business within the market compared to that of its largest competitor, or the combined share of the three largest competitors.

Requirement Contract: An agreement in which a buyer is required to purchase all or part of its needed products from one seller for a defined period of time.

Reseller Strategy: A branding strategy in which the company sells the product under the name of another company.

Retail Mix: The goods and services that an organization offers.

Retail Positioning Matrix: A model for retail positioning based on the breadth of the product line and the value added.

Retrenchment: A consolidation strategy in which a firm withdraws from certain markets.

Robinson-Patman Act (1935): Regulation against price discrimination between different buyers of the same product, where the effect may be to lessen competition and create a monopoly.

Routine Decision Making: A decision-making situation requiring repetitive purchasing.

SWOT Analysis: An examining of the strengths and weaknesses of the organization, and of the opportunities and threats relevant to the organization's future strategy.

Sales Analysis: An approach to monitoring marketing performance that examines the actual sales generated compared to the goals that were established.

Sales/Expense Ratio: A common control method for evaluating salesperson performance that indicates the efficiency of the salesperson in generating output.

Sales Promotion: Any short-term inducement or offer for a particular product or service.

Sample: A collection of data from only a portion of a target population.

Sampling Frame: The means of representing the sampling population.

Sampling Method: The way that sampling units are selected.

Sampling Unit: The elements of the population to be sampled.

Secondary Data: Information that was previously collected for a purpose other than that to which it is being applied.

Selective Comprehension: The way a consumer interprets information in a way that is consistent with past attitudes, beliefs, and knowledge.

Selective Demand: Interest in and preference for a company's products or services.

Selective Exposure: The way a consumer only pays attention to a particular set of advertisements.

Selective Retention: The way consumers only retain a fraction of the material to which they were exposed.

Served Market Share: A measure of the company's sales as a percent of the total sales in the served market.

Services: Intangible activities or processes offered to customers to solve problems, for which the organization is often reimbursed.

Sherman Antitrust Act (1890): Regulation forbidding contracts, combinations, or conspiracies in the restraint of trade.

Shopping Goods: Products in which the customer engages in some significant search to compare alternative brands on selected attributes.

Single Unit Sampling: A sample in which each sampling unit is selected individually.

Situation Assessment: An analysis of the organization's environment and of the organization itself.

Skimming Price: A pricing strategy involving a high initial price relative to competing products or substitutable services.

Social Class: Relatively stable and homogeneous divisions in society in which individuals, families, or groups share relatively similar interests, values, lifestyles, and behaviors.

Source Credibility: The target market's perception that the sender of a message can be believed.

Specialty Items: Products that the consumer specifically seeks out.

Spokesperson: The person who delivers the message in marketing communications.

Stakeholders: Any group with which the firm has, or wants to develop, a relationship.

Standard Industrial Classification (SIC) Code: A federal government classification system that groups organizations based on their major business activity or the major service or product they provide.

Stark II: Regulations published in 1993 by the Health Care Financing Administration that prohibited physician referrals to entities in which they held a financial interest; applies to both Medicare and Medicaid.

Stimulus Response Sales Approach: An approach to selling that is founded in psychology.

Straight Salary: A compensation approach that provides a fixed salary.

Strategic Alliance: A formal arrangement with other companies to operate in a particular market.

Strategic Business Units: Businesses that operate as separate profit centers within a large organization.

Strategic Planning: A process that describes the direction an organization will pursue within its chosen environment and guides the allocation of resources and efforts.

Stress Interview: An interview in which the applicant is placed under stress to assess how he or she will act in similar situations.

Structured Interview: An interview that follows a set list of questions.

Substitutable Goods: Products that satisfy the same basic needs.

Support Goods: Items that are used to assist in the production of other products.

Survey Research: The collection of consumer data by telephone, personal interviews, focus groups, or mail.

Syncratic Decisions: Decisions in which the husband and wife participate jointly.

Syndicated Marketing Research: Commercial secondary data that regularly provides information on a particular question or problem area.

Target Audience: The group to whom an organization is trying to communicate.

Target Market: The group of customers whom the organization wishes to attract.

Target Pricing: A pricing approach that involves setting price to provide a targeted rate of return on investment for a standard level of production or service delivery.

Technology: Innovations or inventions from applied science and research.

Telemedicine: The delivery of health care through interactive audio, video, or data communications.

Total Cost: The total expense that the firm bears in delivering and marketing its product or service.

Trade Name: The commercial name under which a company does business.

Trademark: A *brand* or *trade name* given legal protection.

Trademark Law Revision Act (1988): Legislation granting a company *trademark* protection prior to actual use.

Trial Close: Asking the buyer for an opinion regarding a sales proposal.

Two-Stage Cluster Sample: A sampling method in which sample elements are collected from subsets of the population.

Tying Arrangement: Requirement by the seller of a product that the purchaser also buys another item.

Unstructured Interview: An interview in which the applicant is encouraged to talk freely on a range of subjects.

Utilities: Functions performed by intermediaries in the *channel of distribution.*

Variable Costs: Those costs that vary with the amount of the product or service delivered.

Variance Analysis: A method of evaluating marketing performance that compares actual results to preestablished targets of performance.

Vehicle: The advertising alternative chosen within each medium.

Vertical Integration: A strategy of incorporating products or services that are related to the firm's existing activities and that have usually been developed and offered by others to the marketplace.

Vertical Marketing Systems: Channels in which the intermediaries are integrated so that functions are performed at the most efficient place within the channel.

Volume Discounts: Discounts provided to buyers who purchase the product or service at some predetermined level.

Volume Variance: The difference between expected and real unit sales.

Want: A wish or desire for something.

Wheel of Retailing: A description of the process of how new retail forms enter the market and how they evolve over time.

Workload Method: A method for determining the appropriate size of the sales force based on work effort required to service the market.

Index